Winningham and Preusser's

CRITICAL THINKING

IN MEDICAL-SURGICAL SETTINGS

A Case Study Approach

Winningham and Preusser's

CRITICAL THINKING

IN MEDICAL-SURGICAL SETTINGS

A Case Study Approach

BARBARA A. PREUSSER, PhD, FNPc
Family Nurse Practitioner
Veteran's Administration Medical Center
Salt Lake City, Utah

THIRD EDITION

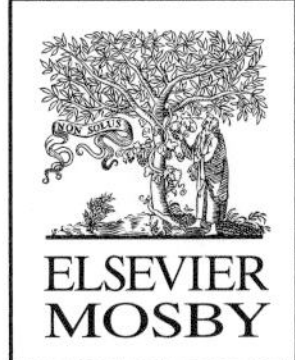

ELSEVIER
MOSBY

11830 Westline Industrial Drive
St. Louis, MO 63146

WINNINGHAM AND PREUSSER'S CRITICAL THINKING IN MEDICAL-SURGICAL SETTINGS: A CASE STUDY APPROACH, THIRD EDITION ISBN: 0-323-02566-8

NOTICE

Pharmacology is an ever-changing field. Standard safety precautions must be followed, but as new research and clinical experience broaden our knowledge, changes in treatment and drug therapy may become necessary or appropriate. Readers are advised to check the most current product information provided by the manufacturer of each drug to be administered to verify the recommended dose, the method and duration of administration, and contraindications. It is the responsibility of the treating appropriately licensed health care provider, relying on experience and knowledge of the patient, to determine dosages and the best treatment for each individual patient. Neither the publisher nor the editor assumes any liability for any injury and/or damage to persons or property arising from this publication.

The Publisher

First Edition 1996. Second Edition 2001.

International Standard Book Number 0-323-02566-8

Executive Editor: Michael S. Ledbetter
Senior Developmental Editor: Laurie K. Gower
Publishing Services Manager: Gayle May
Project Manager: Joseph Selby
Book Design Manager: Gail Morey Hudson

Printed in the United States of America

Last digit is the print number: 9 8 7 6 5 4 3 2

Clinical Consultants

Pharmacy

Tareca Joseph, BS, PharmD
Pharmacist, Primary Care Clinic
Veterans Administration Medical Center
Salt Lake City, Utah

Terri Evans, PharmD, CDE
Pharmacist, Primary Care Clinic
Veterans Administration Medical Center
Salt Lake City, Utah

Nutrition

Linda J. Winningham, MS, RD
Nutritional Consultant
Saline, Michigan

Reviewer

Sheryl Davey, RN, MS
Clinical Professor Emeritus, College of Nursing
University of Utah
Salt Lake City, Utah

Georgianna M. Thomas, EdD, RN
Interim Dean
West Suburban College of Nursing
Oak Park, Illinois

Contributors

Amy Anderson, RN, BSN
Staff Nurse, Emergency/Trauma Department
Banner Good Samaritan Hospital
Phoenix, Arizona

J. Elizabeth Bell, BSN, MSN, ANPc
Primary Care Clinic
Veterans Administration Medical Center
Salt Lake City, Utah

Leslie Black, BSN, MS, ANPc, CWOCN
Urology Clinic
Veterans Administration Medical Center
Salt Lake City, Utah

Kent Blad, MS, FNP, ANCP, CCRN
Assistant Professor
Brigham Young University
Provo, Utah

Stella Blight, BSN, MSN, APRN-BC
Psychiatric Mental Health Specialist
Veterans Administration Medical Center
Salt Lake City, Utah

Jamie K. Burnett, BSN, PAc
Urology Clinic
Veterans Administration Medical Center
Salt Lake City, Utah

Shannon Burton, BS, MS, RN
Assistant Clinical Professor, College of Nursing
University of Utah
Salt Lake City, Utah

Jamie Clinton-Lont, BSN, MSN, ANPc, GNPc
Supervisor, Midlevel Providers in Primary Care
Primary Care Clinic
Veterans Administration Medical Center
Salt Lake City, Utah

LeeAnn Coleman, BSN, MSN, APRN
Psychiatric Mental Health Specialist
Veterans Administration Medical Center
Salt Lake City, Utah

Sheryl Davey, RN, MS
Clinical Professor Emeritus, College of Nursing
University of Utah
Salt Lake City, Utah

Howard T. Diaz, BS, MPAS
Primary Care Clinic
Veterans Administration Medical Center
Salt Lake City, Utah

Angela Deneris, CNM, PhD
Associate Clinical Professor, College of Nursing
University of Utah
Salt Lake City, Utah

Allan Forde, BSN, NPAs, PAc
Director of Clinical Affairs, Utah Physician Assistant Program
University of Utah
Salt Lake City, Utah

Shellagh R. Gutke, BSN, CWOCN
Enterostomal Therapist
Veterans Administration Medical Center
Salt Lake City, Utah

Nancy A. Hayden, BSN, MSN, FNPc
Urology Associates
Nashville, Tennessee

RoxAnn Hauge-Showaker, RN, BSN
Nurse Manager, Surgical Intensive Care Unit
Veterans Administration Medical Center
Salt Lake City, Utah

Laura Hoffman, RN, BSN
Staff Nurse, Surgical Intensive Care Unit
Veterans Administration Medical Center
Salt Lake City, Utah

Lisa A. Jensen, BSN, MS, APRN, CS
Psychiatric Mental Health Specialist
Veterans Administration Medical Center
Salt Lake City, Utah

Penny K. Jensen, BSN, MS, APRN, FNPc
Nonsurgical Impotence Clinic and Primary Care Clinic
Veterans Administration Medical Center
Salt Lake City, Utah

Kathy Jones, RN, MSN, ACNP
General Cardiology—Lipid Clinic, Heart Failure Clinic
Charlotte Cardiology Associates, PA
Charlotte, North Carolina

Marilyn Little, BSN, MSN, APRN-BC
Professor, Salt Lake Community College
Psychiatric Mental Health Specialist
Salt Lake City, Utah

Sally Loken, BSN, MS, FNPc
Primary Care Clinic
Veterans Administration Medical Center
Salt Lake City, Utah

Tom Loken, BSN, MS, FNPc
Home-based Primary Care Specialist
Veterans Administration Medical Center
Salt Lake City, Utah

Holly Martin, BSN, MSN, FNPc
Primary Care Clinic
Veterans Administration Medical Center
Salt Lake City, Utah

Valerie McKee, BS, MS, PAC
Primary Care Clinic
Veterans Administration Medical Center
Salt Lake City, Utah

Katie Morgan, BSN, MSN, ANPc, WHNP
Clinical Instructor, College of Nursing
University of Utah
Salt Lake City, Utah

Jan Marie Peterson, RN, BSN, CDE
Diabetes Educator, Primary Care Clinic
Veterans Administration Medical Center
Salt Lake City, Utah

Deb Plasman, BSN, PAc
Gastrointestinal Clinic
Veterans Administration Medical Center
Salt Lake City, Utah

Barbara A. Preusser, MSN, PhD, FNPc
Primary Care Clinic
Veteran's Administration Medical Center
Salt Lake City, Utah

Kismet Rasmussen, BSN, MSN, FNPc
Heart Failure, Prevention, and Treatment Program
Latter Day Saints Hospital
Salt Lake City, Utah

Kathleen A. Robison, BSN, RN, SW
Nurse Case Manager, Primary Care Clinic
Veterans Administration Medical Center
Salt Lake City, Utah

Craig S. Sandberg, RN, BSN
Staff Nurse, Surgical Intensive Care Unit
Veterans Administration Medical Center
Salt Lake City, Utah

Laura Lee Scott, BSN, MSN, FNPc
Primary Care Clinic
Veterans Administration Medical Center
Salt Lake City, Utah

Marcia A. Scoville, MS, CNS, CNM
All for Women Health Care, Inc
Salt Lake City, Utah

Mary Seegmiller, BSN, MSN
Staff Nurse/Educator
The Orthopedic Specialty Hospital
Salt Lake City, Utah

Sandra Smeeding, MS, CNS, FNP
Director, Integrative Health
Veterans Administration Medical Center
Salt Lake City, Utah

Mikal A. Smoker-Diaz, BS, MS, MPAS
Hematology/Oncology Clinic
Veterans Administration Medical Center
Salt Lake City, Utah

Kristy Van Katwyk, BSN, MSN, FNPc
Cardiology Clinic
Veterans Administration Medical Center
Salt Lake City, Utah

Wendy Whitney, MSN, APRN, FNP, ACNP
Acute Care Nurse Practitioner
Surgical Intensive Care Unit
Veterans Administration Medical Center
Salt Lake City, Utah

Shelley Wood, MEd, Ph.D. PAc
Primary Care Clinic
Veterans Administration Medical Center
Salt Lake City, Utah

Mary Youtsey, BSN, CDE
Diabetes Educator, Primary Care Clinic
Veterans Administration Medical Center
Salt Lake City, Utah

Dedication

To Maryl L.Winningham, APRN, PhD, FACSM, who died February 18, 2001, from complications of breast cancer.

Because this is the first edition of our text to be published since Maryl's death, it seems appropriate to preface it with a few words about Dr. Winningham's professional and personal life. In the interest of brevity we will limit ourselves to an abbreviated recitation of her many and varied accomplishments and particularly to her singular commitment to the ideal of excellence in nursing practice.

With regard to her work life, Maryl was more complex than most of us. She suffered from bipolar disorder; she was internally conflicted regarding how she spent her time and energy. She was caught up in a dilemma that seemed to her to defy resolution. Maryl spent an effective, significant, and meaningful portion of her efforts in two areas: first, educating and training undergraduate nursing students to be consummate professionals, and second, thinking "globally" about cancer-related fatigue (CRF). The dilemma arose from the fact that she was expending considerable effort on those two objectives while her academic situation demanded that she focus her energies on publications in order to garner professional acclaim and advance the careers of herself and her colleagues. Ultimately Maryl chose to abandon the "publication-acclaim" aspect of her career and more fully develop a comprehensive approach to the problem of CRF. The end result of that choice was the publication, less than a year before her death, of *Fatigue in Cancer: A Multidimensional Approach*. This was the first book ever published dedicated solely to the issue of CRF.

Maryl's professional relationships were also complicated. Working at the intellectual level, she could be deeply insightful and penetrating as she delineated difficult to understand theoretical issues to produce innovative, inspired approaches to research clinical nursing interventions. Yet at the same time she struggled very hard to meet deadlines on relatively simple, or even mundane tasks. For those who were driven by their career advancement agendas, Maryl's brilliance seemed incompatible with her less than stellar productivity. Her inconsistent performance was all too frequently misconstrued as lack of commitment. This unfortunate inconsistency in her performance made her colleagues and editors fretful and impatient. Invariably, however frustrated and delayed, for those who stayed the course with her, the ends proved worth the journeys.

Maryl did not fail because of her bipolar disorder; she succeeded in spite of it. She could have pleaded her problems as acceptable sanction waivers for any level of failure. Instead she chose to fight through her problems with the full intent to share her skills and knowledge in ways that ultimately resulted in significant contributions. Perhaps the most positive of all things we can learn from Maryl is that having problems is not a legitimate excuse for not engaging life and making positive things happen.

She was never still. In addition to her many professional and work-related accomplishments, Maryl had a rich and wide-ranging assortment of outside interests and friends with whom she shared those interests. It would not be an unusual occurrence for one of her friends to ask a question or mention a problem and two days later receive a sheaf of papers. Those computer printouts represented many hours of Maryl's time, expended as she ran exhaustive Internet and/or medical database searches for information related to the question or the problem raised by her friend.

One of the most notable of Maryl's outside passions was art. Those of you who may be interested in a clearer picture of her work as a computer graphic artist, a sculptor, and a poet are invited to peruse a memorial written by Dr. Barbara F. Piper. That memorial was published in the *Oncology Nursing Forum* 28(3):437-438, 2001. In a portion of that memorial essay, Dr. Piper gave clear, strong, and sensitive treatment to Maryl's "artistic" side, for which gracious treatment we express our deepest appreciation.

The concept of educating nurses using a case studies method, as employed in this textbook, was to be just the beginning of a rigorous and concerted attempt to bridge the gap between classroom theory and clinical practice. The philosophic positions that inform and underlie this text and that drove the effort to publish it, were held in common between Maryl and her coauthor, Dr. Preusser. That educational philosophy can be summed up in the statement: "Errors in a safe environment." To this day it remains the view of the author that a case studies approach to nursing education creates a situation in which students can make and learn from their mistakes without jeopardizing patients.

It is our hope that students who use this text will strive as diligently for truly professional compassion as they do for technical excellence in the care they administer to their patients.

By Frederick Kesler,
Maryl's dear friend and confidant

Acknowledgments

I would like to thank:

Our patients, who let us learn nursing by practicing on them.

Those nurses we saw in action and told ourselves, "Now *that's* a great nurse!"

The teachers who encouraged us to follow our convictions.

And to those who have bequeathed to us a nursing heritage of integrity, excellence, courage, and service.

To them I humbly acknowledge our gratitude and indebtedness.

This book would never have become a reality if not for the forbearance and help of the following individuals:

Michael Ledbetter, Executive Editor, who made this book a reality and has shared his patience, encouragement, and compassion;

Laurie Gower, Senior Developmental Editor, who tried to keep me on the straight and narrow, patiently listened to me complain, coordinated the review process, and edited this work. Laurie, thank you for the great person you are.

And the consultants, for the creative work they shared and for their sharp eyes that picked up on errors. I thank you for your unflagging support.

I would like to offer a special tribute to the people who said, "It can't be done," "It'll never work," and "We've never done it that way," and thereby challenged us to prove them wrong.

B.A.P.

Contents

Introduction

There is an urgent need for nurses with well-practiced critical thinking skills. As new graduates you will be expected to make decisions and take actions of an increasingly sophisticated nature. You will encounter problems you never saw or heard about during your classroom and clinical experiences. You are going to have to make complex decisions with little or no guidance and limited resources.

We want you to be exposed to as much as possible during your student days but more important, we want you to learn to *think*. You cannot memorize your way out of every situation, but you can *think* your way out of any situation. We know that students often learn more, and faster, when they have the freedom to make mistakes. This book is designed to allow you to experiment with finding answers without the pressure of someone's life hanging in the balance. We want you to do well. We want you to be the best. It is our wish for you to grow into confident, competent professionals. After all, someday we will be one of those people you care for, and when that day comes, we want you to be very, very good at what you do!

What Is Critical Thinking?

Critical thinking is *not* criticizing. Critical thinking is an analytical process that can help you think through a problem in an organized and efficient manner. There are six steps involved in critical thinking (Dressel and Mayhew, 1954). Thinking about these steps may help you when you work through the questions in your cases. In the beginning, it may help for you to write everything down on the Case Study Worksheet (at the end of this section) as you learn the process of discovery. Here are the six steps with an explanation of what they mean.

1. Define the problem by asking the right questions: Exactly what is it you need to know? What is the question asking? Einstein once said that asking the right question was sometimes more important than having the right answer.
2. Select the information or data necessary to solve the problem or answer the question: First you have to ask whether all the necessary data or information is there. If not, how and where can you get additional information? What other resources are available? This is one of the most difficult steps. In real clinical experiences, you rarely have all the information, so you have to learn where you can get necessary data. For instance, patient and family interviews, nursing charting, the patient medical chart, laboratory data on the computer, your observations, and your own physical assessment can help you identify important clues. Of course, information can rapidly become outdated. To make sure you are accessing the most current and accurate information, you will occasionally need to use a computer and the Internet to answer a question.
3. Recognize stated and unstated assumptions; that is, what do you think is or is not true. Sometimes answers or solutions seem obvious; just because something seems obvious doesn't mean it is correct. You may need to consider several possible answers or solutions. Consider all clues carefully and *don't dismiss a possibility too quickly*. Remember *"You never find an answer you don't think of."*
4. Formulate and select relevant and/or promising hypotheses: Think of these as hunches. Try to think of as many possibilities as you can. Consider the pros and cons of each.
5. Draw valid conclusions: Consider all data; then determine what is relevant and what makes the most sense. Only then should you draw your conclusions.
6. Consider the soundness of your decisions: Rethink your conclusions and decisions in light of the whole case. What is the best answer/solution? What could go wrong? This requires considering many different angles. Be willing to revise the conclusions you made in step 5 if new information or clues crop up. In today's health care settings, decision making often requires balancing the well-being needs of the patient with financial limitations imposed by the reimbursement system (this includes Medicare, Medicaid, and insurance companies). In making decisions, you need to take all the relevant issues into account. Remember, you may be asked to explain why you rejected other options.

It may look as if this kind of thinking comes naturally to instructors or experienced nurses. You can be certain that even experienced professionals were once where you are now. (Sometimes they seem to forget that!) The rapid and sound decision making that is essential to good nursing requires years of practice. The practice of good clinical thinking leads to good thinking in clinical practice. This book will help you practice the important steps in making sound clinical judgments again and again, until the process starts to come naturally.

The practice of good clinical thinking leads to good thinking in clinical practice.

Rating Questions

The questions or problems related to cases in this book have been rated according to their level of complexity. Each category requires a more sophisticated level of thinking than the previous. Sometimes different types of questions or problems will be mixed together in the same case. The five categories are as follows.

Knowledge—This represents information, data, or facts and deals with questions like Who? What? When? Where? and How much?

Comprehension—This involves understanding the importance, significance, or meaning of specific information or facts.

Application—This involves understanding the information or facts and implementing or using them. Application also involves figuring out what—of all the information in a given setting—is important and appropriate to the problem and applying that information to a plan of action. Each setting contains a lot of information; some of it is not relevant. In some settings, certain information may even lead us to false conclusions.

Analysis—This involves criticism and evaluation and requires taking a situation or problem apart to figure out what is going on (or going wrong). Analysis involves knowledge, understanding the meaning or significance of that knowledge, and recognizing how it can best be applied. It also involves evaluating ("figuring out") what is wrong or anticipating what can go wrong. In finding out what is wrong, you will encounter one or more assumptions that may lead to false conclusions or something that you don't understand.

Synthesis—This is a more advanced kind of thinking that requires combining, arranging, incorporating, integrating, or coordinating what you know to arrive at a specific result. Synthesis is a creative process that involves pulling everything together. This type of thinking is characteristic of advanced clinicians. In a deeper sense, although the questions in these cases are not synthesis-type questions, your brain is constantly in "synthesis mode." Indeed, that's why case studies help develop your clinical thinking skills—they help you learn to open new brain pathways in a way that memorization cannot.

The "How to" of Case Studies

When you begin each case, read through the whole story once, from start to finish, to get a general idea what it is about. Get out your Case Study Worksheet and write things you had to look up. That way you won't have to look them up a second or third time. This is your "cheat sheet." This will help you move through the case smoothly and get more out of it. How much you have to look up will depend on where you are in your program, what you know, and how much experience you already have. Preparing cases will become easier as you advance in your program.

1 Cardiovascular Disorders

Case Study 1

Name ______________________ Class/Group __________ Date __________

Group Members ____

INSTRUCTIONS: All questions apply to this case study. Your responses should be brief and to the point. Adequate space has been provided for answers. When asked to provide several answers, they should be listed in order of priority or significance. Do not asume information that is not provided. Please print or write clearly. If your response is not legible, it will be marked as ? and you will need to rewrite it.

Scenario

S.L., a 74-year-old woman, has recently moved to your town and is looking for a new primary care provider. For her first appointment she brings all of her medications from her previous provider. You note that she is on warfarin (Coumadin).

1. When you ask her when her last PT (prothrombin time) test was done and the results, she is vague and doesn't seem to know much about it. How would you explain a PT test and why it is important?

2. You ask her why she is on warfarin. Why is it important for her to know?

S.L. reports she has had an irregular heartbeat for many years. There was an unsuccessful attempt at cardioversion and she has been on warfarin ever since. From this story you know that she probably has atrial fibrillation and is on lifelong warfarin therapy. You ask her what education was provided to her about warfarin and she says she was given a booklet but she never read it.

3. What should you do about this lack of education?

Your clinic has an anticoagulation clinic but there is a 6-week admission delay time. The provider asks that you provide some education.

4. Where would you get the information you would need to share with S.L.?

5. During your first education session, S.L. tells you that she remembers being told to avoid all vegetables while on warfarin. How should you respond to this statement?

6. You provide a list of foods that contain vitamin K. During this session she asks if it is OK to drink alcohol. What should you tell her?

7. S.L. informs you she also sees other health care providers who sometimes prescribe medications for her. Does this concern you? How should you respond?

8. S.L. reports that her provider only ordered labs when she saw him every 6 months. She asks if it will be OK to continue the 6-month schedule. What should you tell her?

9. You would want to counsel any patient on warfarin therapy about safety precautions to prevent bruising and bleeding risk. List three precautions you might address.

10. What is a Medic-Alert and why is it important?

Remember to inform patients that their lifestyle, stressors, and illness can affect their anticoagulation. The mechanism of action is unknown. They should report these changes to the anticoagulation provider.

Case Study 2

Name ______________________________ Class/Group __________ Date __________

Group Members ____

INSTRUCTIONS: All questions apply to this case study. Your responses should be brief and to the point. Adequate space has been provided for answers. When asked to provide several answers, they should be listed in order of priority or significance. Do not asume information that is not provided. Please print or write clearly. If your response is not legible, it will be marked as ? and you will need to rewrite it.

Scenario

M.G., a "frequent flier," is admitted to the ED (emergency department) with a diagnosis of heart failure. She was discharged from the hospital 10 days ago and comes in today stating, "I just had to come to the hospital today because I can't catch my breath and my legs are as big as tree trunks." After further questioning you learn she is strictly following the fluid and salt restriction ordered during her last hospital admission. She reports she has been gaining 1 to 2 pounds every day since her discharge.

1. What error in teaching most likely occurred when M.G. was discharged 10 days ago?

You chart the medications M.G. brought with her: Enalapril (Vasotec) 5 mg bid, digoxin 0.125mg qd, rosiglitasone 4 mg, furosemide 40 mg qd, potassium chloride 20 mEq qd. The admitting provider orders all the medications but changes the furosemide to 40 mg intravenous push (IVP) qd and 80 mg IVP now.

2. What is the rationale for changing the method of administering furosemide?

3. You administer 80 mg furosemide IVP. Identify three strategies you would use to monitor the effectiveness of this medication.

Most heart failure admissions are related to fluid volume overload. Patients who do not require intensive care monitoring can most often be treated initially with IVP diuretics, oxygen, and angiotensin converting enzyme (ACE) inhibitors.

4. How do ACE inhibitors help in CHF?

5. M.G.'s symptoms improve with intravenous (IV) diuretics. She is ordered back on oral furosemide once her weight loss is deemed adequate to achieve a euvolemic state. What will determine if the oral dose will be adequate to consider her for discharge?

6. M.G. is ready for discharge. What key management concepts should be taught to prevent relapse and another admission? Hint: use the acronym MAWDS.

Case Study 3

Name ______________________ Class/Group __________ Date __________

Group Members ______________________

INSTRUCTIONS: All questions apply to this case study. Your responses should be brief and to the point. Adequate space has been provided for answers. When asked to provide several answers, they should be listed in order of priority or significance. Do not asume information that is not provided. Please print or write clearly. If your response is not legible, it will be marked as ? and you will need to rewrite it.

Scenario

M.H. is a 70-year-old man who comes to your clinic requesting a routine blood pressure check. When you palpate his radial pulse you notice that it is irregular.

1. What should you do next?

2. M.H. reports that he has been feeling fine. After reviewing the ECG, his provider determines that he is in A-fib (atrial fibrillation). How would you explain A-fib to the patient?

3. Why is the provider concerned about M.H. having A-fib?

4. The provider orders the following studies to further evaluate the A-fib: echocardiogram, Holter monitor, chest x-ray, CBC (complete blood count), thyroid function, and chemistry panel. How would you explain these procedures and why they were ordered for the patient?

The studies showed that M.H. has atrial fibrillation not caused by any identifiable factors. The provider decided to anticoagulate M.H. with warfarin for 3 weeks prior to cardioversion. M.H. has many questions about anticoagulation and cardioversion.

5. Explain the terms anticoagulation and cardioversion to M.H.

6. M.H. is cardioverted successfully and 4 weeks later his warfarin is stopped. You understand that cardioversion is not always successful long term. What patient education should M.H. know regarding atrial fibrillation?

7. M.H. eventually develops chronic A-fib and is placed on lifelong warfarin therapy. You instruct him to monitor and report complications of warfarin therapy. Identify two main areas of concern and list four signs or symptoms for each.

8. What should an anticoagulated patient do if he or she notes any of these signs or symptoms?

9. M.H. asks what he should do if he forgets to take his medication.

10. What can you suggest to help him remember to take his medication?

11. What other factors may influence medication compliance?

Case Study 4

Name ______________________ Class/Group __________ Date __________

Group Members ____

INSTRUCTIONS: All questions apply to this case study. Your responses should be brief and to the point. Adequate space has been provided for answers. When asked to provide several answers, they should be listed in order of priority or significance. Do not asume information that is not provided. Please print or write clearly. If your response is not legible, it will be marked as ? and you will need to rewrite it.

Scenario

M.P. is a lively 78-year-old African-American woman who comes to your clinic for a F/U (follow-up) visit. She was Dx (diagnosed) with HTN (hypertension) 2 months ago and was given a prescription for HCTZ (hydrochlorothiazide) 25 mg qd but stopped taking it because "it made me dizzy and I kept getting up during the night to empty my bladder." She comes to the clinic because her mother died of a CVA (cerebrovascular accident, stroke) at her same age and she is afraid she will suffer the same fate. VS (vital signs) during her initial visit were as follows: VS 160/102-78-16-98.2. She is a lifetime nonsmoker, nondrinker. Father died of a MI (myocardial infarction) at 67 years of age. Mother died of CVA at 78 years of age. One brother is alive but has CAD, DM (diabetes mellitus), and HTN. Her sister is A&W (alive and well) at 62 years of age. Her BMP (basic metabolic panel) and fasting lipids were WNL (within normal limits).

1. After a 10-minute waiting period, you take M.P.'s BP (blood pressure) and get 156/96. According to the most recent JNC (Joint National Committee on Detection, Evaluation, and Treatment of High Blood Pressure) Risk Stratification and Treatment Recommendations, what risk group is she in, and what stage of hypertension does her BP represent?

She goes on to ask whether there is anything else she should do to help with her HTN. Remember, she is 5′ 4″ and weighs 110 pounds. She has never smoked. Her glucose and lipid levels are within normal range.

2. Look up M.P.'s height and weight for her age on a body mass index (BMI) chart. Is she considered overweight? Why or why not? Explain which method you used to determine your answer and where you got your information.

Hint: You can use any one of a number of charts or calculations.

3. What nonpharmacologic lifestyle alteration measures might help someone like M.P. control her BP? List one and explain.

Not everyone responds the same way to lifestyle modifications or medications. There is often a need for "trial and error" in establishing what the best medication or combination of interventions is to manage a health problem. Considerations include (1) how many and what specific side effects are experienced by the individual; (2) how acceptable those side effects are; (3) interactions with medications for other conditions or diseases; (4) cost of the medications; (5) whether the person responds favorably to the medication; and (6) difficulty in taking medications.

4. When someone is taking HCTZ, what laboratory tests would you expect to be monitored? (List at least two.)

Because M.P.'s BP continues to be high, the internist decides to put her on another drug.

5. According to national guidelines, what is another recommended drug category for elderly nondiabetic individuals? Should this be used independently, with her current medication, or with another new drug?

6. The internist decreases her HCTZ to 12.5 mg and adds a prescription for time-released diltiazem XR 120 mg qd. M.P. is told to keep having her BP checked on a weekly basis. In addition, in doing your teaching, what side effects would you ask her to watch for and notify your office if she experiences?

7. It is sometimes difficult to remember whether you've taken your medication. What techniques might you teach M.P. to help her remember to take her medication each day (name at least two)?

You see M.P. 1 month later. She tells you she is feeling fine and does not have any side effects from her new medication. She shows you her calendar where she has been marking her medication record and her BP. Her BP, checked twice at the senior center, measured 136/78 and 134/82.

8. You take M.P.'s BP and get 132/82. She asks whether these BP readings are OK. On what do you base your response?

9. List at least three important things you might help her with in maintaining her success.

M.P. comes in for a routine follow-up 3 months later. She continues to do well on her daily BP drug regimen with average BP readings of 130/78. She participates in a group walking program at the senior center. She admits she hasn't done so well with decreasing her salt intake. She tells you she recently was at a luncheon with her garden club and that most of those ladies take different BP pills than she does. She asks why their pills are different shapes and colors.

10. How can you explain the difference to M.P.?

Bonus Problem: The cost of medications is a critical issue for elderly individuals on a fixed income. To help you develop a sensitivity to the cost of prescriptions, have one person in your study group call to see whether there are generic versions of the medications M.P. is receiving and how much she would pay for a 30-day supply (don't have everybody call the pharmacy at once). Although not all generic drugs are "created equal" in terms of bioavailability (look this one up), see what is the least expensive option for M.P.

Bonus Problem: Remind M.P. that she should continue with her prescribed medications and not make any alterations. Especially emphasize the need to talk with you or the physician before she starts taking any "natural" or herbal remedies, over-the-counter remedies for cold or flu, or nutritional supplements. Name one herbal remedy or natural product that could elevate her BP.

Case Study 5

Name ________________________________ Class/Group ___________ Date ___________

Group Members ____

INSTRUCTIONS: All questions apply to this case study. Your responses should be brief and to the point. Adequate space has been provided for answers. When asked to provide several answers, they should be listed in order of priority or significance. Do not asume information that is not provided. Please print or write clearly. If your response is not legible, it will be marked as ? and you will need to rewrite it.

Scenario

You are a nurse at a free-standing cardiac prevention and rehabilitation center. Your new patient in risk-factor modification is B.J., a 37-year-old traveling salesman, who is married and has three children. During a recent evaluation for chest pain, he underwent a cardiac catheterization procedure that showed moderate single vessel disease with a 50% stenosis in the mid RCA (right coronary artery). He was given a prescription for SL (sublingual) NTG (nitroglycerin), told how to use it, and referred to your cardiac rehabilitation program for sessions 3 days a week. B.J.'s wife comes along to help him with healthy lifestyle changes. You take the following nursing history: B.J.'s father died of sudden cardiac death at age 42, and his mother (still living) had a CABG × 4 (quadruple coronary artery bypass graft) at age 52; his hypertension is controlled on metoprolol 25 mg every 12 hours, which was also prescribed for his coronary disease, as well as taking ASA (aspirin) 325 mg PO daily; he has averaged 1½ packs of cigarettes per day for 20 years; an "occasional" beer ("a six-pack every weekend with the football game"*); and a dietary history of fried and fast foods. His current weight is 235 pounds at 5′8″; he has a waist circumference of 48 inches. His VS are 138/88, 82, 18, 98.4° F.
Note: Be alert to the fact that many individuals tend to underreport their alcohol and drug consumption. Clearly mark patient reports by using quotes to indicate subjective source of information.

1. Calculate B.J.'s smoking history in terms of pack-years.

2. List three nonmodifiable risk factors for CAD.

3. List six modifiable risk factors for CAD.

4. Underline each of the responses in questions 2 and 3 that represent B.J.'s personal CAD risk factors.

5. You would like to know more about B.J.'s hyperlipidemia. What four common laboratory values do you need to know?

B.J. laughingly tells you he believes in the five all-American food groups: salt, sugar, fat, chocolate, and caffeine.

6. Identify health-related problems in this case description; the problem that is potentially life threatening should be listed first.

7. Of all his behaviors, which one is the most significant in promoting cardiac disease?

8. What is the most important priority problem that you need to address with B.J.? Identify the teaching strategy you would use with him.

Hint: What *you* think is the most important may not be what *he* considers the most important, or the one he is willing to work on.

9. What is the second problem you would work with B.J. to change? Identify an appropriate strategy to resolve the problem.

Note: Whenever B.J. and his wife decide to attack dietary changes, try to get a referral to a registered dietitian (RD), who can work with them to develop strategies for long-term nutritional goals to decrease HTN and serum lipids. Many states are requiring dietitians to be licensed the same way nurses are registered. Check to make certain that certain nutritional counseling for a person with specific disease states is not exceeding the nursing standard of practice for your state.

10. B.J.'s wife takes you aside and tells you, "I'm so worried for B. I grew up in a really dysfunctional family where there was a lot of violence. B. has been so good to the kids and me. I'm so worried I'll lose him that I have nightmares about his heart stopping. I find myself suddenly awakening at night just to see if he's breathing." How are you going to respond?

Note: Nightmares about losing a loved one to heart disease are not rare, especially during the time of diagnosis or disease-related crisis. However, a background of childhood violence can have deep roots and often requires special help. Clearly this woman is in distress. Depending on her willingness at this time, it would be good for her to talk with a therapist. If she doesn't think she needs it, try suggesting that it might be good for B.J. and the kids and that it would help her relax and be more responsive to them. At the appropriate point, it would be important for her to be able to share with her husband how she feels. From her description, this sleep disturbance is an unhealthy situation that should be addressed. If she refuses, keep an open relationship; it is important that she keep talking to someone about her fear.

Six weeks after you start working with B.J., he admits that he has been under a lot of stress. He rubs his chest and says, “It feels really heavy on my chest right now.” You feel his pulse and note that his skin is slightly diaphoretic, and that he is agitated and appears to be very anxious.

11. What are you going to do to obtain additional information?

12. B.J. continues to feel symptomatic. Now what are you going to do?

Case Study 6

Name ______________________ Class/Group __________ Date __________

Group Members ____

INSTRUCTIONS: All questions apply to this case study. Your responses should be brief and to the point. Adequate space has been provided for answers. When asked to provide several answers, they should be listed in order of priority or significance. Do not asume information that is not provided. Please print or write clearly. If your response is not legible, it will be marked as ? and you will need to rewrite it.

Scenario

S.P. is a 68-year-old (yo) retired painter who is experiencing right leg calf pain. The pain began approximately 2 years ago but has become significantly worse in the past 4 months. The pain is precipitated by exercise and is relieved with rest. Two years ago S.P. could walk two city blocks before having to stop due to leg pain. Today he can barely walk across the kitchen. S.P. has smoked two to three packs of cigarettes per day for the past 45 years. He has a history of CAD, HTN, PVD (peripheral vascular disease), and osteoarthritis. Surgical history includes CABG x 4V 3 years ago. He has had no further symptoms of cardiopulmonary disease since that time despite the fact that he has not been compliant with the exercise regime his cardiologist prescribed, continues to eat anything he wants, and continues to smoke 2-3 PPD (packs per day). Other surgical history includes ORIF (open reduction internal fixation) of the right femoral fracture 20 years prior.

In clinic today, S.P.'s weight is 261 pounds, height is 5′10″, VS are 163/91, 82, 16, afebrile. His fasting lipids are cholesterol 239 mg/dl, triglyceride150 mg/dl, HDL 28 mg/dl, LDL 181 mg/dl. Medications include lisinopril 20 mg qd, metoprolol 25 mg bid, aspirin 325 mg qd, simvastatin 40 mg qd.

1. S.P. is in clinic today for a routine semiannual follow-up appointment with his primary care provider. You are taking his blood pressure and he tells you that besides the calf pain, he is experiencing right hip pain that gets worse with exercise, doesn't go away promptly with rest, some days it is worse than others, and is not affected by resting position. What are the likely sources of his calf pain and his hip pain?

2. S.P. has several risk factors for claudication. From his history, list two risk factors and explain why they are risk factors.

3. You decide to look at S.P.'s lower extremities. What signs would you expect to find with intermittent claudication? Identify four findings.

4. Where would you expect S.P. to complain of pain if he had superficial femoral artery stenosis? Popliteal stenosis?

His primary care provider has seen S.P. and wants you to schedule the patient for an ankle-brachial index (ABI) test to determine the presence of arterial blood flow obstruction. You confirm the time and date of the procedure and now you call S.P. at home.

5. What will you tell S.P. to do to prepare for the tests?

S.P.'s ABI results showed 0.33 R leg and 0.59 L leg. These results indicate he has severe arterial obstruction in R leg and moderate obstruction in his L leg.

6. You counsel S.P. on risk factor modification. What would you address and why?

7. In addition to risk factor modification, what other measures to improve tissue perfusion or prevent skin damage should you recommend to S.P.?

8. S.P tells you his neighbor told him to keep his legs elevated higher than his heart and ask for compression stockings to keep swelling in his legs down. How should you respond?

9. S.P. recently got hit on the right shin with a softball and now complains of constant right lower extremity pain. What should you be concerned about?

You caution S.P. to avoid repeated injury to his already compromised leg. He assures you he doesn't want to lose his leg and will be more careful in the future.

Case Study 7

Name ______________________ Class/Group __________ Date __________

Group Members ____

INSTRUCTIONS: All questions apply to this case study. Your responses should be brief and to the point. Adequate space has been provided for answers. When asked to provide several answers, they should be listed in order of priority or significance. Do not asume information that is not provided. Please print or write clearly. If your response is not legible, it will be marked as ? and you will need to rewrite it.

Scenario

K.N. is a patient who has a mechanical valve in the mitral position. You know that there are different PT/INR (prothrombin time/International Normalized Ratio) goal recommendations based on the indication for anticoagulation. Mechanical valves in the mitral valve position are considered to be at greater thromboembolic risk than the aortic site. As a result, these valve patients are kept at a higher PT/INR goal range. His INR goal, which is a mathematical calculation to convert PT into an internationally reported unit of measure, is 2.5 to 3.5 INR.

K.N. calls to report a nosebleed that is hard to stop. He is asked to come into the office to check his clotting time. When you get the results his INR is 7.2. The provider has asked you to inform the patient that this level is too high.

1. What should you tell K.N.?

The provider does a brief focused history and physical and some additional labs and determines there are no signs of bleeding. The provider discovered K.N. recently went to the local ED for a sinus infection and had received a prescription for sulfamethoxazole (Septra), an antibiotic that has a significant interaction with warfarin.

2. What could K.N. have done to prevent this problem?

3. The provider gives K.N. a low dose of vitamin K orally and asks him to hold the next two doses of warfarin. What should you tell K.N. about vitamin K?

4. You clarify with K.N. what it means to "hold the next two doses." What should you tell him?

5. The provider then asks you to arrange for K.N. to have his PT rechecked in 2 days. K.N. asks why it needs to be checked again so soon. What do you tell him?

6. K.N.'s INR in 2 days is 3.7. Is this in therapeutic range?

7. The provider made no further changes. He told K.N. to complete his antibiotic course, which will be completed in 2 days and asks that K.N. have his PT checked again in 7 days. Why should it be checked so soon instead of the usual monthly follow-up?

8. K.N. grumbles about all the laboratory tests but agrees to follow through. The next INR is 2.8. The provider instructs him when the next PT is due. What patient education points need to be stressed?

9. Six months later, K.N. informs you that he is going to have a knee replacement next month. What should you do with this information?

You know that sometimes the only needed action is to stop the warfarin several days before the surgery. But other times the provider initiates "bridging therapy," stopping the warfarin and providing anticoagulation coverage with unfractionated heparin or with a low-molecular-weight heparin. After reviewing all his anticoagulation information, the provider decides that he should be on enoxaparin (Lovenox) to provide anticoagulation protection while stopping the warfarin for surgery.

10. What can you tell him about why this is important?

11. You have a discussion with another patient who finally admits that he takes his medications sporadically, whenever he happens to remember. It is not a financial problem or cognitive impairment. You decide to set up an appointment to meet in person with him to brainstorm solutions. At first he doesn't want to be bothered but finally agrees to come. What will you cover at the appointment?

Case Study 8

Name ______________________ Class/Group __________ Date __________

Group Members ____

INSTRUCTIONS: All questions apply to this case study. Your responses should be brief and to the point. Adequate space has been provided for answers. When asked to provide several answers, they should be listed in order of priority or significance. Do not asume information that is not provided. Please print or write clearly. If your response is not legible, it will be marked as ? and you will need to rewrite it.

Scenario

You are working in the internal medicine clinic of a large teaching hospital. Today your first patient is 70-year-old J.M., a man who has been coming to the clinic for several years for management of CAD, hypertension, and anemia. A cardiac catheterization done a year ago showed 50% occlusion of the circumflex coronary artery. He has had episodes of dizziness for the past 6 months and orthostatic hypotension, shoulder discomfort, and decreased exercise tolerance for the past 2 months. On his last clinic visit 3 weeks ago, a chest x-ray (CXR) and 12-lead ECG were done, showing cardiomegaly and a left bundle branch block (LBBB). Results of chemistries (blood studies) drawn at this time were as follows: Na 136 mmol/L, K 5.2 mmol/L, BUN 15 mg/dl, creatinine 1.8 mg/dl, glucose 82 mg/dl, Cl 95 mmol/L, CBC: WBC 4.4 thou/cmm, Hgb 10.5 g/dl, Hct 31.4%, and platelets 229 thou/cmm. This morning his daughter has brought him to the clinic because he has had increased fatigue, significant swelling of his ankles, and SOB for the past 2 days. His VS are 142/83, 105, 18, and 36.6° C.

1. Knowing his history and seeing his condition this morning, what further questions are you going to ask J.M. and his daughter?

J.M. tells you he becomes exhausted and SOB climbing the stairs to his bedroom and has to lie down and rest ("put my feet up") at least an hour twice a day. He has been sleeping on two pillows for the past 2 weeks. He has not salted his food since the physician told him not to because of his high blood pressure (BP), but he admits having had ham and a whole bag of salted peanuts 3 days ago. He denies having palpitations but has had a constant, irritating, nonproductive cough lately.

2. You think it likely that J.M. has congestive heart failure (CHF). From his history, what do you identify as probable causes for his CHF?

3. You are now ready to do your physical assessment. List at least nine things you would assess to confirm your suspicion about the CHF. Also indicate with an "L" or an "R" whether the sign is due to left-sided or right-sided heart failure, or both.

4. The physician confirms your feelings that J.M. is experiencing some CHF. What classes of medications might the physician prescribe?

Note: The hemoglobin (Hgb) and hematocrit (Hct) might be falsely decreased because of hemodilution of the CHF.

5. This is J.M.'s first episode of significant CHF. Before he leaves the clinic, you want to teach him about lifestyle modifications he can make and monitoring techniques he can use to prevent or minimize future problems. List five suggestions you might make and the rationale for each.

6. You tell J.M. the combination of high-sodium foods he had during the past several days may have caused his present episode of CHF. He looks surprised. J.M. says, "But I didn't add any salt to them!" To what health care professional could J.M. be referred to help him understand how to prevent future crises? State your rationale.

7. J.M. receives a prescription for furosemide with a potassium supplement. He wrinkles his nose at the suggestion of potassium and tells you he "hates those horse pills." He tells you a friend of his said he could eat bananas, instead. He says he would rather eat a banana every day than take one of those pills. How will you respond?

8. It's winter and today's temperature is 15° F. J.M. tells you he's been getting cold feet lately. This has never bothered him before. What would you suggest as comfort and safety measures?

9. Researchers sometimes call the legs "the second heart." In view of this statement and J.M.'s cardiac history, explain why "walking would be better than standing" for his circulation.

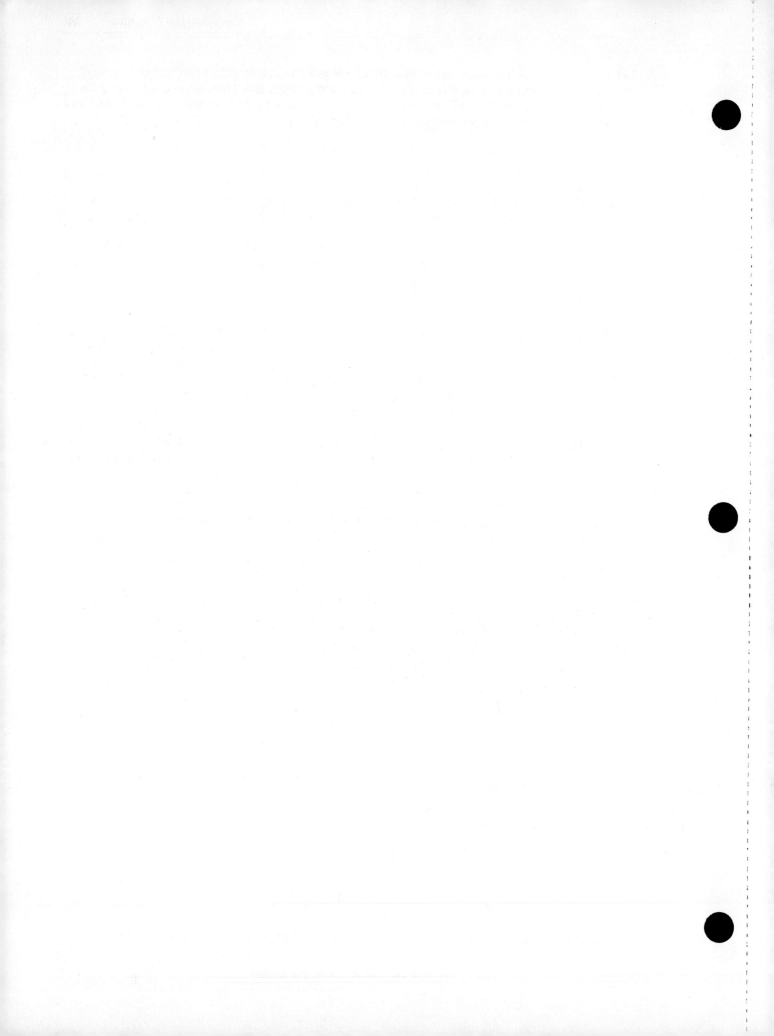

Case Study 9

Name ______________________ Class/Group __________ Date __________

Group Members ____

INSTRUCTIONS: All questions apply to this case study. Your responses should be brief and to the point. Adequate space has been provided for answers. When asked to provide several answers, they should be listed in order of priority or significance. Do not asume information that is not provided. Please print or write clearly. If your response is not legible, it will be marked as ? and you will need to rewrite it.

Scenario

It is midmorning on the cardiac unit where you work, and you are getting a new patient. G.P., a 60-year-old retired businessman, is married and has three grown children. As you take his health history, he tells you that he began feeling changes in his heart rhythm about 10 days ago. He has hypertension and a 5-year history of angina pectoris. During the past week he has had more frequent episodes of midchest discomfort. The chest pain has awakened him from sleep but does respond to NTG, which he has taken sublingually about 8 to 10 times over the past week. During the week he has also experienced increased fatigue. He states, "I just feel crappy all the time anymore." A cardiac catheterization done several years ago revealed 50% occlusion of the RCA (right coronary artery) and 50% occlusion of the LAD (left anterior descending) coronary artery. He tells you that both his mother and father had CAD. He is taking amlodipine, metoprolol, atorvastatin (Lipitor), and baby aspirin 162 mg qd.

1. What other information are you going to ask about his episodes of chest pain?

2. What are common sites for radiation of ischemic cardiac pain?

Note: Patients will tell you what you want to hear, so be careful how you ask your questions.

3. You know that G.P. has atherosclerosis of the coronary arteries but he has not told you about his risk factors. You need to know his risk factors for CAD in order to plan teaching for lifestyle modifications. What will you ask him about?

4. Although he has been taking SL NTG for a long time, you want to be sure he is using it correctly. What information would you make sure he understands about the side effects, use, and storage of sublingual NTG?

When you first admitted G.P., you placed him on telemetry and observed he was in A-fib converting frequently to atrial flutter with a 4:1 block. His VS and all of his lab tests were within normal range, including troponin and creatinine phosphokinase (CK) levels; K was 4.7 mmol/L. He spontaneously converted with medication (diltiazem) from A-fib/atrial flutter to tachycardia/ bradycardia syndrome with long sinus pauses that caused lightheadedness and hypotension.

5. What risks does the new rhythm pose for G.P.?

Because G.P.'s dysrhythmia is causing unacceptable symptoms, he is taken to surgery and a permanent DDI pacemaker is placed and set at a rate of 70/minute.

6. What does the code "DDI" mean?

7. The pacemaker insertion surgery places G.P. at risk for several serious complications. List three potential problems that you will monitor for as you care for him.

8. G.P. will need some education regarding his new pacemaker. What information will you give him before he leaves the hospital?

Note: Information about the Medic-Alert emergency identification system can be obtained by calling 1-800-432-5378.

9. G.P.'s wife approaches you and anxiously inquires, "My neighbor saw this science fiction movie about this guy who got a pacemaker and then he couldn't die. Is that for real?" How are you going to respond to her?

10. G.P. and his wife tell you they have heard that people with pacemakers can have their hearts stop because of theft and security sensors in stores and airports. Where can you help them find more information?

After discharge, G.P. is referred to a cardiac prevention and rehabilitation center to start an exercise program. He will be exercise-tested, and an individualized exercise prescription will be developed for him based on the exercise test.

11. What information will be obtained from the GXT (graded exercise (stress) test), and what is included in an exercise prescription?

Case Study 10

Name ______________________ Class/Group __________ Date __________

Group Members ____

INSTRUCTIONS: All questions apply to this case study. Your responses should be brief and to the point. Adequate space has been provided for answers. When asked to provide several answers, they should be listed in order of priority or significance. Do not asume information that is not provided. Please print or write clearly. If your response is not legible, it will be marked as ? and you will need to rewrite it.

Scenario

You are assigned to care for L.J., a 70-year-old retired bus driver who has just been admitted to your medical floor with right leg DVT. L.J. has a 48-pack-year smoking history, although he states he quit 2 years ago. He has had pneumonia several times and frequent episodes of atrial fibrillation (A-fib). He has had two previous episodes of DVT and was diagnosed with rheumatoid arthritis 3 years ago. Two months ago he began experiencing SOB on exertion and noticed swelling of his right foreleg (lower leg) that became progressively worse until it also involved his thigh to the groin. His wife brought him to the hospital when he C/O increasingly severe pain in his leg. When a Doppler study indicated a probable thrombus of the external iliac vein extending distally to the lower leg, he was admitted for bed rest and to initiate heparin therapy. Significant admission lab values are PT 12.4 sec, INR 1.11, PTT 25 sec, Hgb 13.3 g/dl, Hct 38.9%, cholesterol 206 mg/dl. Basic metabolic panel is normal.

1. Look up the external iliac vein in your anatomy book. List six risk factors for DVT.

2. Identify at least five problems from L.J.'s history that represent his personal risk factors.

3. Something is missing from the above scenario. Based on his history, L.J. should have been taking an important medication. What is it, and why should he be taking it?

4. Keeping in mind L.J.'s health history and admitting diagnosis, what are the most important assessments you should make during your physical examination and assessment?

5. What is the most serious complication of DVT?

Your assessment of L.J. reveals bibasilar crackles with moist cough; normal heart sounds; BP 138/88; P 104; 3+ pitting edema right lower extremity; mild erythema of right foot and calf; and severe right calf pain. He is awake, alert and oriented (AAO) but a little restless. He denies SOB and chest pain.

6. List at least eight assessment findings you should monitor closely for development of the complication identified in question five.

Note: If a pulmonary embolism is massive, the S/S are more like those of myocardial infarction: crushing, substernal chest pain, marked respiratory distress, feeling of impending doom, rapid, shallow breathing, bloody sputum, severe SOB, dysrhythmias, and shock.

L.J. is placed on 72° BR with bathroom privileges (BRP) and given acetaminophen (Tylenol) for pain.

7. Enoxaparin 70 mg (0.7 ml) is prescribed for systemic anticoagulation. L.J. is 5′6″ and weighs 156 pounds. What kind of drug is enoxaparin? Is this dose appropriate? How would it be administered?

8. What instructions will you give L.J. about his activity?

Note: Significant others often want to do something helpful. Having them remind the patient to do their ankle exercises, in particular, can be valuable.

9. What pertinent laboratory values/test results would you expect the physician to order and you to monitor?

10. You identify pain as a key issue in the care of L.J. List four interventions you would choose for L.J. to address his pain.

11. (Optional) This is a copy of one of the ECGs taken from L.J. Identify rate; rhythm; QRS after each P; PR interval; and QRS interval. Are sinus and ventricular rhythm the same? Name this rhythm.

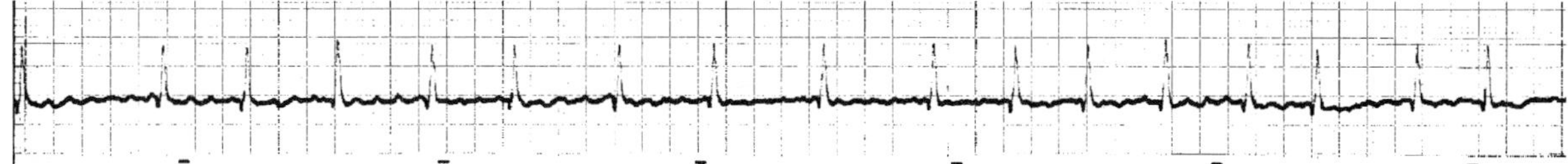

A week has passed. L.J. responded to heparin therapy, was started on warfarin (Coumadin) therapy, and is being discharged to home with home care follow-up. "Good," he says, "just in time to fly out West for my grandson's wedding." His wife, who has come to pick him up, rolls her eyes and looks at the ceiling. You almost drop the discharge papers in disbelief at what you have just heard. (And you thought you did such a good job of discharge teaching!)

12. What are you going to tell him?

L.J. listens to you, and Mrs. J. is quite relieved. (She has been telling her friends about this "wonderful nurse who talked some sense into my husband.") L.J.'s son arranges to videotape the entire wedding ceremony, and guests at the reception tape special greetings for him. It's been 2 weeks, and he seems quite pleased. He watches the tape daily and points out his favorite parts to the home care nurse every time she visits.

Case Study 11

Name ______________________ Class/Group __________ Date __________

Group Members ____

INSTRUCTIONS: All questions apply to this case study. Your responses should be brief and to the point. Adequate space has been provided for answers. When asked to provide several answers, they should be listed in order of priority or significance. Do not asume information that is not provided. Please print or write clearly. If your response is not legible, it will be marked as ? and you will need to rewrite it.

Scenario

J.M. is a 70-year-old retired construction worker who has experienced lumbosacral pain, nausea, and upset stomach for the past 6 months. He has a history of CHF, deep visceral pain, dyspnea, hypertension, sleep apnea, and depression. J.M. has just been admitted to the hospital for surgical repair of a 6.2 cm AAA that is now causing him constant pain. Upon arrival on your floor, his VS are 109/81, 61, 16 and 98.3° F. When you perform your assessment, you find that his apical heart rhythm is regular and his peripheral pulses are strong. His lungs are clear, and he is AAO. There are no abnormal physical findings; however, he hasn't had a bowel movement for 3 days. His electrolytes and other blood chemistries and clotting studies are within normal range, but his Hct is 30.1% and Hgb 9 g/dl.

J.M. has been depressed since the death of his wife 9 years ago. He has no children. His height is 6′2″ and weight 160 pounds. His chronic medical problems have been managed over the years by medications: benazepril 40 mg PO qd, fluoxetine 40 mg PO qd, furosemide 40 mg PO qd, trazodone 50 mg PO qhs, KCl 20 mEq PO bid, and lovastatin 40 mg PO with the evening meal.

1. J.M. has several common risk factors for AAA, which are evident from his health history. Identify and explain three factors.

While J.M. awaits his surgery, it is important that you monitor him carefully for decrease in tissue perfusion.

2. Identify five things you would assess for, and state your rationale for each.

3. What is the most serious, life-threatening complication of AAA, and why?

4. What single problem mentioned in the first paragraph of this case study presents a risk for AAA rupture? Why?

Monitoring urinary output is critical in evaluating shock or for postsurvival problems.

5. What is the minimal acceptable urinary output per hour?

The resection of J.M.'s aneurysm was successful, but for the first 3 postoperative days he was delirious and required one-to-one nursing care and soft restraints before he became coherent and oriented again. He was still somewhat confused when he was transferred back to your floor.

6. What assessments should be made specific to his postoperative care?

7. List five problems that should be high priorities in J.M.'s postoperative care.

8. Postoperative care of the patient undergoing aneurysectomy includes preservation of the graft, preservation of tissue perfusion, and prevention of infection. List three interventions that would address these issues and explain the rationale for each.

When J.M. is being prepared for discharge, you talk to him about health promotion and lifestyle change issues that are pertinent to his health problems.

9. Identify four health-related issues you might appropriately address with him and what you would teach in each area.

10. J.M. will be receiving follow-up visits from the home health care nurse to change his dressing and evaluate his incision. What can you discuss with J.M. before discharge that will help him understand what the nurse will be doing?

11. What link could there be between J.M.'s diet and his depression?

Make sure there is a physician's order for medical nutrition therapy for J.M. He is going to need a lot of help with maintaining a healthy diet specific to his needs. RDs are often aware of community resources that could help someone like J.M.

Case Study 12

Name ______________________ Class/Group __________ Date __________

Group Members ____

INSTRUCTIONS: All questions apply to this case study. Your responses should be brief and to the point. Adequate space has been provided for answers. When asked to provide several answers, they should be listed in order of priority or significance. Do not asume information that is not provided. Please print or write clearly. If your response is not legible, it will be marked as ? and you will need to rewrite it.

Scenario

R.K. is an 85-year-old woman who lives with her husband, 87. Two nights before her admission to your cardiac unit, she awoke with heavy substernal pressure accompanied by epigastric distress. The pain was reduced somewhat when she rolled onto her side but did not completely subside for about 6 hours. The next night she experienced the same chest pressure. The following morning, R.K.'s husband took her to the physician and she was subsequently hospitalized to R/O MI (rule out myocardial infarction).

Labs were drawn in the ED. She was started on O_2 2 L/NC and given nonenteric–coated aspirin 325 mg to be chewed and swallowed. An IV was started.

You obtain the following information from your history and physical exam: R.K. has no history of smoking or alcohol use; has been in good general health with the exception of osteoarthritis of her hands and knees and some osteoarthritis of the spine. Her only medications are ranitidine, ibuprofen for bone and joint pain, and "herbs." Her admission VS are 132/84, 88, 18, 37.2° C. Her weight is 52 kg and height is 163 cm. Moderate edema of both ankles is present, but capillary refill and peripheral pulses are 1+. You hear a soft systolic murmur. You place her on telemetry, which shows frequent premature atrial contractions (PACs) but no ventricular ectopy. She denies any discomfort at present.

1. Give at least two reasons an IV would be inserted. What kind of IV fluid would you expect to be running and at what rate? [k/c/an/ap]

(This question requires a series of mental steps: First, you need to gather your facts, then you need to figure out what they mean. You need to analyze this context, then decide what is appropriate to use.)

2. Why is "nonenteric coated" aspirin specified? What would be a contraindication to administering aspirin?

3. R.K. becomes fatigued during the admission process and you decide to let her sleep. When she awakens, what additional history and physical information should you obtain R/T her admitting diagnosis?

4. List seven lab/diagnostic tests you would expect were drawn or conducted in the ED; suggest what each may contribute.

5. What other source, besides cardiac ischemia, may be responsible for her chest and abdominal discomfort? (specify)

6. Differentiate between pain of cardiac origin and that of noncardiac origin. Be aware that little research has differentiated between the clinical symptoms experienced by women versus those experienced by men.

(***Note:*** There is much individuality in responses. These are merely general guidelines. Older adults, chronically ill patients, diabetics, and women tend to have atypical responses. When in doubt, cardiac disease should be ruled out first. Many patients never experience chest pain or traditional angina with ischemia or an MI.)

Consider:

- Character
- Location
- Provoking factors
- Alleviating factors
- Associated findings

7. Define the concept *differential diagnosis.*

8. Explain how the concept of differential diagnosis applies to R.K.'s symptoms.

9. Florence Nightingale frequently emphasized the value of good observation skills in nurses. Explain how a good nursing assessment can contribute to understanding the cause of her symptoms.

10. Abnormalities on R.K.'s 12-lead ECG were reported as "slight left axis deviation." Serial CKs are 27 units/ml, 24 units/ml, 26 units/ml; troponin is <0.03 ng/ml. A series of tests R/O a noncardiac cause for her chest pain. On the basis of the information presented so far, do you believe she has had an MI? What is your rationale?

11. While you care for R.K., you carefully observe her. Identify two possible complications of CAD and the S/S associated with each.

12. R.K. rings her call bell. When you arrive, she has her hand placed over her heart and tells you she is "having that heavy feeling again." She is not diaphoretic or nauseated but states she is SOB. What can you do to make her more comfortable?

Note: Laboratory tests can be reported in terms of different values. Always read laboratory reports carefully to be sure which units are used in your institution.

R.K.'s husband is very upset. He tells you they have been married for 62 years and he doesn't know what he would do without his wife. One way to help people deal with their anxieties is to help them focus on concrete issues.

13. What information would be useful to get from him? What other health care professional may be able to help with some of these issues?

Case Study 13

Name ______________________ Class/Group ___________ Date ___________

Group Members ____

INSTRUCTIONS: All questions apply to this case study. Your responses should be brief and to the point. Adequate space has been provided for answers. When asked to provide several answers, they should be listed in order of priority or significance. Do not asume information that is not provided. Please print or write clearly. If your response is not legible, it will be marked as ? and you will need to rewrite it.

Scenario

The time is 1900. You are working in a small, rural hospital. It has been snowing heavily all day, and the medical helicopters at the large regional medical center, 4 hours away by car (in good weather), have been grounded by the weather until morning. The roads are barely passable. W.R., a 48-year-old construction worker with a 36-pack-year smoking history, is admitted to your floor with a diagnosis of R/O MI. He has significant male-pattern obesity ("beer belly," large waist circumference), a barrel chest, and reports a dietary history of high-fat food. His wife brought him to the ED after he complained of unrelieved "indigestion." His admission VS were 202/124, 96, 18, 36.8° C. W.R. was put on O_2/NC titrated to maintain Sao_2 (arterial oxygen saturation) >90% and an IV of NTG was started in the ED. He was also given aspirin 325 mg and was admitted to Dr. A's service. There are plans to transfer him by helicopter to the regional medical center for a cardiac catheterization in the morning when the weather clears. Meanwhile you have to deal with limited laboratory and pharmacy resources. The minute W.R. comes through the door of your unit, he announces he's just fine in a loud and angry voice and demands a cigarette.

1. From the perspective of basic human needs, what is the first priority in his care?

2. Are these VS reasonable for a man his age? If not, which one(s) concern(s) you? Explain why or why not.

3. Identify five priority problems associated with the care of a patient like W.R.

4. Which of the following laboratory tests might be ordered to investigate W.R.'s condition? If the order is appropriate, place an "A" in the space provided. If inappropriate, mark with an "I."

____________ CBC
____________ EEG in the morning
____________ Chem 7 (electrolytes)
____________ PT/PTT
____________ Bilirubin q morning
____________ Urinalysis
____________ STAT 12-lead ECG
____________ Type and cross (T&C) for four units packed red blood cells (PRBCs)

5. What significant laboratory tests are missing from the previous list?

6. How are you going to respond to W.R.'s angry demands for a cigarette? He also demands something for his "heartburn." How will you respond?

You phone Dr. A's partner, who is "on call." She prescribes 4 to 10 mg morphine sulfate IV push q1h prn for pain (burning, pressure, angina).

7. Explain two reasons for this order.

8. What special precautions should you follow when administering morphine sulfate IV push?

9. Angina is not always experienced as “pain” (as many people understand pain). How would you describe symptoms you want him to warn you about? Why is this important?

10. What safety measures/instructions would you give W.R. before you leave his room?

11. One of the housekeeping staff asks you, “If the poor guy can’t smoke, why can’t you give him one of those nicotine patches?” How will you respond?

12. If the patch were to be used later to help him quit smoking, how would it be dosed for him?

13. Before leaving for the night, Mrs. R. approaches you and asks, "Did my husband have a heart attack? I'm really scared. His father died of one when he was 51." How are you going to respond to her question?

14. When you come into W.R.'s room at 2200 to answer his call light, you see he is holding his left arm and C/O aching in his left shoulder and arm. What information are you going to gather? What questions will you ask him?

15. Based on your assessment findings, you decide to call the physician. What information are you going to report to the physician, and why?

In the morning, W.R. is transferred by chopper to the medical center and a cardiac catheterization is performed. It is determined that W.R. has CAD. The cardiologist suggests it would be best to treat him medically for now, with follow-up counseling on risk factor modification, especially smoking cessation. He is discharged with a referral for a follow-up visit to his local internist in 1 week.

16. What does it mean to treat him “medically” (conservatively)? What other approaches may be used to treat coronary artery disease?

17. What personality characteristic do you observe in W.R. that places him at high risk for coronary artery disease?

Case Study 14

Name ______________________ Class/Group __________ Date __________

Group Members ____

INSTRUCTIONS: All questions apply to this case study. Your responses should be brief and to the point. Adequate space has been provided for answers. When asked to provide several answers, they should be listed in order of priority or significance. Do not asume information that is not provided. Please print or write clearly. If your response is not legible, it will be marked as ? and you will need to rewrite it.

Scenario

You are working at the local cardiac rehabilitation center and R.M. is walking around the track. He summons you and asks if you could help him understand his recent lab report. He admits to being confused by the overwhelming data on the test and doesn't understand how the results relate to his recent heart attack and need for a stent. You take a moment to locate his lab reports and review his history. Below are the findings.

R.M. is a 61-year-old active male who works full-time for the postal service. He walks 3 miles every other day and admits he doesn't eat a "perfect diet." He enjoys two or three beers every night, he uses stick margarine, eats red meat 2 or 3 times per week, and is a self-professed "sweet eater." His cardiac history includes a recent inferior myocardial infarction, a heart catheterization revealing three-vessel disease: left anterior descending (LAD) coronary artery a proximal 60% lesion; right coronary artery (RCA) proximal 100% occlusion with thrombus, and a circumflex with 40% to 60% diffuse ecctatic lesions. A stent was deployed to the RCA and reduced the lesion to 0% residual stenosis. He has had no need for nitroglycerin. He was discharged on aspirin 325 mg, Plavix (clopidogrel) 75 mg, Lipitor (atorvastatin) 10 mg, Foltx with food, and Altace (ramipril)10 mg qd. Six weeks after his MI and stent deployment, he had a fasting advanced lipid profile report. The results were: total cholesterol 188 mg/dl, HDL 34 mg/dl, triglycerides 176 mg/dl, LDL 98 mg/dl, pattern B LDL typing at 19 nm, homocysteine 18 mg/dl, high sensitivity C-reactive protein (HS CRP) 12 mg/dl, fasting blood sugar (FBS) 101 mg/dl, thyroid-stimulating hormone (TSH) 1.04 mg/dl.

1. Given the information above, which of the following questions is the most important to ask R.M.?
   A. Is he or anyone in his family diagnosed with diabetes?
   B. How long does it take for him to walk 3 miles at home?
   C. His height and weight to calculate BMI (body mass index)?
   D. Does he eat a large quantity of white flour products (white rice, white bread, pasta, sweets, juices, sodas)?

2. When you start to discuss R.M.'s lab values with him he is pleased that his total cholesterol is less than 200 mg/dl and that his LDL is less than 100 mg/dl. He thinks he needs no further alteration in his lipid values. What do you tell him about his triglycerides and pattern B LDL type?

3. R.M.'s physician adds niacin, folic acid, B_{12}, B_6, and omega-3 fatty acids to his list of medications. How do atorvastatin (Lipitor) and the new medications affect lipids?

4. What treatment options are known to decrease CRP?

All these treatments are thought to decrease inflammatory response in the arterial walls and endothelium. Many of these options should be used for primary prevention as well. They will reduce the number of cardiovascular events.

5. HS-CRP is an indicator of:

6. Identify the most common side effect of niacin and statins.

7. Elevated homocysteine can be a factor for what type of vascular complication?

8. Name one food that will increase the homocysteine level.

You enter R.M.'s room and hear the physician say, "There are many options to change the metabolic makeup of your small dense LDL and increased homocysteine. You will need to continue modifying your diet and exercise to enhance your medication regimen." The physician asks R.M. if he has any questions and the patient responds, "No."

9. After the physician leaves the room, R.M. tells you he really didn't understand what the physician said. Explain the necessary lifestyle changes to R.M.

10. A normal homocysteine level is:

Case Study 15

Name ______________________ Class/Group __________ Date __________

Group Members ____

INSTRUCTIONS: All questions apply to this case study. Your responses should be brief and to the point. Adequate space has been provided for answers. When asked to provide several answers, they should be listed in order of priority or significance. Do not asume information that is not provided. Please print or write clearly. If your response is not legible, it will be marked as ? and you will need to rewrite it.

Scenario

L.M. is a 60-year-old woman who is admitted to your telemetry unit in a major medical center after being successfully resuscitated by medics from a cardiac arrest due to ventricular fibrillation (V-fib). L.M., a divorced housewife, had her sudden death experience in the small rural community where she lives and was transported to your facility for evaluation and treatment after she was stabilized. At the time of the arrest, her potassium level was 2.8 mmol/L and magnesium level was 1.3 mg/dl. As you continue to review her medical history, you learn that she had rheumatic fever as a child and over the years has developed severe rheumatic heart disease with mitral and aortic valve involvement and dilated cardiomyopathy. Four years ago she had a percutaneous balloon mitral valvuloplasty (PBMV) for mitral valve stenosis (MVS). She also has probable aortic valve stenosis (AVS). During the past year she has experienced increasing problems with chest pain, SOB, and dyspnea on exertion. Two months ago she developed a severe cough and increasing fatigue. She has been on furosemide 40 mg PO qd, digoxin 0.125 mg PO qd, lisinopril 20 mg PO qd, warfarin (Coumadin) 5 mg qd, and potassium (K-Dur) 20 mEq PO qd. In addition, during the week before her cardiac arrest, she was taking erythromycin 500 mg PO q6h for a lower respiratory tract infection. Although she stopped smoking 4 years ago, she has a 40-pack-year smoking history.

1. What organism causes rheumatic fever?

2. What is a PBMV, and how is it carried out?

3. What medication is commonly used prophylactically to prevent development of rheumatic heart disease when an individual has rheumatic fever?

4. Why would someone like L.M. be given warfarin?

5. Reviewing the above health history, what factors do you think contribute to her current symptoms of chest pain, SOB, dyspnea on exertion, cough, and fatigue? Explain your rationale for each.

6. What factors in the above health history may have precipitated L.M.'s cardiac arrest?

L.M.'s admission VS are 102/60, 84, 16, and 36° C. Her telemetry monitor shows A-fib and frequent PVCs. When you listen to her heart, you hear an S_3 gallop, a grade III/VI systolic murmur, and a soft, blowing diastolic murmur. Her point of maximal impulse (PMI) is displaced laterally. She has no pedal edema. You hear crackles in her lungs. Other assessment findings are normal. She is transferred to the coronary care unit (CCU) and is placed on continuous heparin and lidocaine IV infusions, and started on O_2 at 40% by face mask. Her lab values are drawn. Later in the day during a cardiac catheterization, her CO was found to be 2.3 L/min and her mean pulmonary artery pressure 29 mm Hg.

7. Based on the above assessment, do you believe that L.M. is experiencing some heart failure? Why or why not?

8. L.M.'s lab tests return. Her PT is 23.4 sec/INR = 1.99, PTT 30 sec. What other lab tests would you especially want to monitor?

9. Why is it important to monitor L.M.'s PTT? Is her partial thromboplastin time (PTT) within the therapeutic range? Is the INR within the normal range?

10. What would be the advantages and disadvantages of giving L.M. Pen VK versus erythromycin (list at least one in each category)?

11. List four relevant problems R/T L.M.'s care.

12. In order to prevent serious complications, you will assess and monitor for potential problems. List three significant potential physiologic problems for which L.M. is at risk. Explain.

13. The technologic monitoring and care L.M. receives demands so much time that there has been little opportunity to talk with her about her feelings R/T her sudden death experience. As you plan to approach her, you remind yourself to be sensitive to communication limitations imposed by her pathologic condition. What are two of these limitations, and how will they affect your interaction?

Case Study 16

Name ______________________ Class/Group __________ Date __________

Group Members ____

INSTRUCTIONS: All questions apply to this case study. Your responses should be brief and to the point. Adequate space has been provided for answers. When asked to provide several answers, they should be listed in order of priority or significance. Do not asume information that is not provided. Please print or write clearly. If your response is not legible, it will be marked as ? and you will need to rewrite it.

Scenario

Your patient, 58-year-old K.Z., has a significant cardiac history. He has long-standing CAD with occasional episodes of CHF. One year ago he had an anterior wall MI. In addition, he has chronic anemia, hypertension, chronic renal insufficiency, and a recently diagnosed 4 cm suprarenal AAA. Because of his severe CAD, he had to retire from his job as a railroad engineer about 6 months ago. This morning he is being admitted to your telemetry unit for a same-day cardiac catheterization. As you take his health history, you note that his wife died a year ago (about the same time that he had his MI) and that he does not have any children. He is a current cigarette smoker with a 50-pack-year smoking history. As you talk with him, you realize that he has only minimal understanding of the catheterization procedure. His VS are 158/94, 88, 20 and 36.2° C.

1. Before he leaves for the catheterization laboratory, you briefly teach him the important things he needs to know before having the procedure. List five priority topics you will address.

Several hours later K.Z. returns from his catheterization. The catheterization report shows 90% occlusion of the proximal LAD, 90% occlusion of the distal LAD, 70% to 80% occlusion of the distal RCA, an old apical infarct, and an ejection fraction (EF) of 37%. About an hour after the procedure was finished, you perform a brief physical assessment and find that he now has a grade III/VI systolic ejection murmur at the cardiac apex, crackles bilaterally in the lung bases, and trace pitting edema of his feet and ankles. Except for a soft systolic murmur, these findings were not present before the catheterization.

2. Review the location of these vessels on a diagram of the heart from your anatomy book. Sketch (don't trace) a simple illustration of the anterior heart; label the superior and inferior vena cava, and the aorta. Draw the main coronary arteries on the surface of the heart. Circle the areas of the LAD and RCA that have significant occlusion. Lightly shade the part of the heart where K.Z. had an earlier infarct. Using the illustration as a patient teaching aid, explain, in plain English, how you would teach him what "37% ejection fraction" means and how you would expect it to influence his everyday activity.

3. What is your evaluation of the catheterization results?

4. What problem do the changes in assessment findings suggest to you? What led you to your conclusion?

Note: Patients usually express statements like, "Something is wrong . . . I just don't feel right." The nurse needs to be alert to this and reassure them that he or she is listening to them and monitoring their status. Such statements should never be taken lightly. They should be shared with nurses on the next shift and the patient's physician. If you have a chance, discuss this with your instructor and the rest of the class.

5. List four actions you would take as a result of your evaluation of the assessment and state your rationales.

After assessing him, K.Z.'s physician admits him (with a diagnosis of CAD and CHF) for CABG surgery. Significant lab results drawn at this time are Hct 25.3%, Hgb 8.8 g/dl, BUN 33 mg/dl, and creatinine 3.1 mg/dl. K.Z. is diuresed with furosemide and given two units of PRBCs.

6. Review K.Z.'s health history. Can you identify a probable explanation for his chronic renal insufficiency and anemia?

Five days later, after his condition is stabilized, K.Z. is taken to surgery for CABG × 3V (bypass of three coronary arteries). When he arrives in the surgical intensive care unit (SICU), he has a Swan-Ganz catheter in place for hemodynamic monitoring and is intubated. He is put on a ventilator at Fio_2 0.70 and positive end expiratory pressure (PEEP) 5 cm H_2O. His first hemodynamic readings are as follows: pulmonary artery pressure (PAP) 41/23 mm Hg, central venous pressure (CVP) 13 mm Hg, pulmonary capillary wedge pressure (PCWP) 13 mm Hg, cardiac index (CI) 1.88 L/min/mm^2. ABGs drawn at this time are pH 7.36, $Pco_2$46 mm Hg, Po_2 61 mm Hg, and Sao_2 85%, with a Hgb 10.3 mg/dl.

7. Why are ABGs necesssary in the case of K.Z.? Explain why it would be inappropriate to use pulse oximetry to assess his oxygen saturation status.

8. What is your evaluation of K.Z.'s hemodynamic status based on the previous parameters?

Clinically these values show that the pressures within his heart and lungs are a little high and that his cardiac output is a little low, indicating that his heart is still having difficulty pumping out all the blood that is returned to it and/or that he is a little fluid overloaded. His condition will require careful monitoring.

9. K.Z. is receiving continuous IV infusions of nitroprusside and dobutamine. He also has just received 2 units of fresh frozen plasma (FFP). Given this information, do you think the hemodynamic values reported above reflect poor left ventricular function or fluid overload and why?

10. Why is K.Z. receiving the nitroprusside and dobutamine?

11. What is your responsibility when administering nitroprusside and dobutamine to your patient?

12. Why did he receive the FFP?

13. Is it possible for K.Z. to experience a transfusion reaction when receiving albumin or FFP infusion? Explain your answer.

14. What is your interpretation of his ABGs on 70% O_2?

After 3 days in the SICU (surgical intensive care unit), K.Z.'s condition is stable and he is returned to your telemetry floor. Now, 5 days later, he is ready to go home, and you are preparing him for discharge.

15. List at least two specific areas of teaching that he should receive R/T his cardiac catheterization.

16. List at least four general areas R/T his CABG surgery in which he should receive instruction before he goes home.

Case Study 17

Name ______________________ Class/Group __________ Date __________

Group Members ____

INSTRUCTIONS: All questions apply to this case study. Your responses should be brief and to the point. Adequate space has been provided for answers. When asked to provide several answers, they should be listed in order of priority or significance. Do not asume information that is not provided. Please print or write clearly. If your response is not legible, it will be marked as ? and you will need to rewrite it.

Scenario

C.W., a 70-year-old man, was brought to the ED at 0430 this morning by his wife. She told the ED triage nurse that he had dysentery for the past 3 days and last night he had a lot of "dark red" diarrhea. When he became very dizzy, disoriented, and weak this morning, she decided to bring him to the hospital. C.W.'s VS were BP 70/- (systolic BP 70 mm Hg, diastolic BP inaudible); 110, 20. A 16-gauge IV catheter was inserted and a lactated Ringer's (LR) infusion was started. The triage nurse obtained the following history from the patient and his wife. C.W. has had idiopathic dilated cardiomyopathy (IDCM) for several years. The onset was insidious but the cardiomyopathy is now severe, as evidenced by a left ventricular ejection fraction of 13% found during a recent cardiac catheterization. He experiences frequent problems with CHF because of the IDCM. Two years ago he had a cardiac arrest that was attributed to hypokalemia. He also has a long history of hypertension and arthritis. Fifteen years ago he had a peptic ulcer.

An endoscopy showed a 25 × 15 mm duodenal ulcer with adherent clot. The ulcer was cauterized and C.W. was admitted to the medical intensive care unit (MICU) for treatment of his volume deficit. You are his admitting nurse. As you are making him comfortable, Mrs. W. gives you a paper sack filled with the bottles of medications he has been taking: enalapril (Vasotec) 5 mg PO bid, warfarin (Coumadin) 5 mg PO qd, digoxin 0.125 mg PO qd, KCl 20 mEq PO bid, and tolmetin (a nonsteroidal antiinflammatory drug [NSAID]) 400 mg PO tid. As you connect him to the cardiac monitor, you note that he is in A-fib. Doing a quick assessment, you find a pale man who is sleepy but arousable and oriented. He is still dizzy, hypotensive, and tachycardic. You hear S_3 and S_4 heart sounds and a grade II/VI systolic murmur. Peripheral pulses are all 2+ and trace pedal edema is present. Lungs are clear. Bowel sounds are present, midepigastric tenderness is noted, and the liver margin is 4 cm below the costal margin. A Swan-Ganz catheter and an arterial line are inserted.

1. What medication probably precipitated C.W.'s GI bleeding?

2. What is the most serious potential complication of C.W.'s bleeding?

3. From his history and assessment, identify five S/S (direct and/or indirect) of GI bleeding and loss of blood volume.

C.W. receives a total of 4 units of PRBCs, 5 units of FFP, and many liters of crystalloids to keep his systolic BP above 90 mm Hg. On the second day in the MICU, his total fluid intake is 8.498 L and output 3.660 L for a positive fluid balance of 4.838 L. His hemodynamic parameters after fluid resuscitation are PCWP 30 mm Hg, CO 4.5 L/min.

4. Why will you want to monitor his fluid status very carefully?

5. List six things you will monitor to assess C.W.'s fluid balance.

6. Explain the purpose of the FFP for C.W.

As soon as you get a chance, you look at C.W.'s admission lab results: K 6.2 mmol/L, BUN 90 mg/dl, creatinine 2.1 mg/dl, Hgb 8.4 g/dl, Hct 25%, WBC 16 thou/cmm, and PT 23.4/INR = 4.2. Other results are within the normal range.

7. Are you worried by the elevated potassium? Why, or why not? Explain your answer.

8. In view of the elevated K, what diagnostic test should be performed and why?

9. Why do you think BUN and creatinine are elevated?

10. What do the low Hgb and Hct levels indicate about the rapidity of C.W.'s blood loss?

11. What is the explanation for the prolonged PT/INR?

12. What should be your response to the prolonged PT/INR?

13. What safety precautions should be considered in light of his prolonged PT/INR?

Mrs. W. has been with her husband since he arrived at the ED and is very worried about his condition and his care.

15. List four things you might do to make her more comfortable while her husband is in the MICU.

Case Study 18

Name ______________________ Class/Group __________ Date __________

Group Members ____

INSTRUCTIONS: All questions apply to this case study. Your responses should be brief and to the point. Adequate space has been provided for answers. When asked to provide several answers, they should be listed in order of priority or significance. Do not asume information that is not provided. Please print or write clearly. If your response is not legible, it will be marked as ? and you will need to rewrite it.

Scenario

J.F. is a 50-year-old married homemaker with a genetic autoimmune deficiency; she has suffered from recurrent bacterial endocarditis. The most recent episodes were a *Staphylococcus aureus* infection of the mitral valve 16 months ago and a *Streptococcus mutans* infection of the aortic valve 1 month ago. During this latter hospitalization, an ECG showed moderate aortic stenosis, moderate aortic insufficiency, chronic valvular vegetations, and moderate left atrial enlargement. Two years ago J.F. received an 18-month course of total parenteral therapy (TPN) therapy for malnutrition caused by idiopathic, relentless N/V. She has also had CAD for several years, and 2 years ago suffered an acute anterior wall MI. In addition, she has a history of chronic joint pain.

Now, after being home for only a week, J.F. has been readmitted to your floor with endocarditis, N/V, and renal failure. Since yesterday she has been vomiting and retching constantly; she also has had chills, fever, fatigue, joint pain, and headache. As you go through the admission process with her, you note that she wears glasses and has a dental bridge. She is immediately started on TPN at 125 ml/hr and on penicillin 2 million units IV q4h, to be continued for 4 weeks. Other medications are furosemide 80 mg PO qd, amlodipine 5 mg PO qd, K-Dur 40 mEq PO qd (dose adjusted according to laboratory results), metoprolol 25 mg PO bid, and prochlorperazine (Compazine) 2.5 to 5 mg IVP prn for N/V. Admission VS are 152/48 (supine) and 100/40 (sitting), 116, 22, 37.9° C. When you assess her, you find a grade II/VI holosystolic murmur and a grade III/VI diastolic murmur; 2+ pitting tibial edema but no peripheral cyanosis; clear lungs; orientation × 3 but drowsy; soft abdomen with slight left upper quadrant (LUQ) tenderness; hematuria; and multiple petechiae on skin of arms, legs, and chest.

1. What is the significance of the orthostatic hypotension, the wide pulse pressure, and the tachycardia?

2. What is the significance of the abdominal tenderness, hematuria, joint pain, and petechiae?

3. As you monitor J.F. throughout the day, what other S/S of embolization will you watch for?

4. Three important diagnostic criteria for infectious endocarditis are anemia, fever, and cardiac murmurs. Explain the cause for each sign.

5. On the day after admission, you review J.F.s laboratory test results: Na 138 mmol/L, K 3.9 mmol/L, Cl 103 mmol/L, BUN 85 mg/dl, creatinine 3.9 mg/dl, glucose 185 mg/dl, WBCs 6.7 thou/cmm, Hct 27%, Hgb 9.0 g/dl. Identify the values that are not within normal ranges, and explain the reason for each abnormality.

6. Which laboratory value(s) reflect(s) catabolism of muscle, and why does muscle catabolism occur?

7. If the TPN is scheduled on a 24-hour basis, when would blood glucose be drawn, and why?

8. Why would blood glucose monitoring be important?

9. What is the greatest risk for J.F. during the process of rehydration, and what would you monitor to detect its development?

As you admitted J.F., you were aware that as soon as she became stable, she would be going home in a few days on TPN and IV antibiotics. The home care agency that will be supervising her care is contacted to coordinate discharge preparations and teaching as soon as possible.

10. List five important questions in assessing her home health care needs.

Fortunately, J.F. has a supportive husband and two daughters who live nearby who can function as caregivers when J.F. is discharged. They, as well as the patient, will also need teaching about endocarditis. Although J.F. has been ill for several years, you discover that she and her family have received little education about the disease. You prepare a teaching plan for the family. The home care agency has a PEN-team (parenteral enteral nutrition team) to address her nutritional needs, which will also include vitamins, minerals, and lipids. TPN formulations require complex calculations. The PEN-team takes care of the formulation of the TPN through the pharmacy or dietary staff (depending on local arrangements).

11. List two predisposing causes of bacteremia. Explain.

12. List three other things you would teach.

Your hospital discharge planner facilitates J.F.'s transition to home care.

13. During the initial home visit, the home health nurse evaluates J.F.'s IV site for implementation of the IV therapy program. The nurse interviews the family members to determine their willingness to be caregivers and their level of understanding and enlists the patient's and family's assistance to identify ten teaching goals. What topics would be included on this list?

14. The home health nurse also writes short- and long-term goals for J.F. and her family. Identify two short-term and three long-term goals.

Mr. F. and his two daughters learned to administer J.F.'s TPN during the 18-month treatment. Be aware that IV cases are usually covered by most insurers on a case-by-case basis and with clear documentation.

15. What documentation would be required in order to obtain reimbursement? (Need to clearly document everything that is done and why, in detail.)

Case Study 19

Name ______________________________ Class/Group __________ Date __________

Group Members ____

INSTRUCTIONS: All questions apply to this case study. Your responses should be brief and to the point. Adequate space has been provided for answers. When asked to provide several answers, they should be listed in order of priority or significance. Do not asume information that is not provided. Please print or write clearly. If your response is not legible, it will be marked as ? and you will need to rewrite it.

Scenario

You are just getting caught up with your work when you receive the following phone call: "Hi, this is Deb in the ED. We're sending you M.M., a 63-year-old Hispanic woman with a PMH of CAD. Her daughter reports that she's become increasingly weak over the past couple of weeks and has been unable to do her housework. Apparently she has been C/O swelling in her ankles and feet by late afternoon ("she can't wear her shoes") and has nocturnal diuresis × 4. Her daughter brought her in because she has C/O heaviness in her chest off and on over the past few days but denies any discomfort at this time. The daughter took her to see her family physician, who immediately sent her here. VS are 146/92, 96, 24, 37.2° C. She has an IV of D_5W at KVO in her right forearm. Her labs are as follows: Na 134 mmol/L, K 3.5 mmol/L, Cl 103 mmol/L, HCO_3 23, BUN 13 mg/dl, creatinine 1.3 mg/dl, glucose 153 mg/dl, WBC 8.3 thou/cmm, Hct 33.9%, Hgb 11.7 g/dl, platelets 162 thou/cmm. (Note: The former *mm^3* is currently written *Thou* or *thou/cmm.*) PT/INR, PTT, and urinalysis (UA) are pending. She has had her CXR and ECG, and her orders have been written."

1. What additional information do you need from the ED nurse?

2. How are you going to prepare for this patient?

3. Name three types of sphygmomanometers.

4. Monitoring her BP is going to be very important. What would you do to check the cuff and tubing to make certain they are in good working order? (List at least three things.)

5. M.M. arrives by wheelchair (W/C). As she transfers from the W/C to the bed, what observations should you make? Why?

6. Given the previous information, which of the following orders can you anticipate as appropriate for this patient? Carefully review each order to determine whether it is appropriate or inappropriate as written. If the order is appropriate, place an "A" in the space provided; if the order is inappropriate, place an "I" in the space provided and change the order to make it appropriate. Also provide any other orders that may be appropriate for this patient.

____________ Routine VS
____________ Serum magnesium STAT
____________ Up ad lib
____________ 10 g sodium, low animal fat diet
____________ Change IV to NS at 100 ml/hr.
____________ Cardiac enzymes on admission and q8h × 24 then q AM
____________ CBC (hemogram), chem 7, and lipid profile in morning
____________ Schedule for abdominal CT scan for morning.
____________ Heparin 10,000 units SQ q8h
____________ Docusate sodium 100 mg PO qd
____________ Ampicillin 250 mg IVPB q6h

_____________ Furosemide 200 mg IVP STAT
_____________ Nitroglycerin 0.4 mg 1 SL q4h prn for chest pain

7. When you respond to M.M.'s call light, you observe she is talking rapidly in Spanish and pointing to the bathroom. Her speech pattern indicates she is SOB (she is having trouble completing a sentence without taking a labored breath). You assist her to the bathroom and note that her skin feels clammy. While sitting on the commode, she vomits. On a scale of zero to 10 (zero being no problem, 10 being a code-level emergency), how would you rate this situation and why?

8. Identify at least four actions you should take next, and state your rationale.

9. The physician calls your unit to find out what is happening. What information would you need to convey at this time?

10. The resident is coming to the floor to evaluate the patient immediately. In the meantime she orders furosemide 40 mg IVP STAT. You have only 20 mg in stock. Should you give the 20 mg now, then give the additional 20 mg when it comes up from the pharmacy? Explain your answer.

11. M.M. continues to experience vomiting and diaphoresis that are unrelieved by medication and comfort measures. A STAT 12-lead ECG reveals ischemic changes. The patient is transferred to the CCU. As you give report to the receiving RN, what laboratory value is the most important to report and why?

12. While recovering in the CCU, M.M. slipped in the bathroom and fractured her right humerus. Because of the surgical risks involved, M.M. was treated conservatively and put in a full arm cast. She is placed on prophylactic heparin and is again transferred to your floor. A case manager (CM) has been asked to evaluate M.M.'s home to see whether she can be discharged to her own home or will need to stay in a long-term care facility. Identify at least eight things that the CM would assess.

13. M.M.'s nutritional intake over the past few weeks has been poor. She also has increased nutritional needs because of her fractured arm. What are some of the nutritional needs that should be met? What would you recommend to help her with this?

Because it is determined that Mrs. M.M. lived in an apartment with poor access, she elects to stay with her daughter and five grandchildren in their small home. A home care nurse comes three times a week to check on her. M.M. is easily fatigued, and the children are quite lively. School is out for the summer.

14. Suggest some ways the daughter can ensure that her mother isn't overwhelmed and doesn't become exhausted in this situation.

Case Study 20

Name ______________________ Class/Group __________ Date __________

Group Members ____

INSTRUCTIONS: All questions apply to this case study. Your responses should be brief and to the point. Adequate space has been provided for answers. When asked to provide several answers, they should be listed in order of priority or significance. Do not asume information that is not provided. Please print or write clearly. If your response is not legible, it will be marked as ? and you will need to rewrite it.

Scenario

K.K., a 40-year-old administrative secretary, lost consciousness and slumped to the floor while eating dinner with her husband. He initiated CPR (cardiopulmonary resuscitation). Paramedics arrived within 4 to 5 minutes and found her in V-fib. After successful defibrillation she was transported to the hospital. In the MICU her nurse obtained K.K.'s health history from her husband. She has a long history of rheumatic heart disease (RHD) with MVP and severe left ventricular dysfunction. She has had A-fib/atrial flutter for 6 years. She also has had ventricular arrhythmias for several years that were being treated with various antiarrhythmic drugs. She stopped taking her antiarrhythmic drug prior to the cardiac arrest because she did not like the side effects. Her physician feels she has been noncompliant with her medications and that she is denying her need for mitral valve replacement. For the past 2 months she has had CHF with greatly decreased activity tolerance. Medications she was taking at the time of the arrest were furosemide 80 mg PO qd, KCl 20 mEq PO bid, digoxin 0.125 mg PO qd, lisinopril 5 mg PO qd, and warfarin (Coumadin) 2.5 mg PO qd. On the day of her arrest, she had diarrhea.

1. From K.K.'s history, what factors probably contributed to her cardiac arrest?

On admission to the MICU, K.K. is hypotensive and unresponsive to voice commands. She is intubated and placed on mechanical ventilation. A central line is inserted, and dopamine and lidocaine drips are started. For the first day in the MICU she remains unresponsive to commands, her pupillary reaction is sluggish, eyes deviate slowly to the right, upper extremities have increased tone, and lower extremities are flaccid. Painful stimuli elicit withdrawal and decorticate posturing. Her 12-lead ECG shows A-fib at a rate of 136/min; ST segment depression in leads II, III, AVF, and V_1–V_6; and T wave inversion in leads V_3–V_5.

2. What is the probable cause for her neurologic deficits?

3. Explain how rapid A-fib can cause a decrease in CO and contribute to CHF.

4. What is the significance of the ST segment depression and T wave inversion in her 12-lead ECG?

5. List eight lab results that the MICU nurse should check as soon as possible.

After 4 days in the MICU, K.K.'s condition is stabilized and she is transferred to your telemetry floor. When you first assess her, you find jugular vein distention at 10 cm and hear a grade II/VI systolic murmur and an S_3 sound. A thrill is felt over the precordium, and the S_1 and S_2 can be seen on the chest. She no longer has sensory or motor deficits, and her long-term memory is good. However, she is confused, oriented only to name, and has poor short-term memory. Her lidocaine level in the MICU the day before the transfer (the day the lidocaine was discontinued) was 16.8 mg/L; digoxin level was normal. A cardiac catheterization and ECHO cardiogram showed that K.K. has irreversible heart valve, left ventricle, and left atrium damage and is no longer a candidate for mitral valve replacement. She states she is very fearful about her memory loss and the inoperable heart damage. (K.K. may also be considered as a candidate for a transplant.)

6. List three factors that might be contributing to K.K.'s confusion and disorientation.

7. List four interventions you might implement to relieve K.K.'s fear.

After 2 weeks in the hospital, K.K. is scheduled for placement of an internal cardioverter defibrillator (ICD or AICD) to prevent future cardiac arrest from ventricular fibrillation. You will do her preoperative teaching about ICDs.

8. What is an ICD and how does it work?

9. List four discharge instructions R/T the ICD that you will give K.K.

Case Study 21

Name ______________________ Class/Group __________ Date __________

Group Members ____

INSTRUCTIONS: All questions apply to this case study. Your responses should be brief and to the point. Adequate space has been provided for answers. When asked to provide several answers, they should be listed in order of priority or significance. Do not asume information that is not provided. Please print or write clearly. If your response is not legible, it will be marked as ? and you will need to rewrite it.

Scenario

You are in the middle of your shift in the CCU of a large urban medical center. Your new admission, C.B., a 47-year-old woman, has just flown in to your institution from a small rural community more than 100 miles away. She had an acute anterior wall MI last evening. Her current VS are 100/60, 86, 14. After you make C.B. comfortable, you receive this report from the flight nurse: "C.B. is a full-time homemaker with four children. She has had episodes of 'chest tightness' with exertion for the past year, but this is her first known MI. She has a history of hyperlipidemia and has smoked one pack of cigarettes daily for more than 30 years. Surgical history consists of total abdominal hysterectomy (TAH) 10 years ago after the birth of her last child. She has no other known medical problems. Yesterday at 2000 she began to have severe substernal chest pain that referred down both arms and neck. She rated the pain as 9/10 on a zero to 10 scale. She thought it was severe indigestion and began taking Maalox with no relief. Her husband then took her to the local ED where a 12-lead ECG showed hyperacute ST elevation in the inferior leads II, III, and AVF and V_5–V_6. Before tissue plasminogen activator (TPA) could be given she went into V-fib and was successfully defibrillated after several shocks. She then was given TPA and started on nitroglycerin, heparin, and lidocaine drips. She also was given IV metoprolol and aspirin 325 mg to chew and swallow. This morning she dropped her systolic pressure into the 80s and was placed on a dopamine drip and urgently flown to your institution for coronary angiography and possible PTCA. Currently she has lidocaine going at 2 mg/min, heparin at 1200 μ/hr, and dopamine at 5 μ/kg/min. The nitroglycerin has been stopped due to low blood pressure. Labwork done yesterday showed Na 145 mmol/L, K 3.6 mmol/L, HCO_3 19 mmol/L, BUN 9 mg/dl, creatinine 0.8 mg/dl, WBC 14.5 thou/cmm, Hct 44.3%, and Hgb 14.5 g/dl.

1. Given the diagnosis of acute MI, what other lab results are you going to look at?

2. You find the following lab results in the patient's chart. For each, interpret the result, and evaluate the meaning for C.B.

3. The 12-lead ECG can tell you the location of the infarction. Look at the leads that show ST elevation (see flight nurse's report). What areas of C.B.'s heart have been damaged?

4. What is TPA? Why is it given, and when is it given to a patient having an MI? How is it administered?

5. An hour after her admission, you are preparing C.B. for her PTCA. Evaluate her readiness for teaching and her learning needs. What would you tell her?

The following day you care for C.B. again. During her PTCA procedure yesterday, a circumflex coronary artery lesion was found, but the PTCA failed and a stent was inserted. She is still on the lidocaine and heparin drips. The dopamine has been discontinued. VS are stable. PCWP is 20 mm Hg, and CO is 7.3 L/min. You check her lab results for lidocaine and PTT levels.

6. The lidocaine level is 2.5 μg/ml, and the PTT is 61 sec. Analyze the results and state any actions you would take.

As you work with C.B., you notice that she is extremely anxious. You had observed some anxiety yesterday, which you had attributed to the strange CCU environment, pain, and anticipation of the PTCA procedure. You know that the stent was successful and that she is physically stable. You wonder what is wrong. She tells you that her MI occurred right in the middle of a move with her family from her rural community to an even smaller and unfamiliar town some 500 miles away in a neighboring state. She is dreading the move. Her husband "becomes angry easily and starts lashing out" toward her and the children. She is afraid to move to a community where she will have no friends and family to support her.

7. How can you help your patient? Evaluate the situation and describe possible interventions.

8. C.B.'s husband comes to visit. He is a handsome, well-dressed man who appears to be loving and attentive toward C.B. He brought a bouquet of roses for her and a box of chocolates for the nurses, "Because I appreciate how good you girls have been to my wife." One of your younger colleagues comments to you, "Why, what a nice guy! What is her problem? Every woman would love to be married to a man like that!" How are you going to respond?

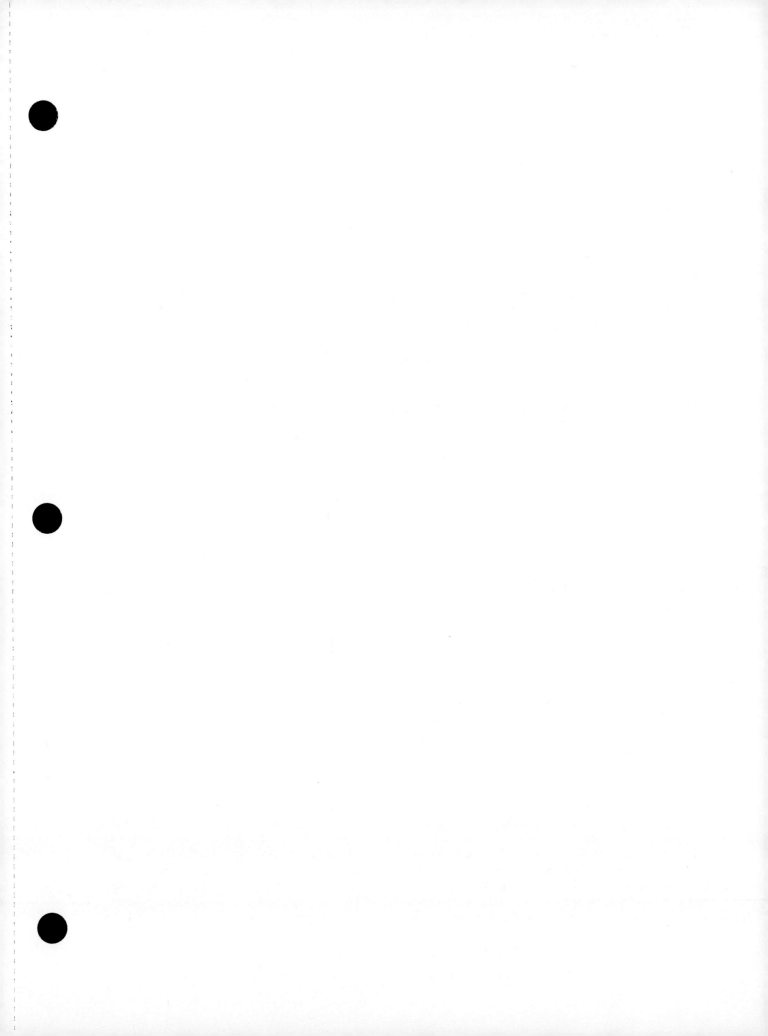

2 Pulmonary Disorders

Case Study 1

Name ____________________ Class/Group __________ Date __________

Group Members ____________________

INSTRUCTIONS: All questions apply to this case study. Your responses should be brief and to the point. Adequate space has been provided for answers. When asked to provide several answers, they should be listed in order of priority or significance. Do not asume information that is not provided. Please print or write clearly. If your response is not legible, it will be marked as ? and you will need to rewrite it.

Scenario

You are a public health nurse working at a county immunization and TB clinic. B.A. is a 61-year-old woman who wishes to obtain a food handler's license and is required to show proof of a negative Mantoux (PPD) test before being hired. She came to your clinic 2 days ago to obtain a PPD test for TB. She has returned to have you evaluate her reaction.

1. What is TB and what microorganism causes it?

Hint: Information and guidelines about preventing and treating TB can be found on the CDC website: www.cdc.gov.

2. What is the route of transmission for TB?

3. The CDC recommend screening people at high risk for TB and providing guidelines for preventive therapy to those at high risk for developing active disease. List five populations at high risk.

4. What is the preferred method for TB screening?

5. When should the individual return to have the test interpreted?

6. How do you determine whether the test is positive or negative?
   - You measure the area of induration (not erythema), which is defined as a hardened area under the skin. The area is measured transverse to the long axis of the forearm.

Note: The American Thoracic Society and the CDC have adopted the following guidelines for positive Mantoux reaction:

- A PPD induration greater than 5 mm is considered positive for persons with, or at risk for, HIV infection; those who have had close, recent contact with someone who has infectious tuberculosis; or persons who have chest x-ray (CXR) that show old, healed TB.
- A PPD induration greater than 10 mm is considered positive for foreign-born persons from high-prevalence countries; IV drug users; medically underserved, low-income populations; residents of long-term care facilities; people with chronic illnesses; and all children and adolescents.
- A PPD induration greater than 15 mm is considered positive for all other persons.

7. What additional information would you want to obtain from B.A. before interpreting her skin test result as positive or negative?

Although B.A. is reluctant to give information, she states that her mother had TB when B.A. was a child, she acknowledges consuming 3 to 4 oz ETOH/day, and has smoked 1½ packs of cigarettes per day for 40 years. She lives with her daughter and becomes angry at the suggestion that she might have TB. She says she feels just fine and doesn't know what all the excitement is about.

8. How would you record B.A.'s smoking history?

9. Three days later, you measure B.A.'s skin test and note that the area of erythema measures 30 mm in diameter and the area of hardness measures 20 mm in diameter. Determine whether B.A.'s skin test is positive or negative.

10. What does a positive PPD result mean?

11. How would you determine whether someone like B.A. has active tuberculosis?

12. According to the CDC, if a person has a positive PPD, what subsequent steps are necessary?

The physician in your TB clinic determines that B.A.'s CXR is clear (shows no signs of any TB). The CDC recommend preventive therapy for adults with evidence of infection but no active disease.

13. According to the American Thoracic Society/CDC (1990) guidelines, what constitutes usual preventive therapy? (Note: Be sure to consult the most recent CDC guidelines. Also note that guidelines for diagnosing and treating TB in individuals who are human immunodeficiency virus (HIV)-positive are different from those for lower-risk populations.)

14. What are the age-related side effects of preventive therapy?

15. Based on the information B.A. gave about her history, what public health follow-up would be warranted?

16. What information should B.A. receive before leaving the clinic?

B.A. is hired under the condition that she must immediately report any S/S of active disease to the county health department or her physician and have a yearly CXR.

Case Study 2

Name ______________________ Class/Group __________ Date __________

Group Members ____

INSTRUCTIONS: All questions apply to this case study. Your responses should be brief and to the point. Adequate space has been provided for answers. When asked to provide several answers, they should be listed in order of priority or significance. Do not asume information that is not provided. Please print or write clearly. If your response is not legible, it will be marked as ? and you will need to rewrite it.

Scenario

M.N., age 40, is admitted with acute cholecystitis, elevated WBC (white blood cells), and a fever of 102° F. She has undergone an open cholecystectomy and has been transferred to your floor. It is the second day postop. She has a nasogastric tube (NGT) to continuous low wall suction, one peripheral IV, and a large abdominal dressing. Her orders are as follows: progress diet to decreased fat diet as tolerated; D_5½NS with 40 mEq KCl at 125 ml/hr; turn, cough, and deep breathe q2h; incentive spirometer (IS) q2h while awake; dangle in AM, ambulate in PM; morphine sulfate 10 mg IM q4h for pain; ampicillin (Omnipen) 2 g IVPB q6h; CXR in AM.

1. Are these orders appropriate for M.N.? State your rationale.

2. What gastrointestinal (GI) complication may result from one of the medications listed in M.N.'s orders?

3. Identify the two most common respiratory-related complications for patients with abdominal or thoracic surgery.

4. What information and assessments would help you differentiate between the two complications in question 3?

5. What procedure is necessary to differentiate between atelectasis and pneumonia?

6. You are assigned to take care of M.N. Her vital signs (VS) are 148/82, 118, 24, 101° F. Her Sao_2 is 88%. Based on these numbers, what do you think is going on with M.N. and why?

7. You know M.N. is at risk for postop atelectasis. What is atelectasis and why is M.N. at risk?

After morning report, you do an assessment and auscultate decreased breath sounds and crackles in the right base posteriorally. Her RML and RLL percuss slightly dull. She splints her right side when attempting to take a deep breath. You suspect that she is developing atelectasis.

8. What most likely accounts for M.N.'s inspiratory-related behavior?

9. What effect will M.N.'s splinting have on potential atelectasis?

10. Identify and clarify five actions you would take next.

11. What four interventions might be used to prevent pulmonary complications?

12. Identify three outcomes that you expect for M.N. as a result of your interventions and her increased activity.

13. M.N.'s sister questions you, saying, "I don't understand. She came in here with a bad gallbladder. What has happened to her lungs?" How would you respond?

14. Radiology calls with a report from the radiologist on the morning CXR. M.N. has atelectasis. Will that change anything that you have already planned for M.N.? Explain what you would do differently if M.N. had pneumonia.

Case Study 3

Name ______________________ Class/Group __________ Date __________

Group Members ____

INSTRUCTIONS: All questions apply to this case study. Your responses should be brief and to the point. Adequate space has been provided for answers. When asked to provide several answers, they should be listed in order of priority or significance. Do not asume information that is not provided. Please print or write clearly. If your response is not legible, it will be marked as ? and you will need to rewrite it.

Scenario

S.R. is a 69-year-old male who owns his own business. The stress of overseeing his employees, meeting deadlines and carrying out negotiations has led to poor sleep habits. He sleeps 3 to 4 hours a night. He keeps himself going by drinking 2 quarts of coffee and smoking three to four packs of cigarettes per day. He weighs 280 pounds and does not use alcohol. His wife complains that his snoring has become difficult to live with.

1. As the clinic nurse, what routine information would you want to obtain from S.R.?

After interviewing S.R. you report the following information to the provider: BP 164/90, P 92, R 18, Sao_2 90% on room air. S.R. is under considerable stress, has gained 50 pounds over the past year, and has a history (Hx) of tobacco and caffeine abuse. He complains of (C/O) difficulty initiating sleep, wakes up with headaches most mornings, and has midmorning somnolence. He is depressed and irritable most of the time and reports difficulty concentrating and learning new things.

Your examination is normal except for multiple bruises over the right ribcage. You inquire about the bruises and S.R. reports that his wife jabs him with her elbow several times every night. In her defense, the wife states, “Well he stops breathing for a long time and I get worried so I jab him to make him start breathing again. If I don’t jab him, I find myself listening for his next breath and I can’t go to sleep.” You suspect sleep apnea.

2. Identify the two main types of apnea and explain the pathology of each.

3. Identify at least five signs or symptoms of OSA and star those symptoms that S.R. has.

4. What test(s) help the provider diagnose OSA?

The primary care provider (PCP) examined S.R. and documented a long soft palate, recessed mandible, and medium size tonsils. S.R.'s screening oximetry study showed 143 episodes of desaturation ranging from 68% to 76% and episodes of apnea were documented. He was diagnosed with OSA with hypoxemia and a full sleep study is ordered.

5. The PCP asks you to counsel the patient about lifestyle changes. What topics should you address with S.R.? Name four.

6. You use the opportunity to develop a teaching handout titled "Preparing for a Good Night's Sleep." You want to share this information with S.R. What would you include in your teaching handout?

Note: Some strategies specifically for OSA are avoid sleeping in a supine position—advise patients to sleep with a pillow-filled back pack on or sew a pocket in the back of a T-shirt and place one or two tennis balls inside.

S.R. returns for a follow-up visit after being diagnosed with OSA. He reports he tried several bedtime strategies and has lost 10 pounds but there has been little improvement in his symptoms. He states he fell asleep while driving to work and wrecked his car. He wants to discuss further treatment options.

7. What are the treatment options for OSA and describe each.

S.R. and the PCP decide on the least invasive treatment—CPAP. The provider writes a prescription for CPAP (the respiratory therapist who sets up the machine will test the patient and determine how much CPAP pressure is needed). The patient has a choice of which durable medical equipment companies he wants to get his equipment from. You help him by giving him the names of three reputable companies and advise him to call his insurance company to find out how much they will pay and how much he will be responsible for.

8. S.R. calls in 2 weeks C/O dry nasal membranes, nosebleeds, and sores behind his ears. What advice would you give S.R.?

Recipe for normal saline spray: 1 quart H_2O plus 1 tsp salt plus a pinch of baking soda. Boil the water for 20 min, let cool and store in the refrigerator for up to 48 hours.

Case Study 4

Name ______________________ Class/Group __________ Date __________

Group Members ____

INSTRUCTIONS: All questions apply to this case study. Your responses should be brief and to the point. Adequate space has been provided for answers. When asked to provide several answers, they should be listed in order of priority or significance. Do not asume information that is not provided. Please print or write clearly. If your response is not legible, it will be marked as ? and you will need to rewrite it.

Scenario

M.N., a 22-year-old man, who lives in a small mountain town in Colorado, is highly allergic to dust and pollen; anxiety appears to play a role in exacerbating his asthma attacks. M.N.'s wife drove him to the clinic when his wheezing was unresponsive to beclomethasone (Vanceril) and ipratropium bromide (Atrovent) inhalers. Upon arrival, his VS are 152/84, 124, 42, 100.4° F. M.N. is started on 4 L O_2/NC, an IV of D_5W at KVO. His ABGs are pH 7.31, $Paco_2$ 48 mm Hg, HCO_3 26 mmol/L, Pao_2 55 mm Hg, Sao_2 88%.

1. Identify the underlying pathophysiology of asthma.

2. The inflammatory response involves what mechanisms?

3. Are M.N.'s VS acceptable? State your rationale.

4. Comment on M.N.'s Sao_2.

5. Identify the drug classifications and actions of Vanceril and Atrovent.

6. Are Vanceril and/or Atrovent appropriate for use during an asthma attack? Explain.

7. The physician orders albuterol 3 mg nebulization treatment STAT (immediately). What is the rationale for this order?

8. What is the rationale for immediately starting M.N. on oxygen?

9. List five short-term interventions that may help relieve M.N.'s symptoms.

After several hours of IV and PO rehydration and a second albuterol treatment, M.N.'s wheezing and chest tightness resolve, and he is able to expectorate his secretions. The physician discusses M.N.'s asthma management with him, and he tells him that his inhalers meet his needs on a day-to-day basis but fail him when he has an asthma attack. The physician discharges M.N. with a prescription for oral steroid "burst" (prednisone 40 mg qd × 5 days), albuterol (Proventil) MDI, and a "spacer" and recommends that he call the pulmonary clinic for follow-up with a pulmonary specialist.

10. What issues would you address in discharge teaching with M.N.?

You ask M.N. to demonstrate the use of his MDI. He vigorously shakes the canister, holds the aerosolizer at an angle (pointing toward his cheek) in front of his mouth, and squeezes the canister as he takes a quick, deep breath.

11. What common mistakes has M.N. made when using the inhaler?

12. What would you teach M.N. about the use of his MDI?

Give him written instructions about follow-up with the pulmonary specialist.

13. M.N.'s wife asks about the possibility of M.N. having another attack. How would you respond?

People with a history of asthma often have special problems with postoperative care. Anesthesia can exacerbate their asthma.

14. If you have a postoperative patient with a history of asthma, what early S/S would indicate respiratory distress? (List at least six.)

15. Identify four S/S of impending respiratory failure.

Tip: To hear lung sounds better, first have the patient turn her or his head to the side (i.e., not facing you) and cough prior to auscultating.
Tip: Often asthmatics have little air movement and therefore lungs sound clear. After beta-agonist wheezing may be heard.

Case Study 5

Name ______________________________ Class/Group __________ Date __________

Group Members ____

INSTRUCTIONS: All questions apply to this case study. Your responses should be brief and to the point. Adequate space has been provided for answers. When asked to provide several answers, they should be listed in order of priority or significance. Do not asume information that is not provided. Please print or write clearly. If your response is not legible, it will be marked as ? and you will need to rewrite it.

Scenario

L.B. is a 30-year-old secretary who presents with 6 weeks of a dry hacky cough after recovering from bronchitis this winter. The cough is worse at night and associated with shortness of breath (SOB). In the past she has experienced coughing spells after running a 5K race. She does have hay fever that seems to be year-round and has eczema in the winter. Both of her children and her maternal grandmother have asthma.

1. As the intake nurse working in the clinic, what routine information would you want to obtain from L.B.?

2. L.B.'s chief complaint is a cough. What are the main causes of chronic cough and what questions should you ask to elicit information about each cause?

L.B. denies symptoms in answer to all of your questions except those given in the initial interview. She is not taking any medication other than a multiple vitamin.

3. What would you include in your physical examination and why?

L.B. was not in acute distress. VS: 110/60,55,18, peak flow was 350 L/min with good effort x 3. Expected peak flow for her height and age was 512 L/min—this is 68% of predicted. She had no sinus tenderness, ears were negative, nasal mucosa was pale and boggy, mouth negative, no cervical adenopathy, lungs were clear to auscultation (CTA) but forced expiration using the PFM seemed to generate a cough. Abdomen soft and nontender. Skin was dry and hands were erythematous in the web spaces but no inflammation in the antecubital, trapezius, or popliteal areas (common location of adult eczema).

4. You need to obtain peak flow readings on L.B. What is the purpose of the PEFR (peak expiratory flow rate) measurement?

5. Give L.B. precise instructions to perform the PFM maneuver.

6. After reviewing the test results, the primary care provider instructs you to give L.B. two puffs of albuterol and take postdilator readings. What is the rationale for the repeat measurement?

7. In order to conduct the postdilator study you must instruct L.B. in the proper use of the MDI using a spacer. How would you explain proper MDI use?

8. The repeat PEFR is 450 L/min, which is 88% predicted. The provider informs L.B. that she has mild asthma and asks you to begin patient education. What topics should you address?

9. The provider ordered triamcinolone (Azmacort) two puffs bid and albuterol two puffs for prn use. What points should you include when teaching L.B. about her medications?

During a follow-up visit, L.B. has mild persistent asthma because her peak flow on the albuterol and triamcinolone has increased to 450, which is 88% predicted. Her cough has subsided and she can again participate in sports without problems. There is no nighttime awakening, no loss of work and no ED visits. She again demonstrates appropriate inhaler technique, has her peak flow record available, and knows that the MDI is empty when the canister floats on its side.

As for triggers, she has noted that wood smoke in the air causes coughing and she will pretreat with albuterol before exercising outdoors in the winter. Finally we have needed to add an antihistamine and nasal steroid to control the allergic rhinitis trigger. She can report her plan for emergent assistance when peak flow does not respond appropriately to exacerbation treatment.

Case Study 6

Name ______________________ Class/Group __________ Date __________

Group Members ____

INSTRUCTIONS: All questions apply to this case study. Your responses should be brief and to the point. Adequate space has been provided for answers. When asked to provide several answers, they should be listed in order of priority or significance. Do not asume information that is not provided. Please print or write clearly. If your response is not legible, it will be marked as ? and you will need to rewrite it.

Scenario

P.R., a 31-year-old woman, contracted an upper respiratory tract infection, developed a high fever, and began to experience progressive ascending paralysis. She was admitted to the local hospital and diagnosed with GBS (Guillain-Barré syndrome). She was intubated and mechanically ventilated. Her VS are 112/68, 134, 12, 101° F. The placement of her percutaneous endoscopic gastrostomy (PEG) tube was confirmed by abdominal x-ray. Her TPN (total parenteral nutrition) was discontinued yesterday, and she was started on EN (enteral nutrition). The consulting dietitian calculated P.R.'s caloric need at 2800 calories/24 hours. P.R. is 5′4″ and weighs 123 pounds. (Note: Registered dietitians prefer the "t" spelling rather than "dietician.")

1. What is ascending paralysis?

2. Identify and discuss at least two factors that would influence the physician's decision to place P.R. on EN.

3. Is 2800 kcal/24 hours a normal caloric requirement for a woman 5′4″, 123 pounds? Compare her provided EN caloric needs with the "ideal" values for a woman of her height and weight. Is it higher or lower? Explain the reason for her current needs.

4. Absolute medical contraindications to enteral feeding are few, and it is preferable to demonstrate failure of EN than to assume that the GI tract is nonfunctional and initiate TPN. Give three examples of medical diagnoses for which EN would be contraindicated.

5. Pulmonary aspiration is a risk with enteral feedings, although the risk is substantially reduced with duodenal placement. Identify four measures that can be taken to minimize the risk for aspiration.

6. Identify five strategies for preventing bacterial contamination of the feeding formula and tubing.

7. Identify two indicators that an EN infusion rate is too rapid.

8. The nurse needs to monitor P.R.'s GI response to EN and steroid therapy. Identify two observations that need to be recorded, and explain the significance of each.

9. It is a common belief that diarrhea (defined as more than three liquid stools per day) is a natural consequence of EN administration. Discuss whether this is a true statement.

10. Identify three factors that could cause diarrhea.

As P.R.'s nurse you are concerned about meeting her needs for fluids, oral hygiene, skin integrity, and activity.

11. Discuss five indicators that would help you assess fluid status.

12. The goal R/T P.R.'s mouth care is to preserve the oral mucosa and dentition. Identify three strategies for providing oral hygiene with an oral endotracheal tube (ETT) in place.

13. What is the rationale for not taking an oral temperature near an ETT?

14. You assess P.R.'s skin every 4 hours. Identify three treatment goals in relation to skin/positioning.

15. What four strategies will facilitate the expected outcome of maintaining skin integrity?

16. You approach P.R. to begin range of motion (ROM) exercises. You ask her whether she is experiencing muscle pain at this time and she nods. You tell P.R. that you will wait until she is pain-free to perform the exercises. Why?

It takes nearly a year for P.R. to make a full recovery. Note that recovery proceeds from proximal to distal muscles.

Case Study 7

Name ________________ Class/Group ________ Date ________

Group Members ________________

INSTRUCTIONS: All questions apply to this case study. Your responses should be brief and to the point. Adequate space has been provided for answers. When asked to provide several answers, they should be listed in order of priority or significance. Do not asume information that is not provided. Please print or write clearly. If your response is not legible, it will be marked as ? and you will need to rewrite it.

Scenario

A.B., a 40-year-old man, is admitted to your medical floor with a diagnosis of pleural effusion. He C/O SOB, pain in his chest, weakness, and a dry, irritating cough. His VS are 142/82, 118, 38 (labored and shallow), 102° F. His CXR shows a large pleural effusion and pulmonary infiltrates in the RLL consistent with pneumonitis. (Note: When the cause of the lung infection is unknown, the condition should be referred to as pneumonitis.)

1. Given his diagnosis, are A.B.'s admission VS expected? Explain.

2. What is pleural effusion?

3. What is the difference between transudate and exudate?

4. List three common causes of pleural effusion.

5. Review the pathophysiology and consequences of pleural effusion and pulmonary infiltrates.

6. How does the underlying pathophysiology give rise to the presenting S/S?

7. How does A.B.'s increased metabolic rate R/T his nutritional needs? Clarify.

The physician performs a thoracentesis and drains 1500 ml of fluid. A specimen for culture and sensitivity (C&S) is sent to the laboratory, and the patient is started on cefuroxime 1 g intravenous piggyback (IVPB) q8h.

8. What is a thoracentesis?

9. What maneuvers would promote the clearance of pulmonary secretions?

10. You enter the room to reposition A.B. If he is on his back, to what side would you turn him and why?

11. The pleural C&S results indicate a large amount of *Klebsiella* growth that is sensitive to cefuroxime. What action should you take next?

12. Because fluid continues to collect in the pleural space, the physician decides to insert a pleural chest tube under nonemergent conditions. What is your responsibility as A.B.'s nurse?

13. Evaluate each of the following statements about chest tube drainage systems. Circle "T" for true of "F" for false. Discuss why the false statements are incorrect.
    a. T F It is the height of the column of water in the suction control mechanism, not the setting of the suction source, that actually limits the amount of suction transmitted to the pleural cavity.
    b. T F A suction pressure of +20 cm H_2O is commonly recommended for adults.
    c. T F Bubbling in the water-seal chamber usually means that air is leaking from the lungs, the tubing, or the insertion site.
    d. T F The rise and fall of the water level with the patient's respirations reflects normal pressure changes in the pleural cavity with respirations.
    e. T F The chamber is a closed system; therefore water cannot evaporate.
    f. T F To declot the drainage tubing, put lotion on your hands, compress the tubing, and vigorously strip long segments of the tubing before releasing.
    g. T F You lower the bed on top of the drainage system and break it. Because you noted an air leak from A.B.'s lung during your initial assessment, you may clamp the chest tube for the short time it takes to reestablish the drainage system.
    h. T F The chest tube becomes disconnected from the drainage system. Because you noted an air leak from the lung during your initial assessment, you can submerge the chest tube 1 to 2 inches below the surface of a 250 ml bottle of sterile saline or water.
    i. T F The collection chamber is full, so you need to connect a new drainage system to the chest tube. It is appropriate to momentarily clamp the chest tube while you disconnect the old system and reconnect the new.
    j. T F The drainage system falls over, spilling the chest drainage into the other drainage columns. The total amount of drainage can be obtained by adding the amount of drainage in each of the columns.

14. How would the nurse appropriately maintain the chest tube system on A.B.?

A.B. receives aggressive antibiotic and pulmonary therapy and is discharged 3 days later with follow-up home care.

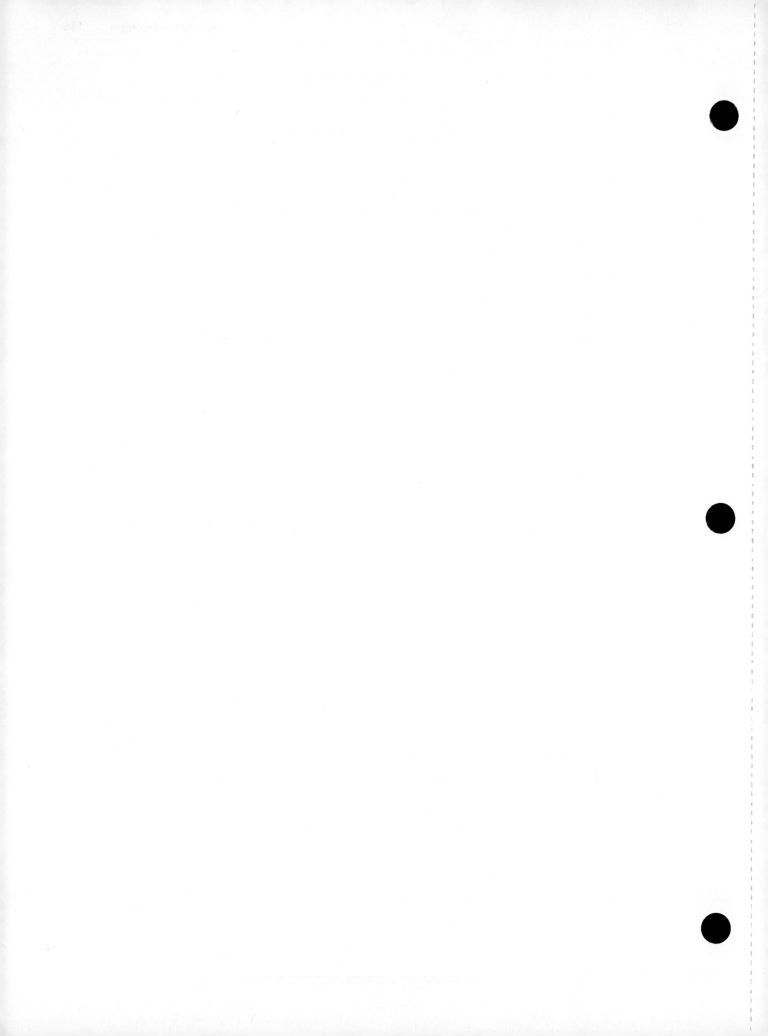

Case Study 8

Name ______________________ Class/Group __________ Date __________

Group Members ____

INSTRUCTIONS: All questions apply to this case study. Your responses should be brief and to the point. Adequate space has been provided for answers. When asked to provide several answers, they should be listed in order of priority or significance. Do not asume information that is not provided. Please print or write clearly. If your response is not legible, it will be marked as ? and you will need to rewrite it.

Scenario

A.W., a 52-year-old woman disabled from severe emphysema, was walking at a mall when she suddenly grabbed her right side and gasped, "Oh, something just popped." A.W. whispered to her walking companion, "I can't get any air." Her companion yelled for someone to call 911 and helped her to the nearest bench. By the time the rescue unit arrived, A.W. was stuporous and in severe respiratory distress. She was intubated, an IV of LR (lactated Ringer's) to KVO (keep vein open) was started, and she was transported to the nearest ED.

On arrival to the ED, the physician auscultates muffled heart tones; no breath sounds on the right, and faint sounds on the left. A.W. is stuporous, tachycardic, and cyanotic. The paramedics inform the physician that it was difficult to ventilate A.W. A STAT portable CXR and ABGs are obtained. A.W. has an 80% pneumothorax on the right, and her ABGs on 100% oxygen are pH 7.25, $Paco_2$ 92 mm Hg, Pao_2 32 mm Hg, HCO_3 27 mmol/L, BE +5 mmol/L, Sao_2 53%.

1. Given the diagnosis of pneumothorax, explain why the paramedic had difficulty ventilating A.W.

2. Interpret A.W.'s ABGs.

3. What is the reason for A.W.'s ABG results?

4. The physician needs to insert a chest tube. What are your responsibilities as the nurse?

5. As the nurse, it is your responsibility to ensure pain control. In A.W.'s case, would you administer pain medication before the chest tube insertion?

6. The ED physician inserts a size 32 chest tube in the second intercostal space, midclavicular line. Many chest tubes are inserted in the sixth intercostal space, midaxillary line. What factor determines where a chest tube is placed?

7. Given the information above, would you expect to observe an air leak when A.W.'s chest drainage system is in place and functioning?

8. Would you expect A.W.'s lung to reexpand immediately after the chest tube insertion and initiation of underwater suction? Explain.

9. The clerk tells you A.W.'s husband has just arrived; A.W. will be admitted to the hospital. How would you address this issue with her husband?

10. You approach A.W.'s bedside and ask about what looks like two healed chest tube sites on her right chest. A.W.'s husband informs you that this is the third time she has had a collapsed lung. He asks whether this trend will continue. How would you respond?

11. A.W. recovers and is discharged home 4 days later with a chest tube and Heimlich valve. The physician connects a one-way (Heimlich) valve between the distal end of the chest tube and a drainage pouch. Discuss the purpose of this device.

A.W. develops several more spontaneous pneumothoraces on the right and eventually has bleomycin instilled over the right lung to induce scarring. She says, "It felt like someone poured kerosene in and threw a lit match in after it. It was the most painful thing I ever went through." Research the scarring procedure so that you know what it does and why it is necessary.
Note: Sclerosing a lung doesn't have to feel like it is burning; it should be managed with adequate pain medication.

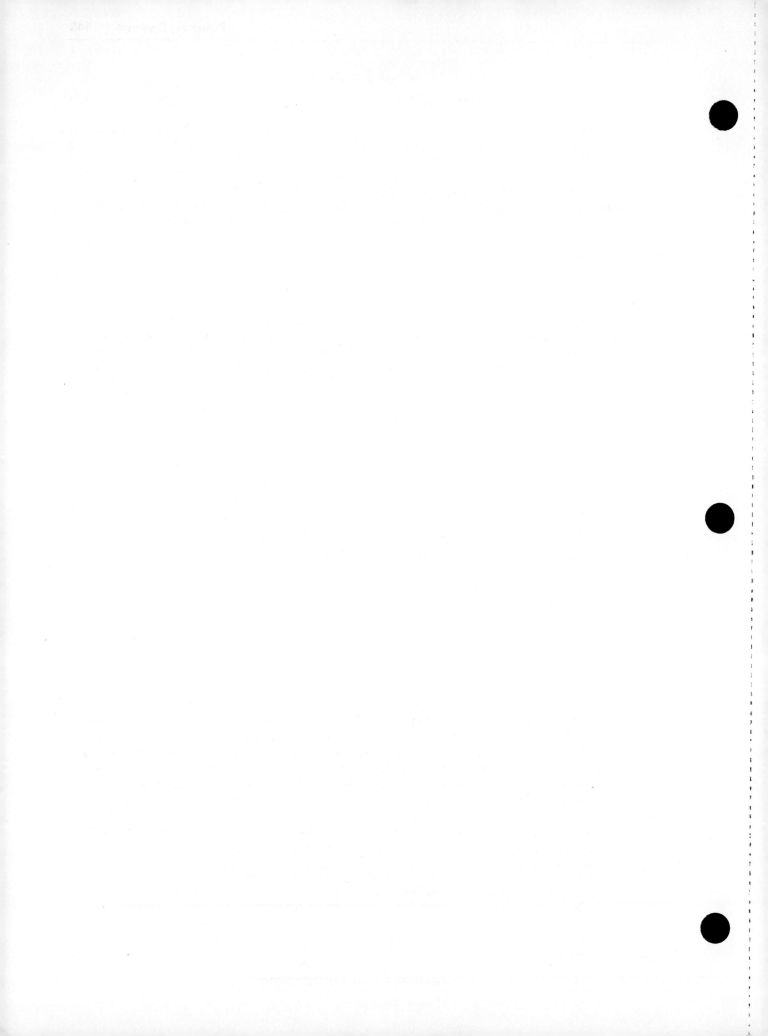

Case Study 9

Name ______________________ Class/Group __________ Date __________

Group Members ____

INSTRUCTIONS: All questions apply to this case study. Your responses should be brief and to the point. Adequate space has been provided for answers. When asked to provide several answers, they should be listed in order of priority or significance. Do not asume information that is not provided. Please print or write clearly. If your response is not legible, it will be marked as ? and you will need to rewrite it.

Scenario

The sister of C.K. called to report her 71-year-old brother came down with a fever 2 days ago. Now he has shaking chills, productive cough, inability to lie down to sleep because "He can't stop coughing." C.K. is examined at the hospital's Primary Care Clinic, is diagnosed (Dx) with community-acquired pneumonia (CAP) and admitted to your floor. The intern is busy and asks you to complete your routine admission assessment and call her with your findings.

1. Identify the four most important things to include in your assessment.

Your assessment findings are as follows: C.K.'s VS are 154/82, 105, 32, 103° F, Sao_2 84% on room air. You auscultate decreased breath sounds in the LLL anteriorly and posteriorly, coarse crackles LUL. His nailbeds are dusky on fingers and toes. He has cough-productive of rust-colored sputum and C/O pain in his left chest when he coughs. C.K. seems to be well nourished and adequately hydrated. He is a lifetime nonsmoker, nondrinker. PMH includes CAD/MI × 2/stent × 3 on metoprolol, amlodipine, lisinopril, furosemide, type 2 diabetes mellitus (DM) on metformin and rosiglitazone. He reports he has not been sexually active for 15 years but was always monogamous with his wife of 49 years. He has never gotten the Pneumovax or flu shot. He does report getting "hives" when he took "an antibiotic pill" a few years ago but doesn't remember the name of the antibiotic (ATB).

2. Which of these assessment findings concern you? State your rationale.

The intern writes the following orders: regular diet; VS with temperature q2h; maintenance IV of D_5½NS at 125 ml/hr; ceftriaxone 1g IV q24h × 10d, doxycycline 100 mg bid × 10d; titrate O_2 to maintain oximeter (Sao_2) >90%; obtain sputum for C&S × 3; draw blood cultures × 2 sites for temperature >102° F; CBC with differential, basic metabolic panel (BMP), and urinalysis with C&S as indicated; CXR on admission and in the morning.

3. Review the orders and determine what you would do first.

4. Is the intravenous fluid of D_5½NS appropriate for C.K.? State your rationale.

5. What is the rationale for ordering oxygen to maintain Sao_2 >90%?

6. What is a C&S test, and why is it important?

7. Why would blood cultures be drawn if the patient spikes a fever?

8. Why are blood cultures drawn from two different sites?

9. What general information can be obtained from a CXR?

10. C.K. recovers from his pneumonia and is preparing for discharge. You know that C.K. is at increased risk for contracting CAP infections. Discuss four strategies for prevention.

11. C.K. confides in you, "You know, my wife died a year ago, and I live alone now. I've been thinking . . . this pneumonia stuff has been a little scary." How will you respond?

Note: Pneumonia, etiology unknown, is properly called "pneumonitis." When pneumonitis is used, it should be defined according to cause, such as viral pneumonia or *Klebsiella pneumoniae*.

Case Study 10

Name ______________________ Class/Group __________ Date __________

Group Members ____

INSTRUCTIONS: All questions apply to this case study. Your responses should be brief and to the point. Adequate space has been provided for answers. When asked to provide several answers, they should be listed in order of priority or significance. Do not asume information that is not provided. Please print or write clearly. If your response is not legible, it will be marked as ? and you will need to rewrite it.

Scenario

P.R., a 31-year-old woman diagnosed with Guillain-Barré syndrome, is being cared for on a special ventilator unit of an extended-care facility because she requires 24-hour-a-day nursing coverage. She has been intubated and mechanically ventilated for 3 weeks and has shown no signs of improvement in respiratory muscle strength. Her ventilator settings are A/C of 12, V_T 700, FiO_2 0.50, PEEP 5. Her VS are 108/64, 118, 12, 100.6° F. She is receiving enteral nutrition by nasal-duodenal tube (2800 calories/24 hours). P.R.'s three children, ages 3, 4, and 6, are staying with her sister because her husband has to keep working his full-time job to maintain their medical insurance.

1. Why is P.R.'s ventilator mode on assist control?

2. P.R. is receiving lorazepam (Ativan) 1 mg slow IVP q4h to reduce her anxiety. Identify two factors that should be considered when choosing lorazepam for P.R.

3. Identify nine nonpharmacologic strategies that you could use to reduce P.R.'s anxiety, increase her comfort, and reduce the need for lorazepam. Be creative!

4. You give P.R. a bath and note that her cheeks billow outward each time the ventilator delivers a breath. What could cause this phenomenon?

5. You try repositioning P.R., place a stopcock in the inflation valve, auscultate the lungs, check the length of the tube at the lip (the tube had not moved), check the cuff and note the air pressure is low. You insert more air in the cuff to seal the leak. Over the next 24 hours the leak becomes worse and the ventilator's low exhaled volume alarm repeatedly sounds. What action should you take?

6. The physician elects to insert a No. 8 Shiley tracheostomy tube with a disposable inner cannula. P.R. becomes increasingly anxious after receiving the news. How would you prepare P.R. and her husband for the tracheostomy?

7. P.R. undergoes the tracheostomy procedure without complications. When you return in the morning and assess the new tracheostomy, you note that the trach tape looks tight. You are unable to insert one finger between P.R.'s neck and the trach tape. Discuss whether or not this is problematic.

8. What should your next actions be?

9. You note that the tissue surrounding the incision is edematous. As you palpate the area, your fingers sink into the skin and you auscultate a popping sound through your stethoscope. Is this to be expected?

10. Based on your decision in question 9, what action should you take?

11. That afternoon, a powerful storm causes a power failure. What should you do?

12. Within minutes of the power failure, the rescue unit arrives at the door. How did they know you needed assistance?

13. You evaluate P.R.'s activity tolerance and note that she desaturates when turned to her right side. You auscultate tubular breath sounds in the entire right lung posteriorally. Based on your knowledge of pathophysiology, explain the probable cause of the desaturation.

You notify the physician of the change in P.R.'s breath sounds. The paramedic unit transports P.R. to the hospital, where she is readmitted for recurring pneumonia.

14. P.R.'s husband arrives shortly after the paramedics transport P.R. to the hospital. He collapses into the nearest chair, tears begin to roll down his cheeks, and he says, "It has been almost a month now. Are you sure she will recover?" How would you respond?

P.R. undergoes aggressive antibiotic therapy and is discharged to extended care facility (ECF) 5 days later. She progresses slowly. It takes nearly 8 months for her to recover, but recovery is complete.

Case Study 11

Name ______________________________ Class/Group __________ Date __________

Group Members ____

INSTRUCTIONS: All questions apply to this case study. Your responses should be brief and to the point. Adequate space has been provided for answers. When asked to provide several answers, they should be listed in order of priority or significance. Do not asume information that is not provided. Please print or write clearly. If your response is not legible, it will be marked as ? and you will need to rewrite it.

Scenario

C.E., a 73-year-old married man and retired railroad engineer, visits his internist complaining: "Whenever I try to do anything, I get so out of breath I can't go on. I think I'm just getting older, but my wife told me I had to come see you about it." His resting Sao_2 registers 83%. He is sent to the local hospital for a CXR and ABGs to be drawn after resting 20 minutes on room air. The next day his physician calls C.E. and informs him that he has severe emphysema and must start on continuous oxygen therapy.

1. How should C.E.'s chief complaint (C/C) be recorded?

2. What is emphysema?

3. What is the most common cause of emphysema? Based on this information, what questions will you ask about health behaviors?

4. List two authoritative Internet resources of professional and patient/family information on lung disease.

5. Locate and print a patient-education handout in Spanish *and* in English on emphysema from one of the Internet sites or a similar resource. Staple it to this assignment.

The physician tells C.E. that his office will have a home health equipment company call him to make arrangements to deliver the equipment and educate him in its use. As an RN working for the company, you are assigned to make the initial home visit.

Note: Diagnosis of emphysema is usually made from the CXR, pulmonary function tests, and ABGs on room air. Insurance companies and Medicare usually pay for oxygen only if room air Pao_2 <55 mm Hg.

For further information, locate HCFA/Medicare on the Internet. Look under U.S. Department of Health and Human Services, Health Care Financing Administration, for the most recent directives.

Look up the Medicare code (number) and information on reimbursement for home treatment of severe emphysema.

6. How would you prepare for the first visit?

7. What issues would you address with C.E. and his wife?

8. The next time you visit, C.E. C/O sores behind his ears. He explains, "That long oxygen tubing seems to take on a life of its own. It twists around and gets caught under doors, chairs, everything. It darn near rips the ears off my head." What can you tell him that could help?

9. You auscultate C.E.'s breath sounds and detect the odor of Vicks VapoRub. When you question C.E. about the use of Vicks, he tells you that he started to apply it in and around his nose to prevent his nose from becoming dry and sore. How would you council C.E. and his wife (safety issues)?

C.E. elected to use liquid oxygen because it offers more freedom and portability. It is also lighter in weight.

10. Over the next 3 weeks, C.E. seemed to adjust well to his liquid oxygen system. However, one evening he walked to the kitchen for a snack and became increasingly SOB. Identify three possible causes.

As per your instructions, C.E. removed the nasal cannula, tested the flow against his check, and felt no oxygen flowing from the catheter. He lacked the force and volume required to yell for help and was too SOB to return to the living room to check his oxygen tank. He bent forward with his elbows on the countertop and struggled to breathe. He became more frightened with each passing second, and his breathing seemed to become increasingly more difficult. A minute later, C.E.'s wife found him and reconnected his oxygen tubing. C.E. sat at the table for 20 minutes before he could walk back to the living room.

11. Why did C.E. assume the peculiar position at the countertop?

12. A week later you receive a call from C.E.'s wife. She relates the incident from the previous week and tells you that C.E. "doesn't want her out of his sight." She asks you to come to the house and "talk some sense into him." What teaching strategies will you use with C.E. and his wife?

13. C.E.'s wife asks you what her husband can do to help her around the house. She says, "The doctor told him to go home and take it easy. He sits in a chair all day. He won't even get up to get himself a glass of water. I've got a bad hip and this has been very hard on me." How would you address her issue?

An OT instructs the couple about energy-saving ways to complete their housework. They both seem satisfied with their new division of labor. In addition, the women's group at their church has volunteered to help once a week with laundry, vacuuming, and other stressful tasks.

14. C.E. states, "You seem to know what you are talking about, so let me ask you something. I wake up with a headache almost every morning. My wife says it's because I snore so loud and don't breathe right when I sleep. Do you know anything about that?" After asking several questions, you inform C.E. that it sounds like he has obstructive sleep apnea. Explain the connection between obstructive sleep apnea and morning headaches.

15. C.E. seems impressed by your explanation. He asks whether there is anything that can be done for his problem. You inform him that there are several treatment modalities for OSA. The most common treatment is CPAP. What is CPAP, and how does it work? What is the difference between CPAP and BiPAP?

You comment that C.E. sounds like he has a cold. He replies, "Oh, our great-grandchildren were over to visit several days ago and they all had snotty noses. I suspect that I'll get it pretty soon. The problem is, every time I get a cold it goes straight to my lungs."

16. What information would you want to review with C.E. and his wife about the S/S of infection and when to seek treatment?

17. What basic hygiene measures can C.E. and his wife take to prevent his developing an infection? (List at least four.)

18. Why is it important for people with lung disease to seek early intervention for infection?

C.E. seemed to be managing his emphysema fairly well. His wife had her hip replaced, made a speedy recovery, and was discharged to home. She suddenly died 4 weeks later from a pulmonary embolus. C.E. was panic-stricken at her loss. A psychiatric nurse practitioner was requested to work with him.

Note: It is important to keep in mind that many home-bound people with chronic illnesses are living a fragile functional independence, depending on the assistance of their partner. When something happens to the partner (death, illness, or stress-related illness), the remaining person is often forced into a nursing home. It is also easier to understand the pressures experienced by the assisting partner: stress-related illnesses, alcoholism, and other forms of substance abuse are not uncommon in these settings, especially where poor community support and inadequate symptom management are factors.

Case Study 12

Name ______________________ Class/Group __________ Date __________

Group Members ____

INSTRUCTIONS: All questions apply to this case study. Your responses should be brief and to the point. Adequate space has been provided for answers. When asked to provide several answers, they should be listed in order of priority or significance. Do not asume information that is not provided. Please print or write clearly. If your response is not legible, it will be marked as ? and you will need to rewrite it.

Scenario

D.Z., a 65-year-old man, is admitted to a medical floor for exacerbation of his COPD (emphysema). He has a PMH of hypertension (HTN), which has been well controlled by enalapril for the past 6 years, and Dx pneumonia yearly × 3 years. He presents as a thin, poorly nourished man who is experiencing difficulty breathing at rest. He reports cough productive of thick yellow-green sputum. D.Z. seems irritable and anxious when he tells you that he has been a two-pack-a-day smoker for 38 years. He C/O sleeping poorly and lately feels very tired most of the time. His VS are 162/84, 124, 36, 102° F, Sao_2 88%. His admitting diagnosis is chronic emphysema with an acute exacerbation; etiology to be determined. His admitting orders are as follows: diet as tolerated; out of bed with assistance; O_2 to maintain Sao_2 90%; maintenance IV of D_5W at 50 ml/hr; I&O; ABGs in AM; CBC with diff., BMP, and theophylline level on admission; CXR q 24h; prednisone 60 mg PO qd; doxycycline 100 mg q12h × 10 days, azithromycin 500 mg IVPB q24h × 2 days then 500 mg PO × 7 days; theophylline (Theo-Dur) 300 mg PO bid; heparin 5000 units sq q12h; albuterol 2.5 mg (0.5 ml) in 3 ml NS and ipratropium 500 fg by nebulizer q4-6h; enalapril (Vasotec) 10 mg PO q AM.

1. Explain the pathophysiology of emphysema.

2. Are D.Z.'s VS and Sao_2 appropriate? If not, explain why.

3. Identify three measures you could try to improve oxygenation.

4. Explain the main purpose of the following classes of drugs: antibiotics, bronchodilators, and corticosteroids.

5. What are the two most common side effects of bronchodilators?

6. You deliver D.Z.'s dietary tray, and he comments how hungry he is. As you leave the room, he is rapidly consuming the mashed potatoes. When you pick up the tray, you notice that he hasn't touched anything else. When you question him, he states, "I don't understand it. I can be so hungry, but when I start to eat, I have trouble breathing and I have to stop." One theory for the increased work of breathing is based on carbohydrate (CHO) loading. Explain this phenomenon based on your knowledge of the breakdown of CHO.

7. Identify four strategies that might improve his caloric intake.

8. Identify three expected outcomes of D.Z.'s treatment.

9. You answer D.Z.'s call light, and he asks for a carton of milk. You remind him that milk causes an increased production of thick mucus. He replies, "Yes, but you told me that I need lots of protein." How should you respond?

10. You notice a box of dark chocolate on D.Z.'s overbed table. He tells you that he wakes at night and eats four or five pieces of chocolate. Several of your COPD patients have identified a craving for chocolate in the past. What is the basis for this craving?

11. What would you do to address dietary and nutritional teaching needs with D.Z. and his wife?

12. List six educational topics that you need to explore with D.Z.

13. What other health care professional would probably be involved in D.Z.'s treatments and how? What is the licensure/certification status of that profession in the state in which you are practicing?

D.Z.'s wife approaches you in the hallway and says, "I don't know what to do. My husband used to be so active before he retired 6 months ago. Since then he's lost 35 pounds. He is afraid to take a bath and it takes him hours to dress—that's if he gets dressed at all. He has gone downhill so fast that it scares me. He's afraid to do anything for himself. He wants me in the room with him all the time, but if I try to talk with him, he snarls and does things to irritate me. I have to keep working. His medical bills are draining all our savings, and I have to be able to support myself when he's gone. You know, sometimes I go to work just to get away from the house and his constant demands. He calls me several times a day asking me to come home, but I can't go home. You may not think I'm much of a wife, but quite honestly, I don't want to come home anymore. I just don't know what to do."

14. How would you respond to her statement?

Case Study 13

Name ______________________ Class/Group __________ Date __________

Group Members ____

INSTRUCTIONS: All questions apply to this case study. Your responses should be brief and to the point. Adequate space has been provided for answers. When asked to provide several answers, they should be listed in order of priority or significance. Do not asume information that is not provided. Please print or write clearly. If your response is not legible, it will be marked as ? and you will need to rewrite it.

Scenario

The ICU nurse calls to give you the following report: "D.S. is a 56-year-old man with a PMH of chronic bronchitis. He quit smoking 12 years ago and exercises regularly. He went to see his physician with C/O increasing exertional dyspnea; a large mass was found in his right lung. Three days ago he underwent a RML and RLL lobectomy; the pathology report showed adenocarcinoma. He has no neurologic deficits and his VS run 120s/70s, 110s, about 30, and he has been running a fever of 100.2° F. His heart tones are clear, all peripheral pulses are palpable, and has an IV of D_5½NS at 50 ml/h in his right forearm. He has a right midaxillary chest tube to PleurEvac drain; there's no air leak, and it's draining small amounts of serosanguineous fluid. He's C/O pain at the insertion site, but the site looks good, and the dressing is dry and intact. He's on 5 L O_2/NC. He refuses pain medication. He's a real nervous guy and hasn't slept since surgery. He'll be there in about 20 minutes."

1. What additional information would you ask the nurse to provide at this time?

D.S. is transported by wheelchair past the nurses' station to a room at the far end of the hall. You enter his room for the first time to find him sitting on the edge of the bed with his left leg in bed and his right foot on the floor. You introduce yourself and tell him that you are going to be his nurse for the rest of the shift. You note that he keeps rubbing his left hand over his right chest.

2. What issues/problems can you already identify?

3. List four things you would do for D.S.

D.S. states, "I have a nephew who rolled his Jeep and busted himself up real bad. He got hooked on those drugs, and I don't want any part of them."

4. How would you respond to D.S.'s statement?

5. Why is D.S. experiencing difficulty using his right arm? Given the type of surgery he underwent, is this expected?

6. You administer 8 mg morphine (MSO_4) IM and tell D.S. that you will return in 30 minutes; 15 minutes later he turns on his call light. When you enter the room D.S. says, "I think I'm going to throw up." What are the next three things you would do?

7. D.S. stated, "I started to feel sick a couple minutes ago. It just kept getting worse until I knew I was going to throw up." Given this information, what do you think is responsible for the sudden onset of nausea?

8. Would it be appropriate to give D.S. a second dose of morphine before reporting his reaction to the physician? State your rationale.

9. D.S.'s pain and nausea are under control an hour later. You remove the chest tube (CT) dressing and note that the area around the insertion site looks slightly inflamed, the tissue immediately around the tube looks white and moist, and there is scant amount of brown drainage. What action would you take next?

The next day, the nurse giving you his report says that D.S. has been driving her crazy all day long. She tells you that he is fine but has been paranoid and very demanding. You enter D.S.'s room to see how he is doing and to tell him you are going to be his nurse again today. You note that his head bobs up and his mouth opens, like a fish taking in water, every time he inhales. He says, "I just can't [breath] seem to [breath] get enough [breath] air."

10. Identify six possible problems that D.S. could have that would account for his behavior.

11. What three actions should you take next? Give your rationale.

D.S.'s RR is 46; you auscultate slight air movement over the large airways and no breath sounds distal to the third ICS. He's sitting on the side of the bed with his arms hunched up on the over-bed table. His gown is in his lap, he is diaphoretic, you note intercostal retractions with inspiration, and all muscles of the upper torso are engaged in respiration.

12. What would you do next?

D.S. is successfully resuscitated and transferred to ICU. The physician returns to your floor and compliments you on your clear thinking and fast action. The nurse who gave you his report comes up to you to apologize. She is relatively new and asks you to explain how you know when a patient is in the early and late stages of respiratory difficulty. She states that she wants to learn from her mistakes so that she doesn't put another patient through what D.S. experienced.

13. How would you distinguish between early and late stages of respiratory failure?

D.S. recovers. His CXR at 5 years shows no recurrence.

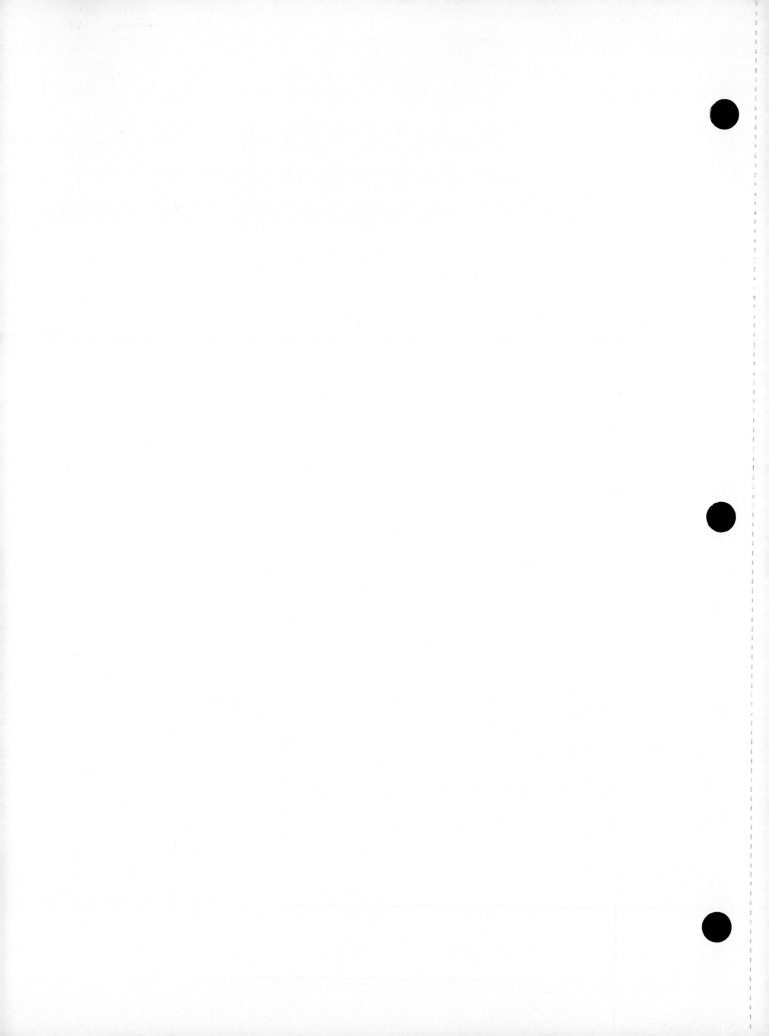

Case Study 14

Name ______________________ Class/Group ____________ Date ____________

Group Members ____

INSTRUCTIONS: All questions apply to this case study. Your responses should be brief and to the point. Adequate space has been provided for answers. When asked to provide several answers, they should be listed in order of priority or significance. Do not asume information that is not provided. Please print or write clearly. If your response is not legible, it will be marked as ? and you will need to rewrite it.

Scenario

G.S., a 36-year-old secretary, was involved in a motor vehicle accident; a car drifted left of center and struck G.S. head-on, pinning her behind the steering wheel. She was intubated immediately after extrication and flown to your trauma center. Her injuries were found to be extensive: bilateral flail chest, torn innominate artery, right hemo/pneumothorax, fractured spleen, multiple small liver lacerations, compound fractures of both legs, and probable cardiac contusion. She was taken to the OR, where she received 36 units of PRC (packed red cells), 20 units of platelets, 20 units cryoprecipitate, 12 units FFP (fresh frozen plasma), and 18 L of LR. She was admitted to the ICU postop, where she developed ARDS (adult respiratory distress syndrome).

1. What is ARDS (adult respiratory distress syndrome)?

G.S. has been in ICU for 6 weeks, and her ARDS has almost resolved. She is transferred to your unit. You receive the following report: Neuro: AAO (awake, alert, and oriented) to person and place, she can move both of her arms and wiggle her toes on both feet; CV: heart tones are clear, VS are 138/90, 88, 26, 99.2° F, bilateral radial pulse 3+, foot pulses by Doppler only; skin: incisions and lacerations have all healed; respiratory: bilateral chest tubes to water suction with closed drainage, dressings are dry and intact; GI: duodenal feeding tube in place; GU (genitourinary): Foley catheter to down drain.

2. What additional information should you require during this report?

You complete your assessment of G.S. You note SOB, crackles throughout all lung fields posteriorly and in both lower lobes anteriorly, and rhonchi over the large airways.

3. What is the significance of crackles and rhonchi in G.S.'s case?

4. The nurse from the previous shift charted the following statement, "Crackles and rhonchi clear with vigorous coughing." Based on your knowledge of pathophysiology, determine the accuracy of this statement.

5. It is time to administer 40 mg furosemide (Lasix) IVP. What effect, if any, will furosemide have on G.S.'s breath sounds?

6. What action should you take before giving the furosemide?

The 0500 laboratory values are as follows: Na 129 mmol/L, K 3.3 mmol/L, Cl 92 mmol/L, HCO_3 26 mmol/L, BUN 37 mg/dl, creatinine 2 mg/dl, glucose 128 mg/dl, calcium 7.1 mg/dl, ABGs on 6 L O_2/NC: pH 7.38, $Paco_2$ 49 mm Hg, Pao_2 82 mm Hg, HCO_3 36 mmol/L, BE +2.2, Sao_2 91%.

7. Keeping in mind that you are about to administer furosemide, which laboratory values concern you and why?

8. Given the laboratory values listed, what action would you take before administering the furosemide, and why?

The physician prescribes the following: draw STAT Mg level; if below 1.4 mg/dl, give $MgSO_4$ 3 g in 100 ml D_5W over 4 hr; give KCl 40 mEq in 100 ml D_5W IVPB over 4 hr NOW; and give $CaCl_2$ g in 100 ml D_5W IVPB over 3 hr. The laboratory is called to draw a STAT Mg level.

9. Given that KCl and CaCl are compatible, would you mix them in the same bag of D_5W? State your rationale.

10. You open G.S.'s medication drawer to draw the furosemide into a syringe. You find one 20 mg ampule. The pharmacist tells you that it will be at least an hour before he can send the drug to you. You realize it is illegal to take medication dispensed by a pharmacist for one patient and use it for another patient. What should you do?

11. While you administer the furosemide and hang the intravenous piggyback (IVPB) medication, G.S. says, "This is so weird. A couple times this morning, I felt like my heart flipped upside down in my chest, but now I feel like there's a bird flopping around in there." What are the first two actions you should take next? Give your rationale.

12. G.S.'s pulse is 66 and irregular. Her BP is 92/70, and respirations are 26. She admits to being "a little lightheaded" but denies having pain or nausea. Your coworker connects G.S. to the code cart monitor for a "quick look." You are able to distinguish normal P-QRS-T complexes, but you also note approximately 22 very wide complexes per minute. The wide complexes come early and are not preceded by a P wave. What do you think has happened to G.S.?

13. What should your next actions be?

14. What are the most likely causes of the abnormal beats?

15. You notice that G.S. looks frightened and is lying stiff as a board. How would you respond to this situation?

G.S.'s PVCs responded well to treatment. Unfortunately, 1 week later she threw a large embolus. All attempts at resuscitation failed.

3 Musculoskeletal Disorders

Case Study 1

Name ______________________________ Class/Group __________ Date __________

Group Members ____

INSTRUCTIONS: All questions apply to this case study. Your responses should be brief and to the point. Adequate space has been provided for answers. When asked to provide several answers, they should be listed in order of priority or significance. Do not asume information that is not provided. Please print or write clearly. If your response is not legible, it will be marked as ? and you will need to rewrite it.

Scenario

M.B. is a 55-year-old woman presenting to the clinic with C/O (complaints of) episodes of feeling "hot and sweaty" during the day and waking up at night soaked with perspiration. Because her sleep is so disrupted, she is tired all day and is having trouble concentrating at work. She says that the episodes are becoming unbearable and is seeking treatment for them.

1. You suspect M.B. is perimenopausal. You obtain her prior medical and surgical history and her current medication regimen. List three questions that would be important to ask in exploring the possibility of menopause being related to (R/T) her symptoms.

2. You are concerned with the possible development of osteoporosis in M.B. List at least eight questions you would ask to determine her risk for development of osteoporosis.

3. M.B. is not currently taking estrogen replacement therapy. What three questions would be important to ask M.B. to determine whether there are any contraindications or precautions to this therapy for her?

4. M.B. says that she does have frequent "backaches." Spinal films (x-rays) are ordered. Later you see a report stating that the films appear normal with no significant findings. What would be an appropriate explanation of these findings?

5. What would be appropriate supportive measures for M.B. to relieve the noninjury-related low back pain in the absence of fracture?

6. M.B. reports that she does not like milk or milk products and rarely includes them in her diet. How can M.B. increase her calcium intake at this time?

7. M.B.'s physician told her that her blood calcium was normal. "If I have enough calcium in my blood, I couldn't have osteoporosis, could I?" she asks you. How will you respond and why?

8. M.B. says she rarely exercises. What advice should be given concerning exercise?

9. M.S. states she still is not certain she has a well-balanced diet with sufficient calcium and vitamin D. What would you suggest to her?

M.S. was given a prescription for 0.625 mg Premarin.

10. What side effects may be experienced with Premarin and what instructions should be given someone receiving it?

Note: Research on this topic changes from week to week. A discussion of the pros and cons of estrogen and progesterone would be helpful.
Note: A recent scientific study found that one third of the individuals in a group who had an MI suffered no chest pain at all.
Note: A lot of osteoporosis in older women, as well as men, develops as secondary to gastric problems, renal disorders, arthritis, and medication intake. Also, deficit in calcium intake is relatively common among low-income people with poor nutrition or in elderly individuals living alone.

Case Study 2

Name ______________________ Class/Group __________ Date __________

Group Members ____

INSTRUCTIONS: All questions apply to this case study. Your responses should be brief and to the point. Adequate space has been provided for answers. When asked to provide several answers, they should be listed in order of priority or significance. Do not asume information that is not provided. Please print or write clearly. If your response is not legible, it will be marked as ? and you will need to rewrite it.

Scenario

J.C. is a 41-year-old man who comes to the ED (emergency department) C/O acute low back pain. He states that he did some heavy lifting yesterday, went to bed with a mild backache, and awoke this morning with terrible back pain. He admits to having had several episodes of similar back pain each year over the past 10 years. In the past the pain has been treated by diazepam, codeine, NSAIDs, and several weeks of bed rest. J.C. has a past medical history (PMH) of a peptic ulcer. He is 6 ft tall, weighs 265 pounds, and has a prominent "potbelly." The ED admitting clerk calls J.C.'s insurance company to authorize payment for treatment at your facility. J.C.'s health maintenance organization (HMO) has identified him as a consumer of "high-cost care" with poor prior outcome. The ED is authorized to perform emergency treatment only and the case manager will make a home visit within 24 hours to devise a treatment plan. The ED physician diagnoses muscular strain of the lower back and orders the following: cyclobenzaprene (Flexeril) 10 mg qid, celecoxib (Celebrex) 200 mg qd; bed rest for 2 days then gradually increase activity; ice packs to the lower back 30 minutes out of every hour.

You are a case manager RN working for Grubabuck HMO and make the initial visit to J.C.'s residence. His wife lets you in and you find J.C. lying on the sofa with his knees flexed and watching videos.

1. What questions would be appropriate to ask J.C. in evaluating the extent of his back pain and injury?

2. What observable characteristic does J.C. have that makes him highly susceptible to low back injury and chronic pain?

3. Why do you think that cyclobenzaprine was prescribed instead of diazepam?

4. J.C. used to take piroxicam 20 mg until he developed his duodenal ulcer. What is the relationship between the two? What S/S would you expect if an ulcer developed?

You determine that J.C. needs an interdisciplinary approach to treatment and rehabilitation for his chronic back problem. Your goal is to minimize J.C.'s long-term health care costs by rehabilitating his back, helping him reduce his weight to reduce stress on his back, and treating his current injury. You coordinate referrals for J.C. to see four health care experts on your team.

5. You refer J.C. to a physiatrist. What is a physiatrist, and what can a physiatrist do to help J.C.?

6. What expert would work with J.C. to help him lose weight? What are this expert's credentials?

7. What kind of expert will work with J.C. using exercise and various treatment modalities to restore his back muscles?

8. What kind of expert will work with J.C. on body mechanics and strengthening him for occupational-and home-related work?

9. A PT teaches J.C. maintenance exercises he can do on his own to promote back health. What three common exercises would be included?

10. What is celecoxib (Celebrex), and how does it work? Name at least one other drug in the same drug family. What advantage/disadvantages do these medications have over the “older” NSAIDs?

11. Why would you want to use an NSAID rather than acetaminophen for pain?

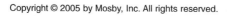

Case Study 3

Name ______________________________ Class/Group __________ Date __________

Group Members ____

INSTRUCTIONS: All questions apply to this case study. Your responses should be brief and to the point. Adequate space has been provided for answers. When asked to provide several answers, they should be listed in order of priority or significance. Do not asume information that is not provided. Please print or write clearly. If your response is not legible, it will be marked as ? and you will need to rewrite it.

Scenario

D.M., a 25-year-old man, hops into the ED C/O right ankle pain. He states that he was playing basketball and stepped on another player's foot, inverting his ankle. You note swelling over the lateral malleolus down to the area of the fourth and fifth metatarsals, and pedal pulses are 3+ bilaterally. His vital signs (VS) are 124/76, 82, 18. He has no allergies and takes no medication. He states he has had no prior surgeries or medical problems.

1. When assessing D.M.'s injured ankle, what should be evaluated?

2. What should initial management of the ankle involve to prevent further swelling and injury to the ankle?

3. You note there is significant swelling over the fourth and fifth metatarsals. How would you further evaluate this finding?

X-rays are negative for fracture, and a third-degree sprain is diagnosed. The physician orders an ankle splint with elastic wrap and crutches with instructions. The physician instructs D.M. not to bear weight on his ankle for 2 days.

4. Describe the technique for applying an elastic wrap. Give the rationale.

5. When instructing D.M. to use crutches, his weight should rest on what part of his body while the crutch is bearing the weight? Explain why.

6. You are to instruct D.M. on application of cold and heat, activity, and care of the ankle. What would be appropriate instructions in these areas?

7. D.M. is given a prescription for acetaminophen/hydrocodone (Lortab) for pain. What instructions concerning this medication should you give him on discharge?

8. Four days later D.M. hobbles into the ED and boldly informs you that he "did it again, only this time it was touch football." He states that the pain pills worked so well, he thought it would be OK. You detect the odor of beer on his breath. What are you going to do?

9. You remove his sock and find a large hematoma forming on the lateral aspect of an already-swollen ankle. The ankle also shows the color of a bruise that is several days old. You inquire about D.M.'s pain perception. He states, "It doesn't feel too bad now, but I sure saw stars when it popped." What is the significance of his statement?

Case Study 4

Name ______________________ Class/Group __________ Date __________

Group Members ____

INSTRUCTIONS: All questions apply to this case study. Your responses should be brief and to the point. Adequate space has been provided for answers. When asked to provide several answers, they should be listed in order of priority or significance. Do not asume information that is not provided. Please print or write clearly. If your response is not legible, it will be marked as ? and you will need to rewrite it.

Scenario

S.P. is admitted to the orthopedic ward. She has fallen at home and has sustained an intracapsular fracture of the hip at the femoral neck. The following history is obtained from her: She is a 75-year-old widow with three children living nearby. Her father died of cancer at 62 years of age; mother died of CHF (congestive heart failure) at 79 years of age. Height 5′3″, weight 118 pounds. She has a 50-pack-year smoking history and denies alcohol use. She has severe rheumatoid arthritis with UGI (upper gastrointestinal) bleed in 1993 and CAD (coronary artery disease) with CABG (coronary artery bypass graft) 9 months ago. Since that time she has engaged in "very mild exercises at home." VS are 128/60, 98, 14, 37.2° C, Sao_2 94% on 2 L O_2/NC. Medications: rabeprazole (Aciphex) 20 mg qd, prednisone (Deltasone) 5 mg PO qd, and methotrexate (Amethopterin) 2.5 mg weekly.

1. List four risk factors for hip fractures.

2. Place a checkmark next to each of the responses in question 1 that represent S.P.'s risk factors.

S.P. is taken to surgery for a total hip replacement. Because of the intracapsular location of the fracture, the surgeon chooses to perform an arthroplasty rather than internal fixation. The postoperative orders include:

- Cefazolin (Kefzol) 2000 mg IV q8h
- Enoxaparin (Lovenox) 30 mg sq q12h
- Warfarin (Coumadin) 1to 10 mg oral per sliding scale (hold day of surgery)
- Peri-Colace 1 cap PO bid
- Trinsicon 1 cap PO with meals
- Complete blood count (CBC) in morning after blood reinfusion

- Hydromorphone (Dilaudid) 25mg IV patient controlled analgesia (PCA) pump
- PT to evaluate postoperative day (POD) 1
- Ketorolac (Toradol) 15mg IM or IV q6h prn
- Hip precautions per protocol
- Ondansetron 4 mg prn nausea
- Toilet seat extension
- Straight catheterization if no void q8h postoperatively

3. Why is the patient receiving enoxaparin and warfarin?

4. What is the difference between arthroplasty and open reduction and internal fixation (ORIF)?

5. List four critical potential postoperative problems for S.P., and explain why you think each is important.

6. How would you monitor for excessive postoperative blood loss?

7. How should a nurse manage a patient using a blood reinfusion system?

8. There are two main goals for maintaining proper alignment of S.P.'s operative leg. What are they, and how are they achieved?

9. Postoperative wound infection is a concern for S.P. Describe what you would do to monitor S.P. for wound infection.

10. Taking S.P's RA into consideration, what interventions should be implemented to prevent complications secondary to immobility?

11. What predisposing factor, identified in S.P.'s medical history, places her at risk for infection, bleeding, and anemia?

12. Briefly discuss S.P.'s nutritional needs.

13. Explain four techniques you can teach S.P. to help her protect herself from infection R/T medication-induced immune suppression.

S.P. was transferred to a long-term care facility for rehabilitation.

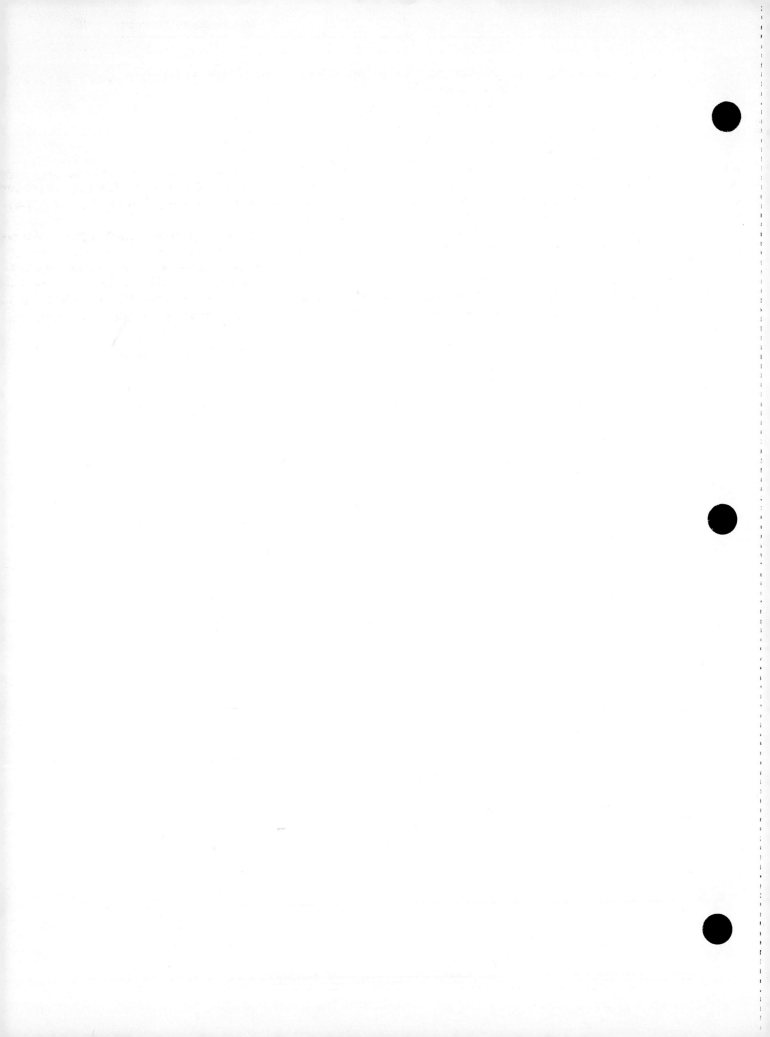

Case Study 5

Name ______________________________ Class/Group __________ Date ___________

Group Members ____

INSTRUCTIONS: All questions apply to this case study. Your responses should be brief and to the point. Adequate space has been provided for answers. When asked to provide several answers, they should be listed in order of priority or significance. Do not asume information that is not provided. Please print or write clearly. If your response is not legible, it will be marked as ? and you will need to rewrite it.

Scenario

H.K. is a 26-year-old man who tried to light a cigarette while driving and lost control of his Jeep. The Jeep flipped and landed on the passenger side. H.K. was transported to the ED with a deformed, edematous right lower leg and a deep puncture wound approximately 5 cm long over the deformity. Blood continues to ooze from the wound.

1. What further assessment should the nurse make of the leg injury and what precautions should she take in making this assessment?

2. What would be the most appropriate method for controlling bleeding at this wound site?

3. From the above information, it is clear that H.K. is a smoker. List at least three issues R/T his smoking that can complicate his care and recovery. What interventions could be instituted to counter these complications? Would using a nicotine patch eliminate these problems?

4. What is the best way to immobilize the leg injury prior to surgery?

H.K. is taken to surgery for ORIF of the tibia and fibula fractures. He returns with a full-leg fiberglass cast with windows over the areas of surgery.

5. Describe assessment of a patient with a long leg cast involving trauma and surgery.

6. In assessing H.K.'s cast on the third day postop, you notice a strong foul odor. Drainage on the cast is extending, and H.K. is C/O pain more often and seems considerably more uncomfortable. VS (vital signs) are 123/78, 102, 18, 39° C. What is your analysis of these findings?

H.K. returns to surgery. The wound over H.K.'s fracture site has become necrotic with purulent drainage. The wound is debrided and cultured; then a posterior splint is applied. H.K. returns to his room with orders for wet- to-moist dressing changes. The physician suspects osteomyelitis and orders nafcillin (Unipen), and gentamicin (Gentak).

7. As you continue to assess H.K. over the following days, what evidence will you look for that antibiotics are effectively treating the infection?

8. What should H.K. be taught concerning the care of his cast?

9. What nutritional needs will H.K. have, and why?

10. To ensure pain management, H.K. is given a 75 μg transdermal fentanyl patch. What therapeutic category does this drug belong to? What S/S would you see if he were to have a toxic or overdose reaction?

11. What is the antidote to toxic narcotic reactions, and how is it administered?

Case Study 6

Name ______________________ Class/Group __________ Date __________

Group Members ____

INSTRUCTIONS: All questions apply to this case study. Your responses should be brief and to the point. Adequate space has been provided for answers. When asked to provide several answers, they should be listed in order of priority or significance. Do not asume information that is not provided. Please print or write clearly. If your response is not legible, it will be marked as ? and you will need to rewrite it.

Scenario

M.M., a 76-year-old retired schoolteacher, underwent ORIF of his right femur. His preoperative control PT was 11 seconds. He has been on bed rest for the first 2 days postoperatively. 0600 VS were 132/84, 80 reg, 18 unlabored, and 37.2° C. He is AAO. No adventitious heart sounds. Breath sounds are clear but diminished in the bases bilaterally. Bowel sounds are present, and he is taking sips of clear liquids. An IV of D_5½NS is infusing to keep open (TKO) in his left hand and should be saline locked in the am if he is able to maintain adequate PO fluid intake. He has orders for O_2 to maintain Sao_2>90%. His labwork shows Hct 34%, Hgb 11.3 mg/dl, K 4.1 mmol/L, PTT 44 sec. Pain is controlled with morphine sulfate 4 mg IV and promethazine (Phenergan) 25 mg IV q3h. He is also taking heparin 5000 units SQ bid, docusate sodium, and wearing a nitroglycerin patch.

At 2330 on the second postoperative day, you answer M.M.'s call light and find him lying in bed breathing rapidly and rubbing his right chest. He is C/O right-sided chest pain and appears to be restless.

1. What are you going to do?

He is slightly hypotensive, tachycardic, tachypneic, restless, and slightly confused. The pulse oximeter reads 86%, so you start him on 3 to 6 L O_2/NC. You identify faint crackles in the posterior bases bilaterally; they were clear this morning. The monitor shows nonspecific T wave changes and tachycardia.

2. Based on your findings, you call the physician. What information are you going to give him or her?

3. The physician orders the patient to be transferred to intensive care unit (ICU), blood coagulation studies, arterial blood gases (ABGs) on room air, continuous pulse oximetry, STAT chest x-ray (CXR), and STAT 12-lead electrocardiogram (ECG). What information will the physician gain from each of the above?

4. Why would the physician order ABGs on room air as opposed to with supplemental O_2?

The ABGs return as follows: pH 7.55, $Paco_2$ 24 mm Hg, HCO_3 24 mmol/L, and Pao_2 56 mm Hg at sea level. Sao_2 is 86% on room air. Chest x-ray shows a small right infiltrate. VS are 150/92, 110, 28, 37.2° C.

5. What is your interpretation of the ABGs, and what do you think the physician will order next?

6. The $\dot{V}/\dot{Q}$ is performed, and the interpretation reads "strongly suggestive of a pulmonary embolus." What are the most likely sources of the embolus?

7. Before the latest partial thromboplastin time (PTT)/INR results are back, the physician orders a heparin bolus of 5000 units IV followed by an infusion of 1200 units/hr. The lab calls with a critical value—the PTT is 120 seconds. Based on these results, what action would you take?

The PTT 4 hours later is 29 seconds.

8. The next day the physician's orders read, "Coumadin 2.5 mg, PT/INR in AM, DC heparin." What is wrong with these orders?

9. Thrombolytics, such as streptokinase and urokinase, have been beneficial in the treatment of PE. Why would this medication be contraindicated in M.M.'s case?

10. List three priority problems R/T the care of M.M. in his current situation.

11. Several days later you hear M.M. requesting his son to bring in a "decent razor" because he is tired of the stubble left by the unit's shaver. How would you address this issue?

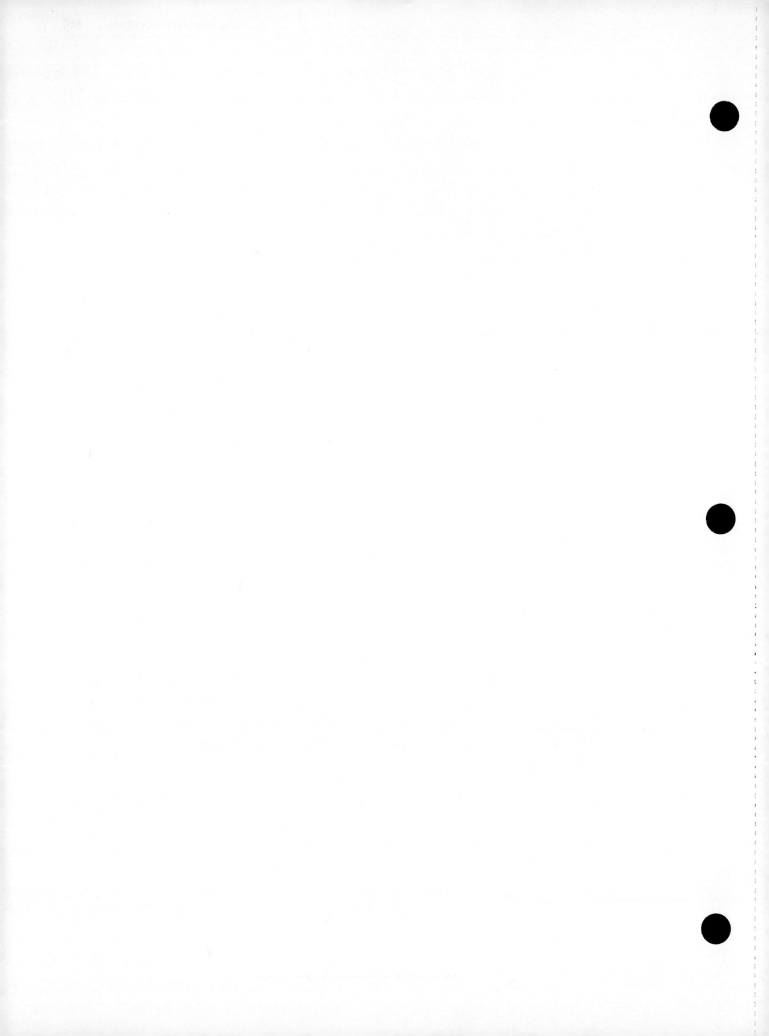

Case Study 7

Name ______________________ Class/Group __________ Date __________

Group Members ____

INSTRUCTIONS: All questions apply to this case study. Your responses should be brief and to the point. Adequate space has been provided for answers. When asked to provide several answers, they should be listed in order of priority or significance. Do not asume information that is not provided. Please print or write clearly. If your response is not legible, it will be marked as ? and you will need to rewrite it.

Scenario

You are working in the ED when a 27-year-old man runs through the door with a blood-soaked towel over his left hand. D.W., a machinist, states he caught his hand in an automatic shear and cut off his left index finger. His coworker has the finger wrapped in a paper towel. You grab a pair of gloves while you direct D.W. to lie on a stretcher, where you remove the towel and apply firm pressure to the stump with sterile sponges. Another nurse takes his VS and announces 196/122, 144, 22. To distract him, you gather information about his PMH, allergies, and tetanus status. He has a history of depression, for which he takes Prozac (fluoxetine), and he is allergic to Darvocet (propoxyphene). He has no significant medical history other than depression.

1. What is your first priority in dealing with D.W.'s amputated finger?

2. D.W.'s stump is bleeding profusely. Would you apply a tourniquet to the end of the finger or not, and why?

3. An x-ray of the index finger reveals an amputation of the distal interphalangeal (DIP) joint. The fracture has left a jagged protruding bone that can be seen from the distal tip. After controlling the bleeding, what would be the appropriate management?

Note: Observe D.W.'s anxiety level and LOC, and assess for shock. Make sure he is in a stable condition in case he goes into shock and/or loses consciousness.

4. What would be suitable treatment of the amputated appendage?

5. D.W. has not had a tetanus shot in the past 10 years. You have run out of adult tetanus/diphtheria (TD) and you only have pediatric DPT available. Would it be suitable to give the pediatric DPT (diphtheria/pertussis/tetanus)?

6. What factors influence the success of the reattached digit?

7. List three issues related to D.W.'s care.

8. You repeat his VS and record the following: 118/86, 78, 18. Do you find the VS changes to be reassuring or distressing, and why?

9. The operating room (OR) calls for D.M. Before he leaves, you need to start an IV. What type of solution would you hang, and why?

10. Why would it be important to further question D.M. about his allergy to Darvocet?

D.M. was prescribed Percocet 1-2 tabs PO q4-6h prn for pain.

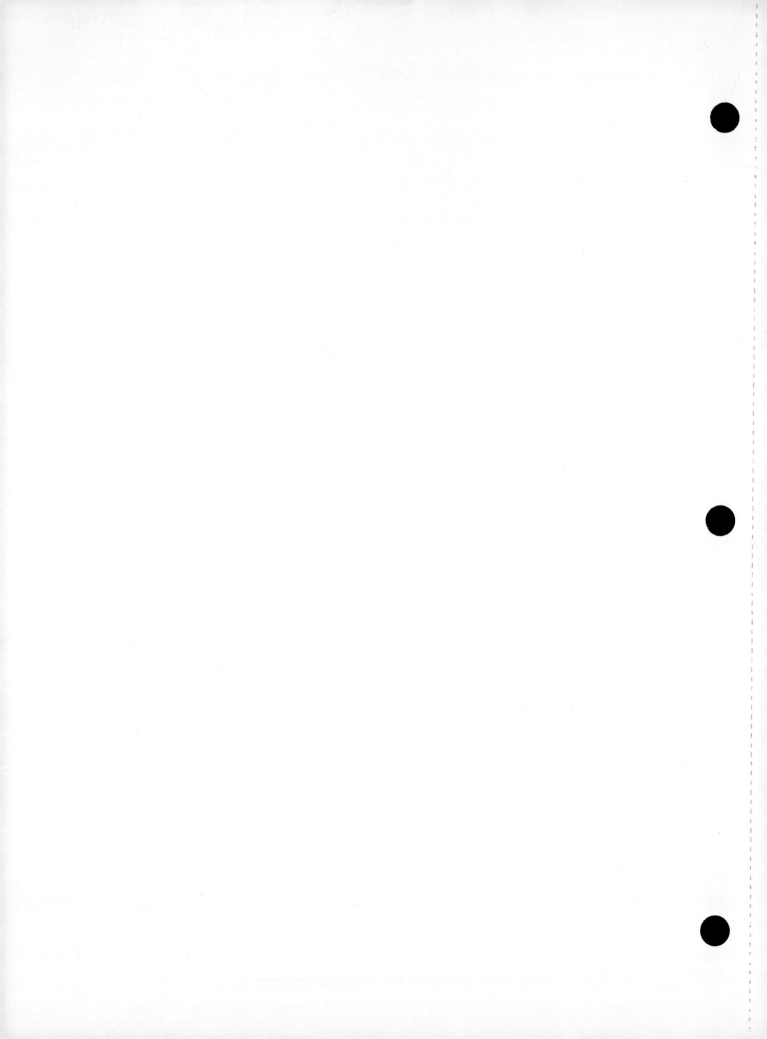

Case Study 8

Name ______________________ Class/Group __________ Date __________

Group Members ____

INSTRUCTIONS: All questions apply to this case study. Your responses should be brief and to the point. Adequate space has been provided for answers. When asked to provide several answers, they should be listed in order of priority or significance. Do not asume information that is not provided. Please print or write clearly. If your response is not legible, it will be marked as ? and you will need to rewrite it.

Scenario

B.G. is struck by a vehicle while riding his motorcycle and is transported to your ED by ambulance. He is found to have a fractured mandible and multiple fractures of the right tibia and fibula.

1. When a patient comes in with facial trauma such as B.G.'s, what two other injuries should you assume exist until ruled out? Explain.

B.G. is taken to the OR for intermaxillary fixation (wiring of the jaw) and pinning of the fractured tibia and fibula.

2. B.G. returns from surgery with his jaws wired. What patient care issue R/T his wired jaws would you be concerned about postoperatively?

Hint: Think in terms of an emergency.

3. What precautions will you take to ensure a patent airway in B.G. if he begins vomiting while his jaws are wired?

4. If B.G. begins vomiting with his jaws wired, what actions should you take?

B.C. is transferred to a rehabilitation facility for treatment of his leg injury.

5. His jaws remain wired. What instructions should you give him concerning oral care and safety?

6. During his stay at the rehabilitation facility, what nutritional teaching does B.G. need to prepare him for discharge?

B.G. has daily dressing changes, antibiotics, and PT; wound debridement is prn.

7. Two weeks after B.G.'s accident, you enter his room to do his afternoon shift assessment. The shades are drawn, he is sitting in the corner with his face to the wall, and you have been told he refused to go to PT this afternoon. He answers your questions in flat, monosyllabic tones. When you ask him what is wrong, he explodes in anger, even more frustrated because his wired jaw keeps him from being able to talk well. What are you going to do?

8. B.G. tells you, "I got a good look at my leg today when the bandage was off. It looks really ugly. I wanted to throw up." What are you going to say?

B.G. was discharged to home but returned to the rehabilitation facility for PT and continued wound management for 3 months. Several months later you see B.G. at the grocery store. You call his name; he waves and walks toward you. You notice that he walks with a slight limp. He tells you that his leg healed, but he has pain in his knee when he walks or hikes any distance.

9. What could be causing pain in B.G.'s right knee? (Remember that his right foreleg had originally been injured.)

10. You suggest B.G. ask his physician about a prescription for a foot evaluation and orthotics. What are orthotics, and what purpose do they serve?

B.G. will be referred to a sports medicine center, orthopedist, podiatrist, or PT to have his gait and foot evaluated.

Case Study 9

Name ______________________ Class/Group __________ Date __________

Group Members ____

INSTRUCTIONS: All questions apply to this case study. Your responses should be brief and to the point. Adequate space has been provided for answers. When asked to provide several answers, they should be listed in order of priority or significance. Do not asume information that is not provided. Please print or write clearly. If your response is not legible, it will be marked as ? and you will need to rewrite it.

Scenario

J.F., a 67-year-old woman, was involved in an auto accident and is life-flighted to your facility. She sustained a ruptured spleen, fractured pelvis, and compound fractures of the left femur. On admission she underwent a splenectomy (5 days ago). Her pelvis was stabilized with an external fixator device 3 days ago, and yesterday her left femur was stabilized using balanced suspension with skeletal traction. She has a Thomas ring with Pearson attachment on her left leg. She has 20 pounds of skeletal traction and 5 pounds applied to the balanced suspension. Her left femur is elevated off the bed at approximately 45 degrees. The foreleg (lower part of her leg) is parallel to the bed and lies in a sling that the nurse adjusts on the frame, and the foot hangs freely. This morning J.F. was transferred to your orthopedic unit for specialized care. You are the nurse assigned to care for her on the night shift.

1. You enter J.F.'s room for the first time. What aspects of the traction would you want to inspect?

2. When inspecting the skeletal pin sites, you note that the skin is reddened for an inch around the pin on both the medial and lateral left leg. What does this finding indicate, and what action would you take?

3. You find J.F.'s body in the lower 75% of the bed, her left upper leg at an exaggerated angle (>45 degrees.) The knot at the end of the bed is caught in the pulley, and the 20-pound weight is dangling just above the floor. What are you going to do?

4. When you lift J.F., you notice that her sheets are wet. Because you have lots of help in the room, you decide to change J.F.'s linen. How would you accomplish this task?

5. J.F. tells you that she feels like she needs to have a bowel movement, but it is too painful to sit on the bedpan. How would you respond?

6. J.F. expels a few small, hard, round pieces of stool. What could be done to promote normal elimination?

You ask J.F. if she is ready for her bath, and she responds positively. You let her bathe the parts she can reach and engage her in a conversation as you attend to the rest of her body. While performing perineal care you notice that the folds of skin around her perineal area are reddened and excoriated.

7. Given that J.F. has been on antibiotics for the past 5 days, what is the likely cause of the problem, and what needs to be done to encourage healing?

8. You ask J.F. what she is doing to exercise while she is confined to bed. She looks surprised and states that she isn't doing anything. What activities can J.F. engage in while on bed rest?

9. You realize that maintaining skin integrity is a challenge in J.F.'s case. What measures will you take to prevent skin breakdown?

10. Although J.F. is recovering nicely, she is becoming increasingly withdrawn. You enter her room and find her crying. She tells you that she is all alone here, that she misses her family terribly. You know that her son is flying into town tomorrow but will only be able to stay a few days. What can be done so that J.F. benefits from her family support system?

Case Study 10

Name ______________________________ Class/Group __________ Date __________

Group Members ____

INSTRUCTIONS: All questions apply to this case study. Your responses should be brief and to the point. Adequate space has been provided for answers. When asked to provide several answers, they should be listed in order of priority or significance. Do not asume information that is not provided. Please print or write clearly. If your response is not legible, it will be marked as ? and you will need to rewrite it.

Scenario

You are working in the ED when M.C., an 82-year-old widow, arrives by ambulance. Because M.C. had not answered her phone since noon yesterday, her daughter went to her home to check on her. She found M.C. lying on the kitchen floor, incontinent of urine and stool, and C/O pain in her right hip. Her daughter reports a PMH of hypertension, angina, and osteoporosis. M.C. takes propranolol (Inderal), nitroglycerin patch, indapamide (Lozol), and Premarin daily. The daughter reports that her mother is normally very alert and lives independently. Upon examination you see an elderly woman, approximately 100 pounds, holding her right thigh. You note shortening of the right leg with external rotation and a large amount of swelling at the proximal thigh and right hip. M.C. is oriented to person only and is confused about place and time. M.C.'s VS are 90/65, 120, 24, 36.4° C; her Sao_2 is 89%. She is profoundly dehydrated. Preliminary diagnosis is fracture of the right hip.

1. In view of M.C.'s history of hypertension and the fact that she has been without her medications for at least 24 hours, explain her current VS.

2. Based on her history and your initial assessment, what three priority interventions should be initiated?

3. M.C.'s daughter states, "Mother is always so clear and alert. I have never seen her act so confused. What's wrong with her?" What are three possible causes for M.C.'s disorientation that should be considered and evaluated?

X-ray films confirmed the diagnosis of intertrochanteric femoral fracture. Knowing that M.C. is going to be admitted, you draw admission labs and call for an orthopedic consult.

4. What laboratory and diagnostic studies would be ordered to evaluate M.C.'s condition, and what critical information will each give you?

5. What are the five Ps that should guide the assessment of M.C.'s right leg before and after surgery?

6. In evaluating M.C.'s pulses, you find her posterior tibial pulse and dorsalis pedis pulse to be weaker on her right foot than on her left. What would be a possible cause of this finding?

7. In planning further care for M.C., list four potential complications for which M.C. should be monitored.

8. M.C. keeps asking about "Peaches." No one seems to be paying attention. You ask her what she means. She says Peaches is her little dog and she's worried about who is taking care of her. How will you answer?

M.C. is placed in Buck's traction and sent to the orthopedic unit until an ORIF can be scheduled. Hydrocodone/acetaminophen (Lortab) is ordered for severe pain with orders for acetaminophen and tramadol for mild and moderate pain, respectively. M.C.'s cardiovascular, pulmonary, and renal status is closely monitored.

9. Tramadol and Lortab are both constipating. What would you do to prevent constipation?

10. What is obstipation?

After her surgery, M.C. is transferred to a long-term care facility for PT/OT rehabilitation. She is placed on prophylactic warfarin (Coumadin).

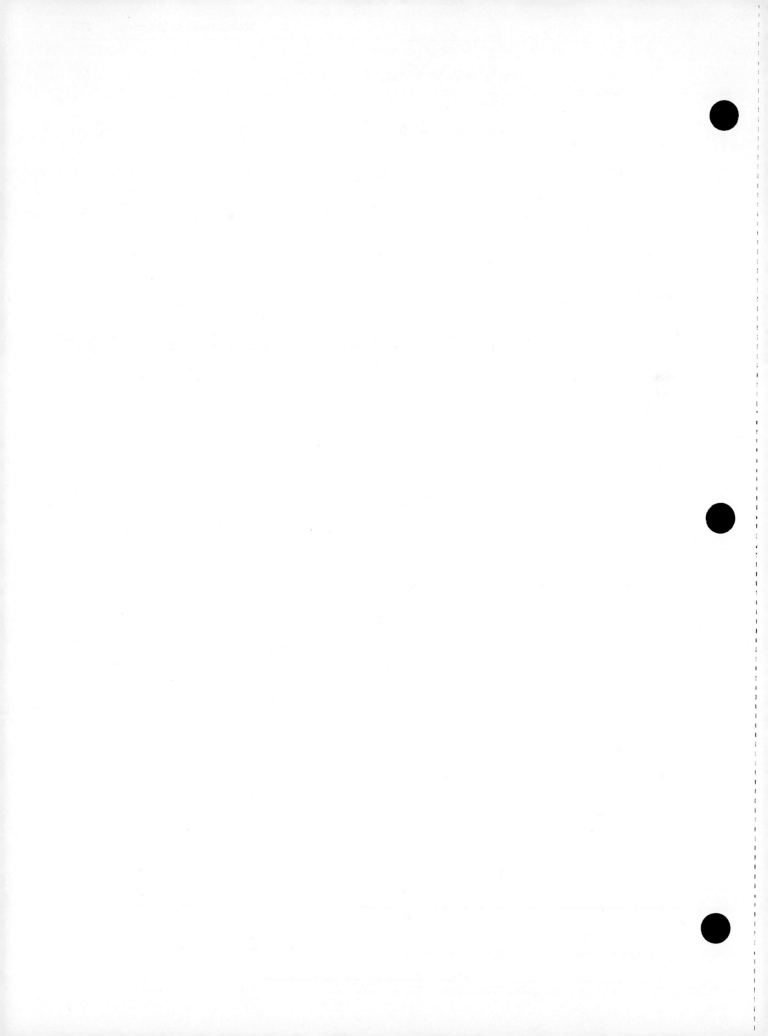

Case Study 11

Name ______________________ Class/Group __________ Date __________

Group Members ____

INSTRUCTIONS: All questions apply to this case study. Your responses should be brief and to the point. Adequate space has been provided for answers. When asked to provide several answers, they should be listed in order of priority or significance. Do not asume information that is not provided. Please print or write clearly. If your response is not legible, it will be marked as ? and you will need to rewrite it.

Scenario

E.B., a 69-year-old man with type 1 DM, is admitted to a large, regional medical center C/O severe pain in his right foot and lower leg. The foot and lower leg are cool and without pulses (absent by Doppler). Arteriogram demonstrates severe atherosclerosis of the right popliteal artery with complete obstruction of blood flow. Despite attempts at endarterectomy and intravascular urokinase over several days, the foot and lower leg become necrotic. Finally, the decision is made to perform an above-the-knee amputation (AKA) on E.B.'s right leg. E.B. is recently widowed and has a son and daughter who live nearby. In preparation for E.B.'s surgery, the surgeons wish to spare as much viable tissue as possible. Hence an order is written for E.B. to undergo 5 days of hyperbaric therapy for 20 minutes bid.

1. What is the purpose of hyperbaric therapy, and what purpose does it serve in a patient like E.B.?

As you are preparing E.B. for surgery, he is quiet and withdrawn. He follows instructions quietly and slowly without asking questions. His son and daughter are at his bedside and they also are very quiet. Finally, E.B. says, "I don't want to go like your mother did. She lingered on and had so much pain. I don't want them to bring me back."

2. You look at his chart and find no advance directives. What is your responsibility?

3. What is your assessment of E.B.'s behavior at this time?

4. What are some appropriate interventions and responses to E.B.'s anticipatory grief?

E.B. returns from surgery with the right stump dressed with gauze and an elastic wrap. The dressing is dry and intact, without drainage. He is drowsy with the following VS: 142/80, 96, 14, 36.6° C, Sao_2 92%. He has a maintenance IV of D_5.9NS infusing at 125 ml/hr in his right forearm.

5. The surgeon has written to keep E.B.'s stump elevated on pillows for 48 hours; after that, have him lie in a prone position for 15 minutes qid. In teaching E.B. about his care, how would you explain the rationale for these orders?

6. In reviewing E.B.'s medical history, what factor may affect the condition of his stump and ultimate rehabilitation potential?

You have just returned from a 2-day workshop on guidelines for the care of surgical patients with type 1 DM. You notice that E.B.'s blood glucose has been running between 130 and 180. The sliding scale insulin intervention does not begin until a blood glucose of 200 is reported. You recognize that patients with blood glucoses even slightly above normal suffer from impaired wound healing.

7. Identify four interventions that would facilitate timely healing of E.B.'s stump.

8. What should the postoperative assessment of E.B.'s stump dressing include?

9. On the evening of the first postoperative day, E.B. becomes more awake and begins to C/O pain. He states, "My leg is really hurting; are you sure it's gone?" How would you respond to E.B.'s question?

E.B. will be discharged to an extended-care facility for strength training; once the patient receives his prosthesis, he will receive balance training. After that he will be discharged to his daughter's home. A PT home evaluation should be ordered.

10. What instructions should be given to E.B.'s daughter concerning safety around the home at this time?

Case Study 12

Name ______________________________ Class/Group __________ Date __________

Group Members ____

INSTRUCTIONS: All questions apply to this case study. Your responses should be brief and to the point. Adequate space has been provided for answers. When asked to provide several answers, they should be listed in order of priority or significance. Do not asume information that is not provided. Please print or write clearly. If your response is not legible, it will be marked as ? and you will need to rewrite it.

Scenario

J.T. has injured his hand at work and is accompanied to the ED by a coworker. You examine his hand and find a piece of a drill bit sticking out of the skin between the third and fourth knuckles of his left hand. There is another puncture site about an inch below and toward the center of the hand. Bleeding is minimal. J.T. is 41 years old, has no significant medical history, and no known drug allergies (NKDA). He states the accident occurred when a mill at work malfunctioned and knocked his hand onto a rack of drill bits. His last tetanus booster was 3 years ago. It is your job to provide the initial care for J.T.'s injury.

1. You examine J.T.'s hand. What should you include in your initial assessment, and why?

You record that J.T.'s fingers are warm with capillary refill <2 seconds. Sensory perception is intact. He is able to flex and extend the distal joints but not the proximal joints of the third and fourth fingers.

2. You notice J.T.'s wedding band and promptly ask him to remove it. Why is this important?

3. J.T. asks you why he can't just pull the bit out and go home. How should you respond to his question?

4. What common diagnostic test will identify fractures and the location of metal fragments in J.T.'s hand?

The drill bit is impaled ½ inch below the surface of the skin, and there are no fractures. Because the hand contains so many blood vessels, nerves, ligaments and tendons, the ED physician decides to consult a surgical hand specialist. A neurologic consult says there is no nerve damage. The surgeon suspects tendon damage and decides to operate immediately.

5. What do you need to do to prepare J.T. for immediate surgery?

6. You record that J.T. has had no food "since 8:00 PM yesterday" and drank "some water" this morning. Based on this information, do you anticipate problems during surgery, and why?

7. Should J.T. be given a tetanus booster before he goes to surgery?

The surgeon repairs two partially severed tendons and wraps the hand in a very large, padded dressing. The distal ½ inch of each digit protrudes from the bulky dressing.

8. While in the short-stay recovery area, J.T. asks the nurse why his fingers look yellowish brown. How should she respond to his question?

The surgeon tells J.T. that he had to repair tendons in his third and fourth fingers and instructs J.T. that he is not to work. He gives J.T. prescriptions for an antibiotic and an antiinflammatory agent. He instructs J.T. to make an appointment to see him in the surgery clinic in 2 days.

9. What instructions should the nurse in the short-stay area discuss with J.T. and his wife before releasing him?

10. J.T. says, "How in the world is the ice supposed to keep my hand cold with this big bandage on it?" How will the nurse reply?

11. J.T. says, "I'll be able to keep my hand up when I'm awake, but what about when I go to sleep?" What suggestion can the nurse make to help J.T. comply with the instructions?

J.T.'s recovery was uncomplicated; he received follow-up occupational therapy and regained the full use of his hand.

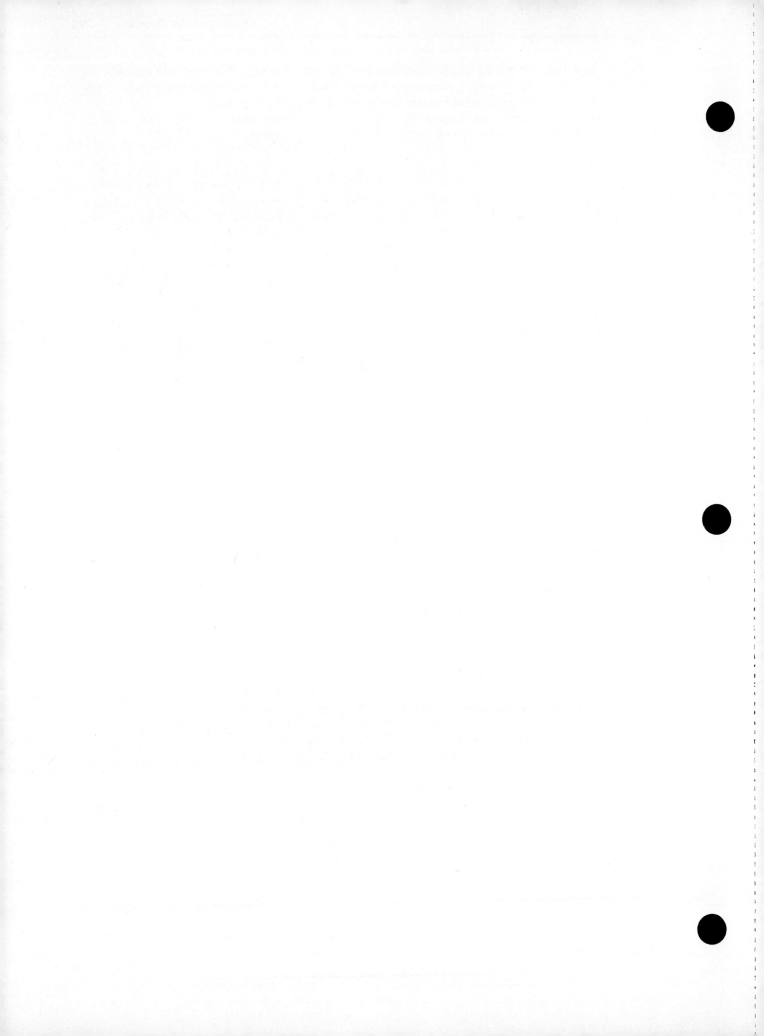

Case Study 13

Name ______________________ Class/Group __________ Date __________

Group Members ____

INSTRUCTIONS: All questions apply to this case study. Your responses should be brief and to the point. Adequate space has been provided for answers. When asked to provide several answers, they should be listed in order of priority or significance. Do not asume information that is not provided. Please print or write clearly. If your response is not legible, it will be marked as ? and you will need to rewrite it.

Scenario

Dr. C., a 53-year-old nursing professor, comes to your chronic fatigue clinic for evaluation of long-term fatigue, weakness, and pain, which have become increasingly disruptive to her lifestyle. Over the years, she sought medical advice about her fatigue but received vague and often conflicting advice such as "get more exercise," "get more rest," "eat better," "exercise more and lose weight," and "pull yourself together." Despite treatment for "depression," the fatigue remains unrelenting. Nothing seems to help. She confides to you that she is so discouraged and tired of dragging through each day that she has thought of suicide, but it violates her belief system.

1. You ask her to describe her symptoms. What questions will you ask about her fatigue, weakness, and pain?

Dr. C. describes her fatigue as daily, unrelenting, and worse in the evening. The overall fatigue, together with muscular weakness ("feels rubbery") and "nervelike" pain, is aggravated by activity and long days. She experiences nausea when extremely fatigued. She has difficulty negotiating inclines and stairs. Although rest makes her feel better, she says she feels guilty about "taking the time." She says she rarely attends social events, is having trouble doing her housekeeping, and has had to give up doing yardwork. She tells you she worries a great deal about her future and whether she'll be able to work until retirement.

You take a detailed history in preparation for a physical and psychosocial evaluation. At age 17 she developed polio. She described this experience as sudden onset (over a 6-hour period) with fatigue, high fever (104.8° F) with shaking chills, weakness, and aching all over. The next day she dragged her feet, experienced constipation, became anorectic, and had chills, indescribable muscle aches, and constant pain. The asymmetric muscular weakness affected all her extremities, especially her legs. This was followed by over 6 months of hospitalization featuring the Sister Kenny method of treatment. The moist, hot packs helped relieve the extreme neuromuscular pain. Together with gentle exercise (swimming pool), they helped prevent contractures. "It was that experience that motivated me to become a nurse," she said and smiled. "It has always been a point of pride that I worked so hard and overcame such a vicious disease." Based on her history and your experience with other patients, you suspect her fatigue, weakness and pain are manifestations of PPS.

2. What comments did Dr. C. make indicating that her functional status (ability to function on a daily basis) is currently compromised? (List five.)

3. What questions do you need to ask to gain an understanding of her support systems?

4. Dr. C. admitted she is used to "pushing herself even when it hurts." Then she asks whether you think an exercise program would be good for her. How would you respond?

5. Dr. C. undergoes some diagnostic tests to confirm the diagnosis of PPS. What type of tests might be used for muscle evaluation?

The diagnosis of PPS as a source of Dr. C.'s fatigue, weakness, and pain is confirmed by the physiatrist. Dr. C. is surprised that she has never heard of PPS and that none of the other physicians have ever suggested it to her. She expresses interest in learning more about her diagnosis.

6. What resources can you suggest to her for further information?

7. On a follow-up visit, you work with Dr. C. on ways to adapt her lifestyle to her limitations. List several prosthetic devices that may help control her fatigue, weakness, and pain, and prevent further loss in muscular functioning.

8. What other suggestions can you make to help Dr. C. adapt to her limitation?

9. On her next visit, Dr. C. tells you she was "shocked" at the idea of thinking of herself as "handicapped." She adds, sadly, "I thought I had beat this years ago, but now my old enemy has come back to haunt me." How do you explain her comments?

In 1952, 20,000 Americans developed paralytic polio. Many of these patients are still alive and seeking health care in clinics and hospitals nationwide. In 1980 people who suffered with polio began reporting new onset of pain, weakness, and fatigue 30 to 40 years after the acute illness. Although the causes are still controversial, it is known that healthy axons sent out "axon sprouts" to innervate orphaned muscles fibers whose motor neurons were destroyed. Biopsies have shown that after 30 to 40 years, the axons stopped sending out sprouts, thus survivors of the original insult are experiencing symptoms of PPS.

Although this case featured someone whose poliomyelitis generally affected the lower body, others experience polio over their entire body, even affecting arm movement and breathing. Many individuals with PPS develop trouble breathing, swallowing, and maintaining an upright posture, so a history of polio should always be a question asked in geriatric populations and immigrants who may have been exposed to polio.

Because many health care providers today have had no experience with PPS, it is important that Dr. C. find someone who can help her identify her unique needs for anesthesia, pain management, and preoperative/postoperative care. Help Dr. C. identify some of these resources.

There are several facts that all PPS patients and their providers should know:

- PPS patients are extremely sensitive to anesthesia due to damage to the reticular activating system (RAS) of the brainstem. Typically, the dose of anesthesia should be cut in half.
- PPS patients require twice as long to recover from the effects of anesthesia because of hypothalamus damage.
- PPS patients have trouble warming up after surgery because of CNS damage. They are unable to vasoconstrict, so they lose heat and remain cold.
- PPS patients are more sensitive to pain than normal D/T damage to endogenous opiate cells in the hypothalamus of the brain. This means that PPS patients need more pain medication for a longer period of time.
- PPS patients require close supervision postoperatively; their respiratory muscles are weak and they may require ventilatory support or supplemental O_2.

4 Gastrointestinal Disorders

Case Study 1

Name ________________________ Class/Group __________ Date __________

Group Members ____

INSTRUCTIONS: All questions apply to this case study. Your responses should be brief and to the point. Adequate space has been provided for answers. When asked to provide several answers, they should be listed in order of priority or significance. Do not asume information that is not provided. Please print or write clearly. If your response is not legible, it will be marked as ? and you will need to rewrite it.

Scenario

The charge nurse on your surgical floor notifies you that your next admission will be H.C., a 70-year-old woman who has an active GI (gastrointestinal) bleed and has just been informed that she has adenocarcinoma of the lung. Her VS are 130/80, 80, 18, 37.2° C.

When H.C. arrives on the floor, no family members are present, she has slightly pink coloring, and she denies pain, although she does appear anxious. Her PMH (past medical history) includes PUD (peptic ulcer disease) with reflux esophagitis, COPD (chronic obstructive pulmonary disease), HTN (hypertension), hypothyroidism, and "fluid retention." PSH (past surgical history) includes TAH (total abdominal hysterectomy) and appendectomy (1965), benign R breast biopsy (1994), and laparoscopic Nissen fundoplication (1994). Her regular medications include ranitidine 150 mg bid, $FeSO_4$ 325 mg qd, potassium chloride (K-Dur) 20 mEq bid, hydrochlorothiazide (HCTZ) 25 mg qd, levothyroxine (Synthroid) 0.1 mg qd, albuterol/ipratropium (Combivent) 2 puffs q6h, and salmeterol (Serevent) disk 1 puff bid.

H.C.'s admission orders brought up from the ED (emergency department) include the following: admit to GI (gastrointestinal) unit; Dx (diagnosis) of gastric ulcer, adenocarcinoma of the lung, longstanding COPD; VS q4h; NPO (nothing by mouth); IV (intravenous) D_5NS with 20 mEq KCl/L at 125 mL/h; I&O (intake and output); PT/PTT (prothrombin time/partial thromboplastin time), CBC (complete blood cell count), and CMP (complete metabolic profile) in AM; UA (urinalysis) on admission; O_2 (oxygen) at 4 L/NC (liters throught nasal cannula) prn (as needed) to keep SaO_2 (arterial oxygen saturation) >92%; pantoprazole 80 mg then drip at 8 mg/h; no NSAIDs (nonsteroidal antiinflammatory drugs) or ASA (aspirin); Hemoccult all stools; call MD (doctor) when husband arrives.

1. Which orders would require some clarification? Why?

O_2 2L?
Route pantoprazol?
Rate of D_5NS infusion?

You put in a call to the physician for clarification of the orders. In the meantime, you proceed with the admission process.

2. What are the major components of the assessment you will perform on H.C.?

Physical Assessment (Head to Toe)
Ask full med list (Inc OTC)/Allergies
Emotional status
Healthcare Proxy

Throughout the assessment, H.C. appears to be SOB (short of breath). Her sentences are getting shorter with pauses in between for breathing. You ask H.C. to stand on the bedside scale. As she stands, she suddenly sits back on the bed, C/O (complains of) dizziness and nausea.

3. H.C. had been admitted for a GI bleed. Review the previous data, and list possible indicators of gastrointestinal hemorrhage.

The physician calls to clarify H.C.'s orders: draw stat H&H (hematocrit and hemoglobin), change IV to D_5½NS at 100 mL/h, titrate O_2 to maintain Sao_2 between 88–90%, stat PT/PTT, CBC, CMP. The lab work returns: Hgb 10 g/L, Hct 30%, K 3.4 mmol/L.

4. Based on these laboratory findings, what are you going to do?

Dr. B. arrives and completes an emergent EGD (esophagogastroduodenoscopy) but was unsuccessful in his attempt to stop the bleeding. Dr. B. discusses the options with H.C. and her husband. A decision is made to go ahead with partial gastrectomy to remove the ulcer. The pulmonary consultant indicates that H.C.'s adenocarcinoma has metastasized to adjacent tissues to the extent that H.C. is not a candidate for lung resection. Radiation is planned to begin as soon as possible following this GI surgery.

5. What preop care would you expect to give?

Vitals.
NPO
NG tube teaching
IV/meds
Incentive Spirometry
Importance of turning to prevent skin breakdown
Pain meds.

6. In view of H.C.'s history, which part of your preoperative teaching do you think will be most necessary for H.C., and why?

H.C. returns to the floor after surgery. She has had a large wedge resection of her stomach with a partial selective vagotomy and a pyloroplasty. She is quite lethargic with stable VS. Her EBL (estimated blood loss) during surgery was minimal (100 mL). Her postop orders are as follows: Monitor H&H q8h. Transfuse 2 U PRBC (packed red blood cells) slowly (each over 4 h) and give furosemide 20 mg IVP (intravenous push) between units. Check HGB/HCT after second unit and call MD. CXR (chest x-ray) in AM with CBC, CMP, PT/PTT.

7. What is the rationale for ordering furosemide 20 mg IVP between units of PRBCs?

8. Why did the MD order a CXR in the morning?

9. The second postop day, H.C. still has a nasal O_2 cannula and a pulse oximeter. Where might you expect H.C. to have some skin breakdown?

10. How can the nurse best prevent skin breakdown?

H.C. has no postoperative complications and is discharged to her home with her husband on the fifth POD (postoperative day).

11. What warning signs would you teach H.C. to call her surgeon for?

12. H.C. is preparing for discharge when she turns on her call light. As you enter the room, she says, "I'm leaking." You examine her incision and note that her surgical wound has opened slightly (dehiscence). What action should you take?

After examining H.C., the physician instructs you to dress the wound with a wet- to-moist dressing. You contact the home health nurses for follow-up care for H.C., and she is discharged to her home.

13. In addition to dressing changes, what related services might the home health nurses provide for H.C. and her husband?

Three weeks later, H.C. was discharged from home care and started her radiation treatments.

Case Study 2

Name ______________________ Class/Group __________ Date __________

Group Members ____

INSTRUCTIONS: All questions apply to this case study. Your responses should be brief and to the point. Adequate space has been provided for answers. When asked to provide several answers, they should be listed in order of priority or significance. Do not asume information that is not provided. Please print or write clearly. If your response is not legible, it will be marked as ? and you will need to rewrite it.

Scenario

T.H., a 57-year-old stockbroker, has come to the gastroenterologist for treatment of recurrent mild to severe cramping in his abdomen and blood-streaked stool. You are the RN doing his initial work-up. Your findings include a mildly obese (male-pattern obesity) man who demonstrates moderate guarding of his abdomen with both direct and rebound tenderness, especially in the LLQ (left lower quadrant). His VS are 168/98, 110, 24, 38.0° C, and he is slightly diaphoretic. T.H. reports that he has periodic constipation. He has had previous episodes of abdominal cramping, but this time the pain is getting worse. He has NKDA (no known drug allergies).

PMH (past medical history): T.H. has a "sedentary job with lots of emotional moments"; he has smoked a pack of cigarettes a day for 30 years and has had "two or three mixed drinks in the evening" until 2 months ago. He states, "I haven't had anything to drink in 60 days." He denies regular exercise: "Just no time." His diet consists mostly of "white bread, meat, potatoes, and ice cream with fruit and nuts over it." Denies Hx (history) of cardiac or pulmonary problems and no personal Hx of cancer, although his father and older brother died of colon cancer. He takes no "regular" medications and denies the use of any other drugs.

1. Identify four general health risk problems T.H. exhibits.

2. Identify a key factor in his family history that may have profound implications for his health and present state of mind?

3. Identify three key findings on his physical exam, and indicate their significance.

The physician ordered a KUB (x-ray of the kidneys, ureters, bladder), CBC (complete blood cell count), CMP (complete metabolic profile). Based on x-ray and lab findings, physical exam and history, the physician diagnoses T.H. as having acute diverticulitis and discusses an outpatient treatment plan with him.

4. What is diverticulitis? What are the consequences of untreated diverticulitis?

5. While the patient is experiencing the severe crampy pain of acute diverticulitis, what interventions would you perform to help him feel more comfortable?

6. What is the rationale for ordering bed rest and anticholinergics?

7. What classes of medications would be prescribed for someone hospitalized for acute diverticulitis?

Metronidazole (Flagyl) or clindamycin (Cleocin) are antibiotics used in conjunction with a broad-spectrum penicillin, cephalosporin, or aminoglycoside to treat diverticulitis. T.H. is being sent home with prescriptions for metronidazole (Flagyl) 500 mg PO (by mouth) q6h and amoxicillin/clavulanate (Augmentin) 875 mg PO bid.

8. Given his history, what questions must you ask T.H. before he takes the initial dose of metronidazole? State your rationale.

9. What is a disulfiram reaction?

10. Aside from warning T.H. about the interactions just described, what instructions should you give him regarding his metronidazole prescription?

11. What information would you want to know before starting T.H. on ampicillin?

12. What are the signs and symptoms of an allergic reaction?

13. What will you do if the patient indicates a history of an allergic reaction to penicillin (PCN)?

14. In order to prevent future episodes of constipation, what dietary changes would the RD discuss with T.H.?

You obtain a referral for T.H. to work with an RD about nutritional issues.

15. What measures do you think the RD will discuss with T.H. to avoid recurrent acute diverticulitis?

T.H. returns for a check-up 14 days later; all S/S of diverticulitis are gone. He is working on his lifestyle changes and reports he is walking 30 min qd (every day). Only 10% to 25% of patients with diverticulitis require any surgery (usually a colectomy). Those who do often suffer recurrent, uncontrollable diverticulitis.

Case Study 3

Name ______________________ Class/Group __________ Date __________

Group Members ____

INSTRUCTIONS: All questions apply to this case study. Your responses should be brief and to the point. Adequate space has been provided for answers. When asked to provide several answers, they should be listed in order of priority or significance. Do not asume information that is not provided. Please print or write clearly. If your response is not legible, it will be marked as ? and you will need to rewrite it.

Scenario

A healthy 14-year-old boy, R.K., is admitted to an outpatient clinic. About 4 hours ago, he was rollerblading and fell while jumping over some obstacles. His left arm was caught under him as he fell. He had a "sharp" pain in the LUQ (left upper quadrant) immediately after the fall. This pain eased off gradually but is returning. His mother brought him to the clinic because he fainted every time he tried to stand up. He C/O (complained of) nausea and has vomited twice. R.K. appears somewhat pale and slightly diaphoretic. He denies being SOB (short of breath) or dizzy when lying down. VS are 104/52 (supine), 92, 24, afebrile.

1. What are R.K.'s key symptoms?

2. What organs lie in the LUQ (left upper quadrant)?

3. What are the assessment priorities? (list in order of priority).

4. The clinic is not equipped to care for R.K. What should they do next?

5. While the clinic nurses are waiting for the transport unit, what interventions would they initiate?

6. R.K. is sent by ambulance to your ED, which is 5 miles away. You are the RN receiving R.K. What do you do first?

7. R.K. does not have SOB, dizziness, or N/V while lying down. Given the circumstances of the accident, what is the significance of this statement?

8. R.K.'s CT (computed tomography) scan reveals a ruptured spleen; he needs immediate surgery. What additional information do you need to obtain before he goes to the OR (operating room)?

9. What is the greatest danger of a splenic rupture?

10. Before surgery, which lab tests should be drawn?

R.K. is taken to OR (surgery) and undergoes an exploratory laparotomy and splenorrhaphy. Estimated blood loss (EBL) is 1600 mL, most of which was infused by means of the Cell Saver.

11. What is a splenorrhaphy, and why should this be done instead of a splenectomy?

12. R.K. is 14 years old, and he heals rapidly. He is discharged on the fifth postoperative day after having his sutures removed. What factors may have favored his wound healing?

Case Study 4

Name ______________________ Class/Group __________ Date __________

Group Members ____

INSTRUCTIONS: All questions apply to this case study. Your responses should be brief and to the point. Adequate space has been provided for answers. When asked to provide several answers, they should be listed in order of priority or significance. Do not asume information that is not provided. Please print or write clearly. If your response is not legible, it will be marked as ? and you will need to rewrite it.

Scenario

T.B., a 60-year-old retiree, is admitted to your unit from the ED (emergency department). Upon arrival you note that he is trembling and nearly doubled over with severe abdominal pain. T.B. indicates that he has severe RUQ (right upper quadrant) pain that radiates to his back, and he is more comfortable walking bent forward than lying in bed. He admits to having had several similar bouts of abdominal pain in the last month but "none as bad as this." He feels only slightly nauseated but has experienced N/V (nausea and vomiting) during previous episodes. T.B. experienced an acute onset after eating fish and chips at a fast-food restaurant. His daughter insisted on taking him to the hospital.

Assessment findings are AAO (awake, alert, oriented) × 3 and MAEW (moves all extremities well). Moves restlessly and continually, C/O of notable fatigue. Breath sounds clear throughout, anterior and posterior. Heart sounds clear without adventitious sounds, heart rate regular, all pulses 3+ bilaterally. Bowel sounds audible, abdominal guarding noted with exquisite tenderness to light palpation over R side, especially RUQ (right upper quadrant). Has sharp inspiratory arrest with palpation of the RUQ. Reports light-colored stools × 1 week. Voids medium amber urine per urinal without difficulty. Skin and sclera slightly jaundiced. Admit VS are 164/100, 132, 26, 36° C.

36°C = 96.8 F

1. What structures are located in the RUQ of the abdomen?

   Gallbladder, pancreas, liver

2. Which of the above mentioned organs are palpable in the RUQ?

   -Liver borders

Abdominal ultrasound demonstrates several retained stones in the common bile duct. T.B. is admitted to your floor and is scheduled for a laparoscopic cholecystectomy with T-tube insertion in the AM. The doctor plans to retrieve stones from the common bile duct during an ERCP (endoscopic retrograde cholangiopancreatography) with sphincterotomy within 24–48 hours of the "lap-chole." The T-tube will be removed after the ERCP.

3. Given T.B.'s diagnosis, what laboratory values would be important to evaluate?

   Bilirubin, amylase, CBC c̄ dif, ~~[illegible]~~ urinalysis, electrolytes, cardio work up, bleeding studies.

4. List four preop preparations that need to be done.

   NPO; pre-op teaching, foley, NG, pain control, pulmonary teaching.

5. T.B. is medicated with morphine 8–10 mg IM q4h for pain. He reports that, on a scale of 1 to 10, his pain has decreased from 10 to 4 in 1 hour. What else could be done for T.B.'s pain?

Δ Positioning
Nausea meds
Patient teaching
PCA pump

6. What data charted in the assessment are consistent with common bile duct obstruction?

RUQ pain with radiation to his back; guarding; jaundice, red amber urine (+) murphy's sign; ↑ VS; steatorrhea

7. At 23:30, T.B. spikes a temperature to 38.6° C (tympanic). A CXR is ordered and he is started on a broad-spectrum antibiotic: imipenem/cilastatin 500 mg IV q6h (check renal function—medication must be dose-adjusted or there is an increased risk for seizure). What, if anything, needs to be done before the antibiotic is begun?

Urine/Sputum culture
Allergies
Check weight

8. T.B. undergoes a laparoscopic-cholecystectomy. Why is a T-tube drain installed during common bile duct surgery?

Allows for bile to pass incision and having stone taken out later.

The first day after surgery, T.B. has a small amount of bloody drainage on the dressing and approximately 500 mL in the drainage bag. When you remove the tape to change the dressing, you note that T.B.'s skin is blistered and reddened.

9. In order to protect the blistered area from further damage, you apply a hydrocolloid dressing, such as DuoDERM, HydraPad, Restore, or Ultec, to the damaged skin. What are the benefits of this type of dressing?

Give you barrier. Keeps bile from damaging skin

10. T.B. recovers uneventfully and will be discharged home. If T.B. had an open cholecystectomy and was being discharged with a T-tube, what would he need to know about this drain?

- Monitor ~~d~~ drainage.
- skin care as needed
- Clamping around meals
- signs of distress.

11. What discharge teaching does T.B. need?

Case Study 5

Name ______________________ Class/Group __________ Date __________

Group Members ____

INSTRUCTIONS: All questions apply to this case study. Your responses should be brief and to the point. Adequate space has been provided for answers. When asked to provide several answers, they should be listed in order of priority or significance. Do not asume information that is not provided. Please print or write clearly. If your response is not legible, it will be marked as ? and you will need to rewrite it.

Scenario

W.T., a 22-year-old white male, presented to the ED (emergency department) complaining of "bad" abdominal pain. The generalized abdominal pain started 24 hours ago but seemed to "ease up" after he vomited. Several hours later the pain returned but had shifted to the RLQ (right lower quadrant) and has remained there. The pain is steadily getting worse. W.T. reports marked nausea and "dry heaves," and he has no appetite. He has also had diarrhea for the last day. VS are 124/76, 92, 16, 38.8° C. W.T. works in a bar, has no health insurance, and his history is positive for tobacco ("1½ packs a day"), ETOH (alcohol) ("six-pack of beer a day"), and marijuana ("couple of hits a day"). He is allergic to PCN (penicillin) ("It makes me itch all over").

1. What organs are located in the RLQ?

2. In what order will the ED nurse examine this patient's abdomen?

3. Next, the patient's abdomen is checked for rebound tenderness. How is this done, and what does it indicate?

You note no masses and localized rebound tenderness in the RLQ. W.T.'s lab work returns: WBC 15.5/mm^3 with a left shift, Hgb 14.6 g/dL, Hct 43.8%, platelets 280,000/mm^3; the UA is unremarkable.

4. One of these lab findings is markedly abnormal and, when combined with the physical findings, is usually indicative of a specific diagnosis. Identify the abnormal lab value, the assessment findings, and probable diagnosis.

W.T. is given ceftriaxone (Rocephin) 1 g IVPB and is sent to the OR for an open exploratory laparotomy for probable acute appendicitis. He undergoes an appendectomy for a purulent but unruptured appendix and is admitted to your unit at 23:30. His VS are stable and his orders include: D_5½NS with 20 mEq KCl/L at 100 mL/h; diet as tolerated; up ad lib; morphine sulfate 8–10 mg q4h prn for pain; when tolerating PO fluid, change pain medication to Tylenol No. 3, 1–2 PO q4h prn for pain; Inapsine ¼ to ½ mL IV/IM q6h prn.

5. Which of the preceding orders need to be clarified before a dose is given? Explain.

6. How will you determine the seriousness of W.T.'s allergic reaction to PCN?

7. What type of reaction is considered an allergic reaction?

8. During the morning report, you are told that W.T. had an uneventful night; his VS are stable, and his IV of D_5½NS at 100 mL/h is infusing on time. He received his second and final dose of prophylactic cefoxitin, and he had no signs of allergic reaction. He will probably be discharged this morning. What questions do you want to ask the night nurse before she leaves?

9. Indeed, W.T. appears stable, and discharge orders are written the afternoon after surgery. What key issues need to be addressed in his discharge teaching?

Many inherent individual factors will affect the scope and direction of patient teaching. Consider W.T.'s background: he works in a bar, and his history is positive for tobacco, ETOH, and marijuana use. These factors should not be ignored. To address them would ensure the best chance of a full recovery.

10. Outline patient teaching on pain that would address these issues.

11. What additional areas for teaching are not addressed in the previous questions?

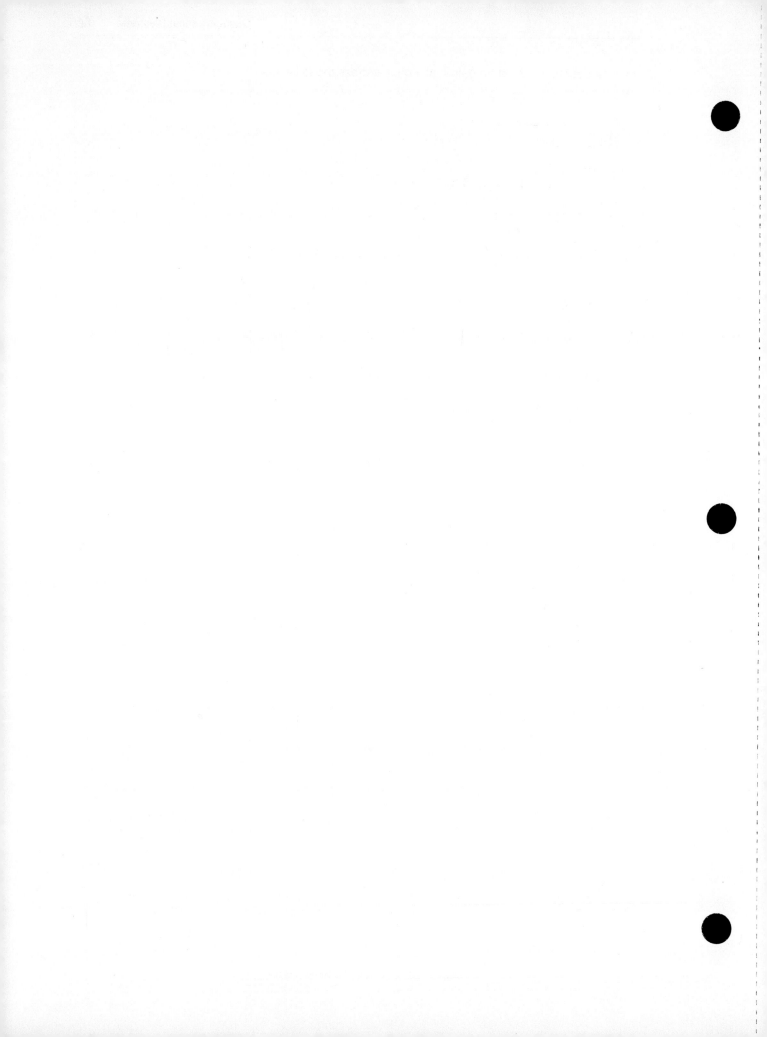

Case Study 6

Name ______________________ Class/Group __________ Date __________

Group Members ____

INSTRUCTIONS: All questions apply to this case study. Your responses should be brief and to the point. Adequate space has been provided for answers. When asked to provide several answers, they should be listed in order of priority or significance. Do not asume information that is not provided. Please print or write clearly. If your response is not legible, it will be marked as ? and you will need to rewrite it.

Scenario

J.S., a 57-year-old salesman, has come to his practitioner's office with a moderate amount of chest pain. He says this pain comes and goes and is worst at night, when it wakes him up. He looks haggard, with dark circles under his eyes, stating "I've got to get more sleep than this."

1. What are some common causes of "chest pain"?

2. What will you ask J.S. to better evaluate his pain?

3. J.S. says the pain has been waking him up for 3 months. What would you want to know about J.S.'s lifestyle?

J.S. indicates that he has tried taking antacids and some other medicine he bought at the drug store just in case the pain was due to ulcers, but he gets no relief. He tried some sleeping pills, but he just woke up groggy with a headache in addition to the chest pain.

4. What tests will be done to help determine the source of the problem?

5. A barium swallow confirms a large sliding esophageal hiatal hernia. J.S. asks, "What is a hiatal hernia, and what do you mean it's sliding?" How would you explain this to him?

6. J.S. asks, "Is heartburn always caused by a hiatal hernia?" How would you respond?

7. J.S. would rather try more conservative medical treatment before having surgery. What measures can he try to minimize his pain? List at least five.

J.S. writes down all your instructions and is determined to conquer his problem without surgery.

8. What medications are most likely to be prescribed for J.S.? What will he need to know about them?

Two months later J.S. reappears at your office, looking even worse than before. “I just can’t keep the pain controlled, especially when I’m on the road.”

9. After discussion, J.S. agrees on a date to have his hiatal hernia repaired. As he does this, he looks doubtful but desperate. What do you want to ask him right now?

10. J.S. wants to know how the minilaparotomy (minilap) surgery is different from the larger laparotomy surgery. Using a picture you explain the following:

11. J.S. is to have a minilaparotomy. What preoperative teaching will he need?

J.S. went to surgery for an NFP by means of a minilaparoscopy. The surgery was successful, and J.S. went home on the second postoperative day. Two months later he stops back in when he comes in for an appointment with his surgeon. He has had complete relief of his gastric reflux and can sleep flat at night without waking up.

Case Study 7

Name ____________________ Class/Group __________ Date __________

Group Members ____

INSTRUCTIONS: All questions apply to this case study. Your responses should be brief and to the point. Adequate space has been provided for answers. When asked to provide several answers, they should be listed in order of priority or significance. Do not asume information that is not provided. Please print or write clearly. If your response is not legible, it will be marked as ? and you will need to rewrite it.

Scenario

While you are working as a nurse on a GI/GU floor, you receive a call from your affiliate outpatient clinic notifying you of a direct admission, ETA (estimated time of arrival) 60 minutes. She gives you the following information: A.G. is an 87-year-old woman with a 3-day history of intermittent abdominal pain, abdominal bloating, and N/V. A.G. moved from Italy to join her grandson and his family only 2 months ago and she speaks very little English. All information was obtained through her grandson. PMH: colectomy for colon cancer 6 years ago, ventral hernia repair 2 years ago. No Hx of CAD, DM, or pulmonary disease. She takes only ibuprofen occasionally for mild arthritis. Allergies include sulfa drugs and meperidine. A.G.'s tentative diagnosis is small bowel obstruction (SBO) secondary to adhesions. A.G. is being admitted to your floor for diagnostic work-up. Her VS are stable, she has an IV of D_5½NS with 20 mEq KCl at 100 mL/h, and 3 L O_2/NC.

1. Based on the nurse's report, what signs of bowel obstruction did A.G. present?

2. Are there other S/S that you should observe for while A.G. is in your care?

3. A.G. and her grandson arrive on your unit. You admit A.G. to her room and introduce yourself as her nurse. As her grandson interprets for her, she pats your hand. You know that you need to complete a physical examination and take a history. What will you do first?

4. The grandson, an attorney, tells you elderly Italian women are extremely modest and may not answer questions completely. How might you gather information in this case?

5. What key questions must you ask this patient while you have the use of an interpreter?

6. How would the description of A.G.'s pain differ if she has a small versus large bowel obstruction?

7. With some difficulty, you insert an NGT into A.G. and connect it to intermittent LWS (low wall suction). How will you check for placement of the NGT?

8. List, in order, the structures through which the NGT must pass as it is inserted.

9. What comfort measures are important for A.G. while she has an NGT?

10. You note that A.G.'s NGT has not drained in the last 3 hours. What can you do to facilitate drainage?

11. The NGT suddenly drains 575 mL; then it slows down to about 250 mL over 2 hours. Is this an expected amount?

12. You enter A.G.'s room to initiate your shift assessment. A.G. has been hospitalized 3 days and her abdomen seems to be more distended than yesterday. How would you determine whether A.G.'s abdominal distention has changed?

After 3 days of NGT suction, A.G.'s symptoms are unrelieved. She reports continued nausea, cramps, and sometimes very strong abdominal pain; her hand grips are weaker; and she seems to be increasingly lethargic. You look up her latest laboratory values and compare them with the admission data. Her Na has changed from 136 to 130 mmol/L, K has changed from 3.7 to 2.5 mmol/L, Cl from 108 to 97 mmol/L, CO_2 25 to 31 mmol/L, BUN (blood urea nitrogen) from 19 to 38 mg/dL, creatinine from 1 to 2.2 mg/dL, glucose from 126 to 65 mg/dL, albumin from 3.0 to 2.1 g/dL, and protein from 6.8 to 4.9 g/dL.

13. Which lab values are of concern to you? Why?

14. What measures do you anticipate to correct each of the imbalances described in Question 13?

In view of A.G.'s continued slow deterioration, the surgeon meets with the patient and her family and they agree to surgery. The surgeon releases an 18-inch section of proximal ileum that has been constricted by adhesions. Several areas looked ischemic, so these were excised, and an end- to-end anastomosis was done. A.G. tolerated the procedure well and recovered rapidly from the anesthesia in the PACU (postanesthesia care unit). Once on the unit, her recovery was slow but steady. A.G. went home in the care of her grandson and his wife on the seventh postoperative day. Discharge plans included walking several times per day in the house; importance of C&DB (cough and deep breathing) and use of the IS (incentive spirometer) q2h; and observing the wound for S/S of infection.

In reviewing the beginning of this case, it is clear that A.G.'s nutritional status had been poor. It would be appropriate for her to have medical nutrition therapy regarding long-term nutrient needs. Be sure the grandson is included in any plans.

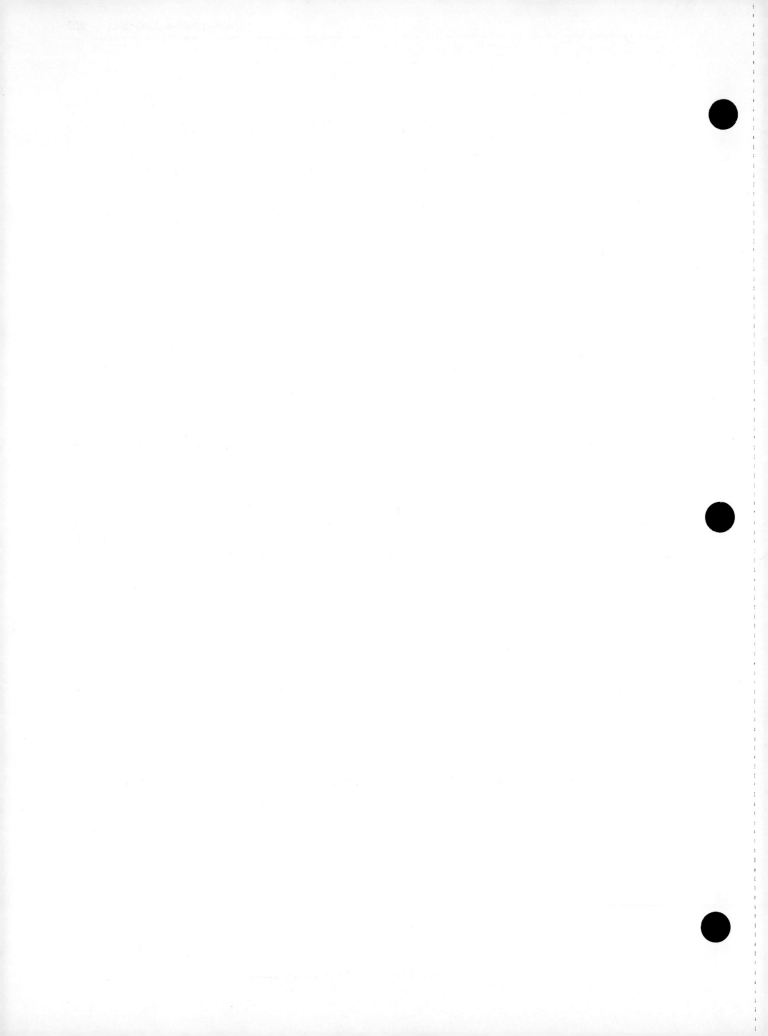

Case Study 8

Name ______________________ Class/Group __________ Date __________

Group Members ____

INSTRUCTIONS: All questions apply to this case study. Your responses should be brief and to the point. Adequate space has been provided for answers. When asked to provide several answers, they should be listed in order of priority or significance. Do not asume information that is not provided. Please print or write clearly. If your response is not legible, it will be marked as ? and you will need to rewrite it.

Scenario

P.M., a 24-year-old house painter, has been too ill to work for the last 3 days. When he arrives at your outpatient clinic, he seems an alert but acutely ill young man of average build, with a deep tan over exposed areas of skin. He reports headaches, severe myalgia, a low-grade fever, cough, anorexia, and N/V, especially after eating any fatty food. P.M. describes vague abdominal pain that started about the same time as the other problems. PMH: no health problems, nonsmoker, drinks a "few" beers each evening to relax. Assessment: VS are 128/84, 88, 26, 38.1° C; AAO × 3, MAEW except for aching pain in his muscles; very slight scleral jaundice present; heart tones clear and without adventitious sounds; breath sounds clear throughout A&P; abdomen soft and palpable without distinct masses. You note moderate hepatomegaly; liver edge is easily palpated and tender to palpation. P.M. mentions that his urine has been getting darker over the last 2 days.

P.M. is presenting with the key signs of hepatitis. Lab work is sent for identification of his precise problem. Results: Na 140 mmol/L, K 3.9 mmol/L, Cl 102 mmol/L, CO_2 26 mmol/L, BUN 10 mg/dL, creatinine 1.0 mg/dL, platelets 86/mm^3, direct bilirubin 1.6 mg/dL, total bilirubin 2.3 mg/dL, albumin 3.8 g/dL, total protein 6.2 g/dL, ALT (SGPT) 66 U/L, AST (SGOT) 52 U/L, LDH 205 U/L, ALP 176 U/L, PT 12 s, INR 1.06, PTT 32 s. Urine urobilinogen 1.6 EU/L, albuminuria 160 mg/dL, + bilirubinuria, + for anti-HAV (hepatitis A virus) IgM.

1. Which key diagnostic tests will determine exactly what type of hepatitis is present?

2. A CBC, BMP, LFT (liver function test), PT/PTT was drawn. Which of the lab values listed above specifically indicates liver disease?

3. List three drugs that can cause increased ALT levels.

4. Considering that the basic pathology of hepatitis involves inflammation, degeneration, and regeneration of the hepatocyte, what type of diet will you strongly encourage P.M. to follow?

5. Differentiate between hepatitis A, B, and C on the basis of the mode of transmission and prevention.

6. Name three major activities that can be done in a community to prevent the spread of hepatitis (all types).

7. In P.M.'s case, the IgM class anti-HAV antibody is positive. This result indicates that P.M. is infected with hepatitis A and is in the acute or early convalescent period of the disease. Is this disease contagious? What precaution would you take?

8. Pruritus is usually associated with jaundice. What will you do to ease this problem for P.M.?

9. How would you explain to P.M. the likely progression of his disease? (This approach requires not only knowledge of disease and its progression but an ability to figure out P.M.'s thought processes.)

10. P.M. is living at home with his parents and four younger siblings. The youngest is a 4-year-old. His parents ask how to prevent the rest of the family from getting hepatitis. What specific instructions will you give? How will you know that these instructions are understood?

11. Given P.M.'s lifestyle, what specific patient teaching points must you emphasize?

Case Study 9

Name ______________________________ Class/Group __________ Date __________

Group Members ____

INSTRUCTIONS: All questions apply to this case study. Your responses should be brief and to the point. Adequate space has been provided for answers. When asked to provide several answers, they should be listed in order of priority or significance. Do not asume information that is not provided. Please print or write clearly. If your response is not legible, it will be marked as ? and you will need to rewrite it.

Scenario

John Doe #6, approximately 50 years old, is admitted to your floor from the ED. He is lethargic, has a cachectic appearance, does not follow commands consistently, and is mildly combative when aroused. He smells strongly of alcohol and has a notably swollen abdomen and lower extremities. This man was sent to the ED by local police who found him lying unresponsive along a rural road. He was aroused somewhat in the ED. Examination and x-rays are negative for any injury, and he is admitted to your unit for observation. He has no ID and is not awake or coherent enough to give any history or to answer questions. Admitting orders are: admit to E3 with R/O hepatic encephalopathy with ETOH intoxication; IV D_5½NS with 20 mEq KCl at 75 mL/h; add 1 amp MVI (multivitamins) to 1 L of IVF/d (IV fluid/day); NTG to LWS (low wall suction); Foley catheter to DD (down drain); HOB at 30 to 45 degrees at all times; lactulose 45 mL PO qid until three soft stools; abdominal ultrasound in AM; CBC with diff, BMP, LFT, PT/PTT, NH_3 now and in AM; soft restraints prn; vitamin K 10 mg IV or PO qd × three doses; thiamine 100 mg IM qd; folic acid 5 mg IM qd; pyridoxine 100 mg PO qd; once patient is able to take PO – low-protein diet, eat with assistance only; call HO for any sign of GI bleed, DTs, or SBP >140 or <100, DBP <50, P >120.

1. Which of the preceding orders must be done by the RN? By the aide? By the clerk?

2. The lab work drawn in the ED has come back. The blood alcohol level (BAL) is 320 mg/dL, and the blood ammonia (NH_3) level is 155 μg/dL. What do these values indicate?

While you are getting John Doe #6 settled, you continue your assessment. Neuro: PERRL, MAE sluggishly pulling away during assessment, follows commands sporadically. CV: P regular but tachycardic without adventitious sounds. All peripheral pulses palpable and 3+ bilat, 3+ pitting edema in lower extremities. IV of D_5½NS with one amp MVI and 20 mEq KCl/L at 75 mL/h in L forearm. Resp: breath sounds decreased to all lobes, no adventitious sounds audible, patient does not cooperate with C&DB, on RA (room air) with Sao_2 at 90%. GI: tongue and gums are beefy red and swollen, abdomen enlarged and protuberant, girth is 141 cm (64 in), abdominal skin is taut and slightly tender to palpation. NTG patent, BS positive with NTG clamped. GU: Foley to DD with 75 mL dark amber urine since admission (2 h). Skin: pale torso and LEs (lower extremities), heavily sunburned to UEs (upper extremities) and head. Skin appears thin and dry. Numerous spider angiomas on upper abdomen with several dilated veins across abdomen. VS are 120/60, 104, 32, 37.3° C. His protein is 5.2 g/dL, and albumin is 2.1 g/dL. A toxicology screen and electrolytes have been drawn.

3. What is the significance of the spider angiomas, dilated abdominal veins, peripheral edema, and distended abdomen?

4. How would you further assess the distended abdomen, and what is the clinical name for your findings?

5. What is your concern about John Doe's nutritional status? What are your objective findings?

6. Why isn't John Doe on a high-protein diet?

7. How might you respond to fellow staff nurses' remarks, "Why are we wasting time with this 'wino'? He isn't worth the time or money. Why don't they let him die?"

8. A nursing problem relative to John Doe's care is "risk for injury." Ensuring safety is a critical part of the nursing role. Consider at least three areas of injury risk, and identify actions you will take to ensure his safety.

9. What are the S/S of delirium tremens (DTs)?

10. Falls are particularly dangerous for someone in this patient's situation. Why?

John Doe #6 survives a rocky course of hepatic encephalopathy and near-renal failure. After 27 days, including a week in the ICU, he is discharged to a drug and alcohol rehabilitation facility. He is employed as a longshoreman; fortunately, his insurance covers his month of in-house intense rehabilitation.

Case Study 10

Name ______________________ Class/Group __________ Date __________

Group Members ____

INSTRUCTIONS: All questions apply to this case study. Your responses should be brief and to the point. Adequate space has been provided for answers. When asked to provide several answers, they should be listed in order of priority or significance. Do not asume information that is not provided. Please print or write clearly. If your response is not legible, it will be marked as ? and you will need to rewrite it.

Scenario

J.D., with 2 years of sobriety behind him, has been promoted from longshoreman to nightshift foreman in a warehouse. He has new hope and new friends in his AA groups. Unfortunately, his cirrhotic liver has not recovered from 20 years of heavy drinking, and he still has residual effects. During the past 2 days he has had a "bad cough." This morning he coughed up bright red blood (BRB) and came into the ED. His coughing and bleeding have subsided for now. An IV of D_5½NS with 20 KCl/L at 100 mL/h is started and baseline lab samples are drawn. He is sent to the floor for observation. Shortly after you admit J.D., you hear coughing while passing his room. You enter and see BRB all over his gown and bed. He looks very frightened.

1. What needs to be done at once?

2. What specific tasks must be done?

3. What do you think J.D.'s emotional state is? How would his body respond to this emotion?

4. Recognizing his emotional state, what can you do to intervene?

5. What treatment options exist for esophageal varices? List in the order in which they are most likely to be tried.

6. The gastroenterologist comes to the unit to perform an endoscopic exam. How will you prepare J.D. for this?

7. The gastroenterologist performs the fiberoptic endoscopic examination. Neither cauterization nor sclerotherapy is successful for more than a few minutes and J.D.'s bleeding intensifies. The physician elects to use balloon tamponade to hold pressure on the varices until J.D. can more safely undergo surgery. What key rule will you observe with this tube?

8. What is the major complication of balloon tamponade, and how can you help prevent this?

9. J.D. looks at you and asks, "Am I going to die?" You know that the operative mortality rate is 5% to 15% in elective cases and 50% in emergency cases. Even the survivors have a curtailed lifespan because of an increased rate of hepatic encephalopathy and liver failure. How would you respond?

10. What is shunt surgery and why is it done?

11. J.D.'s current H&H is 8.6/26. He is to receive 2 U PRBCs and 2 U of salt-poor albumin (SPA). How will you know if J.D. is having any negative reactions to the transfusion, and what would you do to intervene?

12. How much will you expect the hematocrit to rise after the transfusion of 2 U of PRBCs?

The blood has infused without evidence of reaction, and his VS are stable. J.D. talked to the hospital chaplain at length and then was sent to OR for a portacaval shunt. He will be transferred to ICU afterward for recovery.

Case Study 11

Name ______________________ Class/Group ____________ Date ____________

Group Members ____

INSTRUCTIONS: All questions apply to this case study. Your responses should be brief and to the point. Adequate space has been provided for answers. When asked to provide several answers, they should be listed in order of priority or significance. Do not asume information that is not provided. Please print or write clearly. If your response is not legible, it will be marked as ? and you will need to rewrite it.

Scenario

C.W., a 36-year-old woman, was admitted several days ago with a diagnosis of recurrent inflammatory bowel disease (IBD) and possible SBO (small bowel obstruction). C.W. is married, and her husband and 11-year-old son are very supportive, but she has no extended family in-state. She has had IBD for 15 years and has been on mesalamine (Asacol) for 15 years and prednisone 40 mg qd for the last 5 years. She is very thin; at 5′2″ she weighs 86 lb and has lost 40 lb over the last 10 years. She has an average of five to ten loose stools per day. C.W.'s life has gradually become dominated by her disease (anorexia; lactase deficiency; profound fatigue; frequent nausea and diarrhea; frequent hospitalizations for dehydration; and recurring, crippling abdominal pain that often strikes unexpectedly). The pain is incapacitating and relieved only by a small dose of diazepam (Valium), Pedialyte, and total bed rest. She confides in you that sexual activity is difficult, "It always causes diarrhea, nausea, and lots of pain. It's difficult for both of us." She is so weak she cannot stand without help. You write CBR (complete bed rest) with side rails up on the Kardex. (You also make a mental note of the probability that she has osteoporosis secondary to long-term steroid use.)

1. Identify six priority problems for C.W.

2. You enter C.W.'s room and note that she has been crying. You ask what's wrong, and she explains that the nurse who admitted her to the hospital the last time said, "Welcome to death row!" C.W. says that she is knowledgeable about her condition, but she still can't seem to shake that "death row" feeling. She was afraid to come to the hospital this time. What can you do to help this woman?

C.W. replies, "Treat me with respect, and as a person, not a disease. Act like I have the right and intelligence to understand my condition. Recognize that I probably know what I'm talking about when I try to refuse a delicious milkshake. When I'm either NPO or nauseated, please don't pop popcorn where I can smell it! It's pure torture!"

3. Considering C.W.'s weakness, chronic diarrhea, and lower-than-desired body weight, what interventions should minimize skin breakdown?

C.W.'s condition deteriorates on the third day postadmission; she experiences intractable abdominal pain and unrelenting N/V. C.W. is taken to the OR for probable SBO and is readmitted to your unit from the postanesthesia care unit (PACU). During surgery, 38 inches of her small bowel were found to be severely stenosed with two areas of visible perforation. Much of the remaining bowel is severely inflamed and friable. A total of 5 feet of distal ileum and 2 feet of colon have been removed and a temporary ileostomy was established. She has a Jackson-Pratt (JP) drain to bulb suction in her RLQ and her wound was packed and left open. She has two peripheral IVs, an NGT, and a Foley. Her VS are 112/72, 86, 24, 38.2° C (tympanic).

4. You begin a thorough postoperative assessment of C.W.'s abdomen. What does your assessment include? List these steps in the order in which the assessment should be completed.

5. A nursing student enters C.W.'s room and auscultates her abdomen. She looks at you and excitedly announces that she hears good bowel sounds. You take the opportunity to teach her the proper method of auscultating bowel sounds on a patient who has NGT to continuous LWS. How would you correct her error?

The nursing student follows your advice and listens again. She says "You're right, I didn't hear a thing." You tell her that she can impress her classmates while educating them in the correct technique.

6. C.W. is 4 days postop. During the routine dressing change, you note a small pool of yellow-green drainage in the deepest part of the wound. You realize the physician will want a wound culture. How will you culture C.W.'s wound?

7. You obtain a wound culture, complete the dressing change, obtain a full set of VS, and note a temp of 38.1° C, and assess increased tenderness in C.W.'s abdomen. You call to notify the physician and ask for additional orders. What orders do you anticipate?

8. What information do you need to send to the lab with the wound culture specimen?

9. The physician calls back and asks you to describe C.W.'s wound. What key aspects of the wound should be included?

10. The physician asks you how C.W.'s stoma and drainage look. What should a healthy stoma and usual drainage look like?

11. Will any aspect of C.W.'s history significantly affect the wound healing process? How?

12. With a fairly significant wound infection developing, why is C.W.'s temperature relatively low?

13. The physician tells you that she will be over to examine C.W. As you tell C.W. that her doctor is coming to talk to her, C.W. says that she feels something wet running down her side. You find some leakage of intestinal drainage onto the skin. What should you do?

You change the ileostomy appliance before the physician arrives. C.W. is evaluated, and it is determined that she should return to surgery for exploratory laparotomy.

Case Study 12

Name ______________________ Class/Group __________ Date __________

Group Members ____

INSTRUCTIONS: All questions apply to this case study. Your responses should be brief and to the point. Adequate space has been provided for answers. When asked to provide several answers, they should be listed in order of priority or significance. Do not asume information that is not provided. Please print or write clearly. If your response is not legible, it will be marked as ? and you will need to rewrite it.

Scenario (Continuation of Case Study 11)

C.W. is a 36-year-old woman admitted 7 days ago for IBD with SBO. She underwent surgery 3 days postadmission for a colectomy and ileostomy. She developed peritonitis and 4 days later returned to the OR for an exploratory laparotomy, which revealed another area of perforated bowel, generalized peritonitis, and a fistula tract to the abdominal surface. Another 12 inches of ileum were resected (total of 7 feet of ileum and 2 feet of colon). The peritoneal cavity was irrigated with NS, and three drainage tubes were placed: a JP drain to bulb suction, a rubber catheter to irrigate the wound bed with NS, and a sump drain to remove the irrigation. The initial JP drain remains in place. A R subclavian triple lumen catheter was inserted.

1. C.W. returns from PACU on your shift. What do you do when her bed is rolled into her room?

2. You pull the covers back to inspect the abdominal dressing and find that the original surgical dressing is saturated with fresh bloody drainage. What should you do?

3. C.W. has a total of four tubes in her abdomen as well as an NGT. What information do you want to know about each tube?

Note: For safety, all tubes should be clearly labeled.

4. The sump irrigation fluid bag is nearly empty. You close the roller clamp, thread the IV tubing through the infusion pump, check the irrigation catheter connection site to make sure it is snug, and then discover that the nearly empty liter bag infusing into C.W.'s abdomen is D_5W, not NS. Does this require any action? If so, give rationale for actions, and explain the overall situation.

The physician arrives on the unit and removes C.W.'s surgical dressing. There is a small "bleeder" at the edge of the incision, so the physician calls for a suture and ties off the bleeder. You take the opportunity to ask her about a morphine PCA pump for C.W., and the physician says she will write the orders right away.

5. Postoperative pain will be a problem for C.W. after the anesthesia wears off. How do you plan to address this?

6. Pharmacy delivers C.W.'s first bag of TPN. The physician has instructed you to start the TPN at a rate of 60 mL/h and decrease the maintenance IV rate by the same amount. What is the purpose of this order?

7. The physician did not specifically order glucose monitoring, but you know that it should be initiated. You plan to conduct a finger stick blood test q2h for the first several hours. What is your rationale?

8. C.W.'s blood glucose increased temporarily, but by the next day it dropped to an average of 70 to 80 mg/dL and has remained there for 2 days. Her VS are stable, but her abdominal wound shows no signs of healing. She has lost 1 kg over the last 3 days. What do these data mean?

You discuss your concerns with C.W.'s physician, and she agrees to request a consult from an RD. After gathering data and making several calculations, the RD makes recommendations to the attending physician. The TPN orders are adjusted, C.W. begins to gain weight slowly, and her wound shows signs of healing. Nutritional problems in clinical populations can be complex and often require special attention.

9. You and a coworker read the following in C.W.'s progress notes: "Wound healing by secondary closure. Formation of granular tissue with epithelialization noted around edges. Have requested dietitian to consult on ongoing basis. Will continue to follow." Your coworker turns to you and asks whether you know what that means. How would you explain?

10. Both of you start to discuss what specific digestive difficulties C.W. is likely to face in the future. What problems might C.W. be prone to develop after having so much of her bowel removed?

11. The RD consults with C.W. about dietary needs. You attend the session so that you will be able to reinforce the information. What basic information is the dietitian likely to discuss with C.W.?

12. After 3 days of dressing changes, C.W.'s skin is quite irritated, and a small skin tear has appeared where tape was removed. How can you minimize this type of skin breakdown and help this area heal?

13. What specifics of ostomy teaching do you plan to do?

C.W. successfully battled peritonitis. Gradually, tubes were removed as she grew stronger with TPN and time. C.W. learned how to change her ostomy appliance and was discharged home.

Case Study 13

Name ______________________ Class/Group __________ Date __________

Group Members ______________________________________

INSTRUCTIONS: All questions apply to this case study. Your responses should be brief and to the point. Adequate space has been provided for answers. When asked to provide several answers, they should be listed in order of priority or significance. Do not asume information that is not provided. Please print or write clearly. If your response is not legible, it will be marked as ? and you will need to rewrite it.

Scenario

B.B., a 72-year-old woman, is admitted from the ED with C/O constant, severe abdominal and lower back pain for 2 days and SOB over the last 24 hours. "I've had to rest four or five times gettin' back to the house from the shed. It's gotten real hard to manage all by myself." A niece stopped by and insisted B.B. come into the county hospital ED. B.B. has never received any medical care of any kind. She lives by herself "up the mountain" off of a dirt road in rural Pennsylvania. She is restless, nauseated, and in pain. Everything around her in the hospital is new and frightening to her. VS are 108/72, 128, 30, 37.9° C (tympanic), Sao_2 84% on 2 L O_2/NC. B.B. is admitted to your unit at 19:00.

1. What possible diagnoses would you suspect with a presentation of severe abdominal pain?

2. The ED nurse giving you the report says that B.B.'s admitting diagnosis is R/O pancreatitis. You know that pain control is difficult in patients with pancreatitis. What information will you want to ask the ED nurse before hanging up?

3. B.B. arrives on your unit. As she is getting into bed, you notice that her eyes are very wide and she is looking all around. She seems totally overwhelmed in response to the ED nurse's instructions about how to operate the bed. What parts of her background information may be used to guide the manner in which you approach B.B.?

4. What approach would you use to obtain a psychosocial history and complete your assessment?

You complete an assessment and note the following abnormalities: restless, prefers to sit on side of bed, leaning forward and tightly clutching her handbag. States pain has decreased "some after that lady jabbed me with that needle downstairs." Skin is cool, diaphoretic, and pale. Heart rate irregular and tachy. Peripheral pulses weakly palpable x 4 extremities. Resp rapid but unlabored on 2 L O_2/NC, Sao_2 85%, breath sounds absent at the base of the LLL (left lower lobe) posteriorly. Reports marked nausea without emesis. BS hypoactive x four quads. Abdomen distended and exquisitely tender throughout to light palpation, guarding noted. Has not voided but states that she has "made less water than usual." Poor skin turgor, dry mucous membranes, mild scleral jaundice.

5. How are you going to assess B.B.'s pain?

B.B.'s admission labs return: Na 148 mmol/L, WBC 17,200/cmm, amylase 200 U/L, K 4.2 mmol/L, Hgb 12.5 g/dL, Hct 38%, lipase 375 U/L, Cl 114 mmol/L, LDH 160 U/L, HCO_3 98 mmol/L, platelets 306/mm^3, AST 54 U/L, BUN 26 mg/d, ALT 46 U/L, creatinine 1.0 mg/dL, ALP 96 U/L, glucose 185 mg/dL. You make a mental note that calcium is missing from the list and an order for a calcium level should be obtained.

6. Which lab values are important in the diagnosis of pancreatitis?

7. Review the CBC and BMP results. What results are consistent with your observations on her physical exam?

8. B.B. voids 150 mL dark brown urine 2 hours after admission to your unit. What will you do?

9. The physician orders a 500-mL bolus of NS and Foley to down drain. What do these orders mean, and why are they appropriate at this time? What priority assessment must be done when a fluid bolus is given?

You deliver the NS bolus over an hour and insert a Foley catheter. You are surprised that the color of B.B.'s urine is dark amber, instead of the dark brown urine that you saw in the commode. You send a specimen to the lab.

10. The next time you answer B.B.'s call light, she states that her pain is, "Getting bad again." You are puzzled because she is not used to taking narcotics and it has been only 2 hours since her last injection of morphine 5 mg. What can be done to improve her pain management?

NSAIDs are added to the pain regimen. You administer the first dose and notice that her bedpan is under the covers and it contains the same dark brown fluid that you noted in the commode. You ask B.B. about it and she states, "Aw honey, that's just my chewing tobacco." She spits, and the dark fluid lands in the pan.

11. Is there any connection between heavy tobacco use and the effectiveness of medications?

12. Based on your discovery, what action would you take?

13. B.B.'s oximeter alarms at 83% saturated, her respiratory rate is 34, and the IV bolus has infused. You auscultate no breath sounds from the scapula down on the L. You percuss B.B.'s lung posteriorly and hear a dull thud up to the scapula on the L and percuss resonant on the R. What is the significance of your findings?

14. What two actions would you take next and why?

The physician orders a stat CXR, which shows a significant pleural effusion developing over the LLL.

15. Based on the diagnosis of pleural effusion, what treatment will the physician likely perform next, and what is your responsibility throughout the treatment?

Patients with subdiaphragmatic inflammatory processes frequently present with pneumonia or pleural effusion. Cloudy, yellow fluid (250 mL) was removed. B.B. was placed on broad-spectrum antibiotics until the cultures returned. She was found to have acute pancreatitis and was eventually released to return home. As she is wheeled out of the hospital, B.B. tells you, “I'll die up on my mountain before I'll come back here.” She probably did.

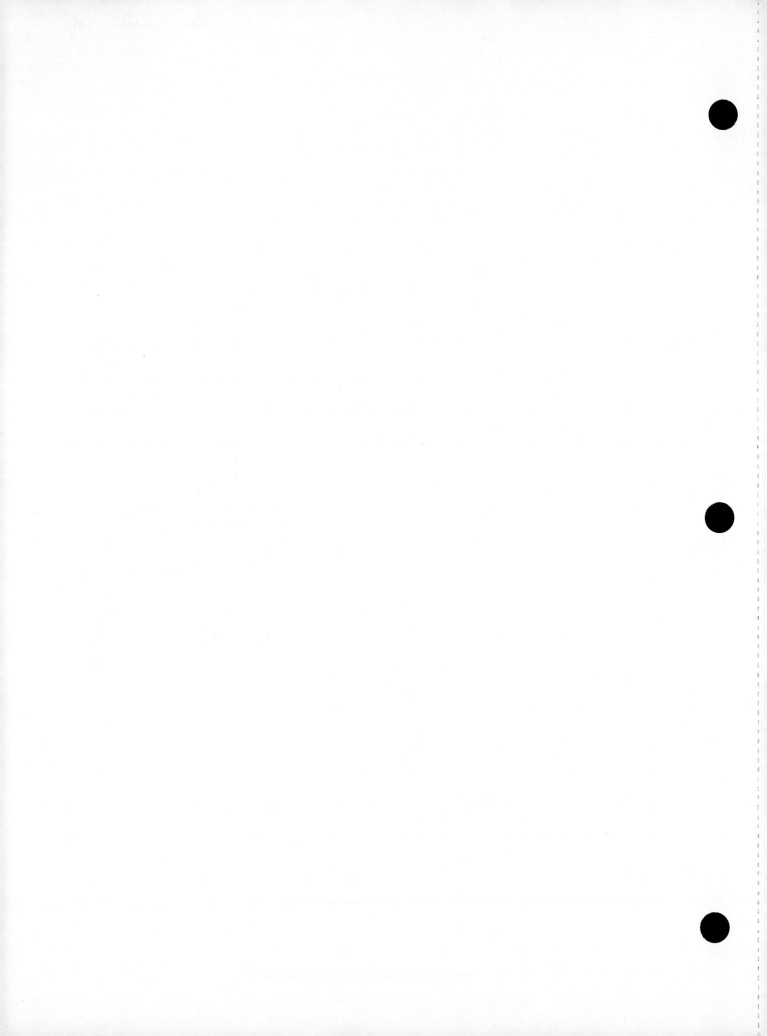

Case Study 14

Name ______________________________ Class/Group __________ Date __________

Group Members ____

INSTRUCTIONS: All questions apply to this case study. Your responses should be brief and to the point. Adequate space has been provided for answers. When asked to provide several answers, they should be listed in order of priority or significance. Do not asume information that is not provided. Please print or write clearly. If your response is not legible, it will be marked as ? and you will need to rewrite it.

Scenario

You are a nurse working on a surgical unit and take the following report from the RN in the ED. "We are sending you a direct admit with R/O SBO (small bowel obstruction) and/or food blockage. Dr. N. the GI (gastrointestinal) doctor is on his way in to see the patient. D.S. is a 78-year-old obese male, C/O sudden onset of severe abdominal cramping, distention, N/V and denies passing of flatus or stool within the last 12 hours. PMH includes CHF, HTN, colon cancer, ulcerative colitis. He underwent a total colectomy 16 years ago, and had an enterocutaneous fistula 12 years ago. Lab samples have been drawn and the results will be sent to your floor. We started an IV and placed an NGT. His VS are 143/76, 82, R 26 and slightly labored, and T 101.2° F. He is on his way up."

1. Given that D.S. had a total colectomy, you know he has an ileostomy. What is the difference between a colostomy and ileostomy, where would the stoma be located, and what type of drainage should you expect from each?

D.S. is brought to the floor. He is quite agitated and complaining of severe abdominal cramping, pain, and nausea.

2. What are two priority issues that need to be addressed immediately?

After D.S. is settled into his room, the NGT and IV are functioning well, and he has received pain medication, you begin your admission assessment. His abdomen in extremely large, firm to touch, with multiple scars and an ileostomy pouching system in his RLQ.

3. What are the more common complications of an ileostomy?

4. How would you determine if the stoma is healthy?

5. What stoma changes would you report to the doctor immediately?

6. Why are transparent ostomy pouches recommended postop or when patients are hospitalized?

7. Will the stoma present visual clues of blockage/obstruction?

8. Why is a peristomal hernia a problem?

D.S. continues to C/O abdominal pain and cramping and becomes increasingly restless. You notice that the abdomen behind/around his stoma and pouch appears larger when compared to the other side of his abdomen.

9. How would you assess for a possible hernia?

You note that the ostomy pouch has liquid brown effluent along the lateral edge of the wafer. You check to see that the pouch is properly attached to the barrier and discover that stool is indeed leaking from under the barrier. D.S. apologizes for not bringing any supplies with him, stating “my ostomy nurse told me to always carry extra supplies for times like this.”

D.S. does not remember what size he needs, but you note he is wearing a two-piece system with a plastic ring/flange that attaches somewhat like a Tupperwear seal.

10. How will you determine the correct pouching size and system?

You have finished with your general head- to-toe assessment and order the appropriate pouching products for D.S. You have already taken clean towels, washcloths, and chucks into his room, along with a hamper to receive dirty/used laundry. You gather scissors, skin-prep, and adhesive remover to assist with the pouching change.

11. As you return to his room you review the steps for changing an ostomy pouch. What are the three steps you need to remember?

You have gathered all needed supplies and D.S. is as comfortable as possible. You begin the pouching change. Using the adhesive remover, with the push-pull method, you gently remove the wafer/barrier. As you lift the wafer, you note that the peristomal skin has severe erythema directly encircling the stoma. There is denudation (partial-thickness breakdown) at the medial stoma-skin edge.

12. How should the skin around the stoma look?

13. Generally there are four different causes of erythema or skin breakdown. Identify two.

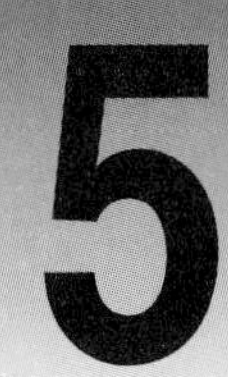

Genitourinary Disorders

Case Study 1

Name ______________________ Class/Group __________ Date __________

Group Members ____

INSTRUCTIONS: All questions apply to this case study. Your responses should be brief and to the point. Adequate space has been provided for answers. When asked to provide several answers, they should be listed in order of priority or significance. Do not asume information that is not provided. Please print or write clearly. If your response is not legible, it will be marked as ? and you will need to rewrite it.

Scenario

You are working in an ECF (extended-care facility) when M.Z.'s daughter brings her mother in for a week stay while she goes on vacation. M.Z. is an 89-year-old widow with a 4-day Hx of dysuria, back pain, incontinency, severe mental confusion, and loose stools. Her MD had recently discontinued her HRT (hormone replacement therapy) 1 month ago. Her most current VS are 118/60, 88, 18, 99.4° F. The medical director ordered several lab tests on admission. The results were as follows: WBC 11/cmm, CMP (complete metabolic profile) WNL (within normal limits). Postvoiding catheterization yielded 100 mL and UA showed WBC 100+/HPF (high powered field), RBC 3–6, bacteria rare. The urinary C&S (culture and sensitivity) results were as follows: *E. coli* (*Escherichia coli*) > 100,000 colonies, sensitive to ciprofloxacin, trimethoprim/sulfamethoxazole, nitrofurantoin.

1. The medical director makes rounds and writes to start an IV of D_5.25NS @ 75mL/h and insert a Foley to DD (down drain). Because M.Z. is unable to take oral meds, the MD ordered ciprofloxacin 200 mg bid IVPB (intravenous piggy back). Is the type of fluid and rate appropriate for M.Z.'s age and condition? Explain.

2. What S/S will you look for in a patient receiving IV ciprofloxacin?

3. You enter the room to start the IV and insert the Foley catheter but find the aide has taken the patient to the bathroom for a BM. You open the door to observe the patient wiping herself from back to front. You realize this is a teaching moment and take the aide aside and instruct her. What is the association between M.Z.'s UTI and the organism found in her urine culture?

4. As you insert the Foley catheter you note the introitus is red and dry; no vaginal discharge is noted. You inform the managing physician that M.Z. has atrophic vaginitis and get an order for vaginal estrogen replacement (Estrace cream). M.Z.'s daughter will need to be instructed how to insert the cream for her mother. Outline your teaching plan.

5. What should you instruct the daughter to look for and report to M.Z.'s doctor?

6. The aide comes to you to report that M.Z. is picking at her IV and asks if she can apply wrist restraints. How should you respond?

7. If M.Z. develops diarrhea, what special instructions should you give the nursing assistant assigned to give basic care to M.Z.?

8. You are the nurse assigned to M.Z.'s care. You notice that the nursing assistant emptying the gravity drain is not wearing personal protection devices. You also observe that the spout is contaminated during the process. What issues need to be considered in protecting M.Z.'s safety? Describe your actions in working with the nursing assistant.

9. The nursing assistant reports that M.Z.'s 8-hour intake is 520 mL and the output is 140 mL. Is this significant? Generate at least two possible factors that could account for the difference. For each factor, identify which item would be assessed and how.

10. M.Z. has completed her ATB therapy, her mental status has cleared, and she is ready for discharge. What instructions should you discuss with the daughter?

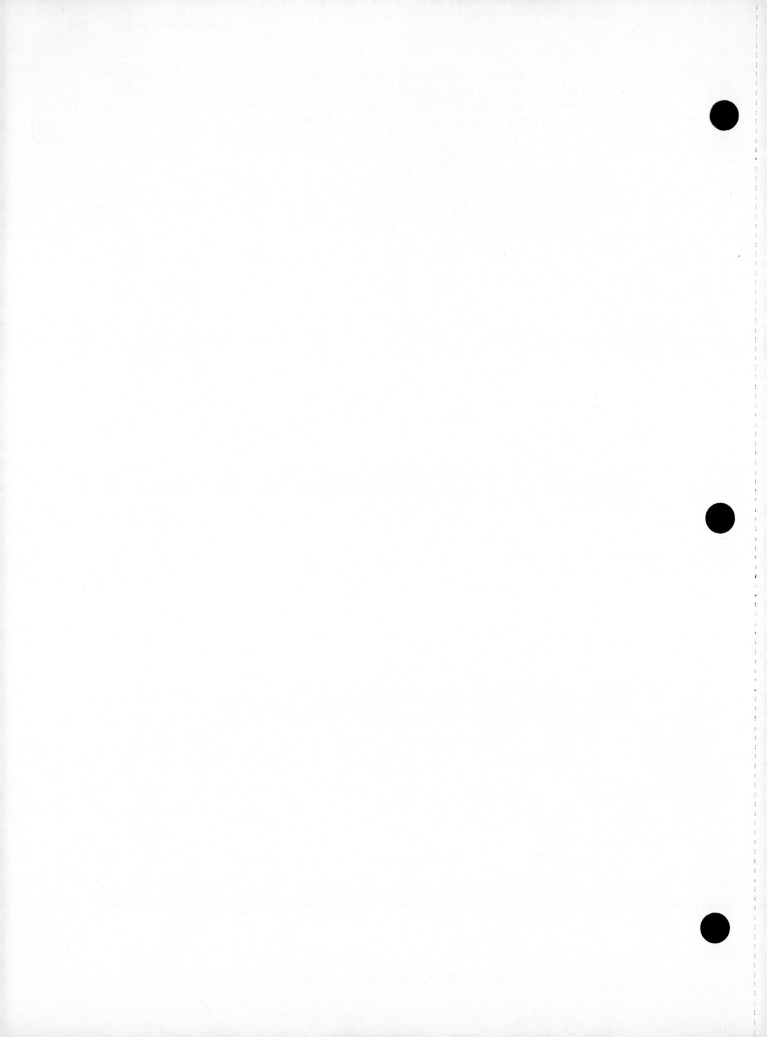

Case Study 2

Name ______________________________ Class/Group __________ Date __________

Group Members ____

INSTRUCTIONS: All questions apply to this case study. Your responses should be brief and to the point. Adequate space has been provided for answers. When asked to provide several answers, they should be listed in order of priority or significance. Do not asume information that is not provided. Please print or write clearly. If your response is not legible, it will be marked as ? and you will need to rewrite it.

Scenario

J.T., a 26-year-old female, comes to your urology clinic for the first time. She has been referred by her PCP for recurrent UTI (urinary tract infection) with hematuria. She C/O abdominal pain, L>R, and intense vaginal pain, especially with intercourse. She reports she has IBS (irritable bowel syndrome), seasonal allergies, a lot of stress in her life, and eats a lot of spicy foods, fruits, and caffeine. J.T. brought a letter from her referring MD stating that although her UA (urinalysis) with C&S (culture and sensitivity) have always been negative, she has been Tx with Levaquin and Diflucan without resolution of symptoms. She had a CHB (cystoscopy hydrodistention of bladder) that showed "petechiae, glomerulations, inflammatory changes, and Hunner's ulcer." Her Bx (biopsy) showed "chronic cystitis with edema, vascular congestion, and increased mast cells."

1. You are the intake nurse working in the clinic. Based on J.T.'s Hx, operative note, and Bx, what would be the most likely Dx and why?

2. What is interstitial cystitis?

3. What are the most common symptoms of IC?

4. J.T. is concerned she may have received or could pass on her IC to her husband. What should you tell her to calm her fears?

5. What therapy would be appropriate for J.T.? Indicate whether each following statement is true (T) or false (F); then correct all false statements.

   ______ A. Modify diet to exclude or reduce caffeine, ETOH (alcohol), spicy foods, and fruits and vegetables that are high in potassium acids.

   ______ B. Recommend antihistamines W/O decongestants or ephedrine to block histamine release and decrease inflammation.

   ______ C. Reduce fluids to limit urinary frequency.

   ______ D. Recommend a daily MVI, especially one high in vitamin C.

   ______ E. Physical therapy, biofeedback, and Kegel exercises may help to relieve pelvic pain.

   ______ F. IC is not affected by stress.

   ______ G. Pentosan polysulfate (Elmiron) is not a reasonable first-line drug.

   ______ H. Six to 8 weeks of bladder instillation of dimethyl sulfoxide (DMSO), triamcinolone (Kenalog) liquid, and heparin may dramatically reduce symptoms.

   ______ I. Cystectomy with urinary diversion is effective in eliminating IC pain.

Case Study 3

Name ______________________ Class/Group __________ Date __________

Group Members ____

INSTRUCTIONS: All questions apply to this case study. Your responses should be brief and to the point. Adequate space has been provided for answers. When asked to provide several answers, they should be listed in order of priority or significance. Do not asume information that is not provided. Please print or write clearly. If your response is not legible, it will be marked as ? and you will need to rewrite it.

Scenario

You are working in the ED when M.B., a 72-year-old man, enters with a C/C (chief complaint) of inability to void. His initial VS are 168/92, 70, 20, 98.2° F.

1. Are M.B.'s VS appropriate for a man his age? If not, what are the abnormalities? Offer possibilities for the abnormality.

While taking M.B.'s Hx, you discover he believes he is generally in good health and leads an active life. His current medications include finasteride (Proscar) 5 mg daily and vitamin supplements. He reports that he has been unable to void for 12 hours and is very uncomfortable. He asks you to help him.

2. During your initial assessment, what physical/emotional findings would you expect in regard to his C/C?

3. What are your priorities for this patient?

4. After examining M.B., the ED physician asks you to insert an indwelling Foley catheter. What should you include in M.B.'s teaching before placing the Foley?

5. After 2 unsuccessful attempts to advance the catheter into the bladder, you stop. What is your next intervention? Why?

6. The ED physician completes the catheterization and writes orders to discharge M.B. with instructions to see his PCP the following day. It is your responsibility to give discharge instructions. Outline your plan of care.

Case Study 4

Name ______________________ Class/Group __________ Date __________

Group Members ____

INSTRUCTIONS: All questions apply to this case study. Your responses should be brief and to the point. Adequate space has been provided for answers. When asked to provide several answers, they should be listed in order of priority or significance. Do not asume information that is not provided. Please print or write clearly. If your response is not legible, it will be marked as ? and you will need to rewrite it.

Scenario

You are working on a postoperative surgical floor and are assigned to A.T., a 65-year-old female with a 30-year smoking history who has recently had a radical cystectomy with ileal conduit for invasive bladder cancer.

1. You begin your assessment and look at the transparent urostomy pouch covering the ileal conduit. The stomal opening is red and is draining urine with mucus. Is this normal?

2. The patient asks you to explain the difference between an ileal conduit and an ileostomy. How should you explain this to her?

3. A.T. is learning how to change her appliance. She tells you the stoma feels wet and it has no feeling when she touches it. Educate A.T. about the stoma.

4. What additional topics need to be addressed when doing ileal conduit teaching?

5. A.T. is very quiet and sullen the third postoperative day. You ask her if something is wrong and she confides she is concerned about whether or not her husband will find her attractive after he sees her "rosebud." What is the underlying problem?

You ask A.T. if her husband or children had a physical problem that required a surgical repair, would she love them any less. She quickly tells you "No, of course not." You suggest that her family will likely respond the same way to her surgery. You suggest that someone from the "ostimate" program come and talk to her.

6. What is the ostimate program?

7. A.T is well enough to begin self-care but asks you if you will change her pouch because she "doesn't want to look at it." Is there anyone on the hospital staff who could help teach A.T. ostomy self-care and offer more support?

8. A.T.'s urine looks cloudy and another nurse suggests that you send a specimen from her pouch to the lab for analysis. Her urine does not smell foul, she has no fever or flank pain. Should you follow through on this suggestion? Why or why not?

9. What are the S/S (signs and symptoms) of a UTI in a patient with an ileal conduit?

10. You walk into the room and notice that A.T.'s pouch has sprung a leak and she has placed a washcloth over the pouch to absorb the urine. She asks you for tape to attach the washcloth to the bag. How should you respond to her request?

A.T. eventually masters the pouch application and is discharged home. She returns to the Urology Clinic in 6 months for a follow-up visit. She has lost 24 lb and presents with a smaller stoma surrounded by a half inch ring of wart-like skin. The nurse explains to A.T. that her stoma has shrunk and the bag no longer fits properly; alkaline urine washing over unprotected skin from too large an appliance opening causes a skin reaction that can either appear smooth or wart-like. The wart-like skin buildup is referred to as hyperkeratotic, hyperplastic, epitheliomatous hyperplasia, metaplasia, or acanthosis.

11. What can be done once a hyperkeratotic lesion forms around a stoma?

12. What is the proper size for an appliance for an ileal conduit?

A.T. mastered her ileal conduit and became a very popular ostimate.

Case Study 5

Name ______________________ Class/Group __________ Date __________

Group Members ______________________________________

INSTRUCTIONS: All questions apply to this case study. Your responses should be brief and to the point. Adequate space has been provided for answers. When asked to provide several answers, they should be listed in order of priority or significance. Do not asume information that is not provided. Please print or write clearly. If your response is not legible, it will be marked as ? and you will need to rewrite it.

Scenario

S.M. is a 68-year-old man who is being seen at your clinic for routine health maintenance and health promotion. He reports that he has been feeling well and has no specific complaints except for some trouble "emptying his bladder." He had a CBC and CMP completed 1 week before his visit, and the results are as follows: Na 140 mmol/L, K 4.2 mmol/L, Cl 100 mmol/L, HCO_3 26 mmol/L, BUN 22 mg/dL, creatinine 0.8 mg/dL, glucose 94 mg/dL, RBC 5.2 million/mm^3, WBC 7,400/mm^3, Hgb 15.2 g/dL, Hct 46%, platelets 348,000/mm^3. PSA (prostate-specific antigen) 0.23 ng/mL, and UA was WNL. VS at this visit are 148/88, 82, 16, 96.9° F.

1. What can you tell S.M. about his lab work?

While obtaining your nursing history, you record no family history of cancer or other genitourinary problems. S.M. reports frequency, urgency, nocturia × 4; he has a weak stream and has to sit to void. These symptoms have been progressive over the past 6 months. He reports he was diagnosed with a large prostate a number of years ago.

2. S.M. is curious why his BPH would affect his urination. He is concerned he has prostate cancer. What would you teach him?

3. The PCP asked for a PVR (postvoiding residual urine). You document that S.M. voids 60 mL and his PVR is 110 mL. What is the significance of his PVR?

4. You report the PVR to the PCP. The three most commonly ordered medications to treat BPH (benign prostatic hypertrophy) are doxazosin, terazosin, and tamsulosin. What is the purpose of these medications?

5. The PCP ordered tamulosin (Flowmax) 0.4 mg PO qd. You enter S.M.'s room to teach him about this medication. What points should you include?

6. S.M. asks, "What is retrograde ejaculation?" Explain this concept.

7. "Will this condition affect my relationship with my wife?" What should you tell him?

8. What would you expect S.M. to report if the medication was successful?

S.M. returns in 8 months to report his symptoms are worse than ever. He has tried several different medications, but medication management failed, and he is told surgical intervention is necessary.

9. What surgical options are available to S.M.?

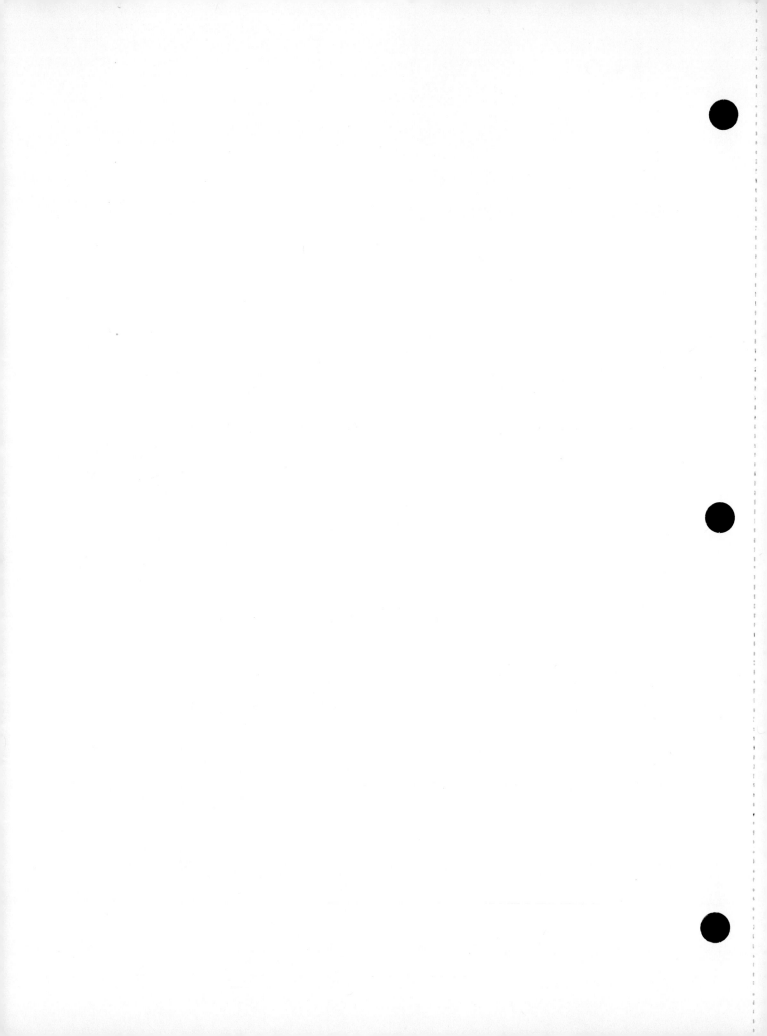

Case Study 6

Name ______________________ Class/Group __________ Date __________

Group Members ____

INSTRUCTIONS: All questions apply to this case study. Your responses should be brief and to the point. Adequate space has been provided for answers. When asked to provide several answers, they should be listed in order of priority or significance. Do not asume information that is not provided. Please print or write clearly. If your response is not legible, it will be marked as ? and you will need to rewrite it.

Scenario

K.B. is a 32-year-old woman being admitted to the medical floor for C/O fatigue and dehydration. While taking your history you discover that she has diabetes and has been insulin-dependent since the age of 8. She has undergone hemodialysis for the past 3 years. Your initial assessment of K.B. reveals a pale, thin, lethargic woman in NAD (no acute distress). Her admitting chemistries are Na 145 mmol/L, K 6.0 mmol/L, Cl 93 mmol/L, HCO_3 27 mmol/L, BUN 48 mg/dL, creatinine 5.0 mg/dL, glucose 238 mg/dL. Her skin is warm and dry to touch with poor skin turgor, and her mucous membranes are dry. Her VS are 140/88, 116, 18, 99.9° F. She tells you she has been nauseated for 2 days so she has not been eating or drinking. She reports severe diarrhea. Serum calcium, phosphate, and magnesium have been drawn but are not yet available.

1. What aspects of your assessment support her admitting diagnosis of dehydration?

2. Identify two possibilities for K.B.'s low-grade fever.

The rest of K.B.'s physical assessment is within normal limits. She tells you she has an AV (arteriovenous) fistula in her left arm.

3. What is a fistula? Why does K.B. have one?

4. In assessment of an AV fistula, what physical findings would you expect during auscultation and palpation? Why?

Over the next 24 hours, K.B.'s nausea subsides, and she is able to eat normally. Her physician believes her nausea to be R/T her elevated Cr/BUN. While you are helping her with her AM care, she confides in you that she has never really understood what "diet I'm supposed to be on anyway."

5. What information would you seek from K.B. now?

6. Because K.B. is on hemodialysis, what are her special nutritional needs?

K.B.'s CBC (complete blood cell count) yields the following results: WBC 7,600/mm^3, RBC 3.2 million/mm^3, Hgb 8.1 g/dL, Hct 24.3%, and platelets 333,000/mm^3.

7. Are these values normal? If not what are the abnormalities?

8. K.B.'s physician notes that she is anemic, which is most likely the cause of her increasing fatigue. Why is K.B. anemic?

The following day K.B. is discharged feeling much better and with a good understanding of her dietary restrictions. Her iron stores have been evaluated and found to be adequate. Her physician has instructed her to resume her preadmission medications, except for the addition of recombinant human erythropoietin 50 units/kg three times a week with dialysis.

9. What information would you give K.B. about her new medication?

Case Study 7

Name ______________________________ Class/Group __________ Date __________

Group Members ____

INSTRUCTIONS: All questions apply to this case study. Your responses should be brief and to the point. Adequate space has been provided for answers. When asked to provide several answers, they should be listed in order of priority or significance. Do not asume information that is not provided. Please print or write clearly. If your response is not legible, it will be marked as ? and you will need to rewrite it.

Scenario

A.B. is a 55-year-old male who was referred to the Urology Clinic by his PCP (primary care provider) for an elevated PSA (prostate-specific antigen). He reports that he has been feeling well and has no specific complaints. He had a CBC, BMP, UA, lipid profile, and screening PSA completed the week before when he was seen by his PCP. His CBC, lipid profile, urinalysis, and blood chemistries are all within normal limits, but his PSA is slightly elevated at 4.92 ng/mL.

1. A.B. wonders if he has prostate cancer. What can you tell A.B. about his PSA?

2. A.B. is scheduled for a prostate biopsy. He wonders what he needs to do to prepare for this test. Explain a prostate biopsy procedure and how to prepare for the procedure.

A.B.'s prostate biopsy is positive for cancer. He has discussed his diagnosis with the urologist. He is now thinking about his treatment options and asks you to clarify some of the questions he has. He was told about his Gleason grade but is not sure what this is.

3. What is a Gleason grade?

4. The urologist discusses possible treatment options with A.B. Identify three treatment options for prostate cancer.

A.B. has decided to have his prostate removed. He is planning on having surgery in 2 weeks but is concerned about the possible consequences of surgery.

5. Identify the major immediate postoperative concern for A.B.

6. Identify the two main long-term consequences of prostatectomy?

7. The urologist you work for has asked you to give A.B. preoperative instructions. What should you tell him?

A.B. returns S/P radical prostatectomy. Initial postoperative orders include:

A. VS per hospital protocol
B. Inspect, reinforce, and change dressing according to hospital protocol.
C. NPO until after first BM or passing flatus.
D. Notify MD if UOP (urine output) <30 mL/h, absent BS (bowel sounds), SOB (short of breath)
E. Up ad lib
F. Overhead irrigation as needed to maintain patent Foley catheter
G. If Foley clots, change Foley catheter.
H. SCDs (sequential compression devices) per hospital protocol
I. H/H with PT/PTT q6h × 24h
J. RN to maintain change dressing and observe epidural insertion site
K. JP (Jackson-Pratt) to suction drain

8. Review the list of postoperative orders. Place a star next to incorrect orders and correct them.

9. A.B. returns for his 6-month F/U (follow-up) visit. He reports he can get an erection but has difficulty maintaining an erection for sexual relations. You discuss alternative erectile aides. What options should you address?

Case Study 8

Name ________________________________ Class/Group __________ Date __________

Group Members ____

INSTRUCTIONS: All questions apply to this case study. Your responses should be brief and to the point. Adequate space has been provided for answers. When asked to provide several answers, they should be listed in order of priority or significance. Do not asume information that is not provided. Please print or write clearly. If your response is not legible, it will be marked as ? and you will need to rewrite it.

Scenario

It is a hot summer day, and you are an RN in the ED. S.R., an 18-year-old woman, presents at the ED with severe L flank and abdominal pain, and N/V. S.R. looks very tired, her skin is warm to touch, and she is perspiring. She paces about the room doubled-over and is clutching her abdomen. S.R. tells you that the pain started early this morning and has been pretty steady for the last 6 hours. She gives a history of working outside as a landscaper and takes little time for water breaks. Her PMH includes 3 kidney stone attacks, all during summer months. Exam findings: her abdomen is soft and without tenderness, but her L flank is extremely tender to touch/ palpation/percussion. You place S.R. in one of the exam rooms and take the following VS: 188/98, 90, 20, 99° F. Urinalysis shows RBC 50–100 on voided specimen, WBC zero.

1. It is very common for drug seekers to present with blood in their urine. What should you do to ensure the urinalysis is correct?

2. The MD orders an IVP (intravenous pylegram). What question do you need to ask S.R. before the test is conducted?

3. S.R. states she had an allergic reaction during her last IVP and was instructed "Don't let anyone give you dye for any testing." The MD cancels the IVP; what alternative test should be conducted?

The abdominal CT scan shows a L 2 mm UVJ (ureteral vesicle junction) stone.

4. What are the two most common types of stones?

5. What is the most likely cause of S.R.'s stone?

6. Identify two methods of treating a patient with an UVJ stone?

S.R. was discharged with instructions to strain all urine and return if she experienced pain unrelieved by the pain medication or increased N/V (nausea and vomiting).

7. What specific instructions will you give S.R. about her urine, fluid intake, medications, and activity?

S.R. returns to the ED in 6 hours with C/O pain unrelieved by the pain medication and increased blood in her urine. She is being held in the ED until she can be transported to surgery.

8. What is the plan of care for S.R.?

A 2-mm calculus was removed by basket extraction. Pathologic examination reported the stone to be calcium oxalate.

9. If S.R continues to form stones, what recommendations would an MD make for this patient?

10. Because S.R.'s stone has been reported as calcium oxalate, what type of diet would be recommended?

Case Study 9

Name ______________________ Class/Group __________ Date __________

Group Members ____

INSTRUCTIONS: All questions apply to this case study. Your responses should be brief and to the point. Adequate space has been provided for answers. When asked to provide several answers, they should be listed in order of priority or significance. Do not asume information that is not provided. Please print or write clearly. If your response is not legible, it will be marked as ? and you will need to rewrite it.

Scenario

K.B. is a 45-year-old male who presents to his primary care provider with the complaint of erectile dysfunction. He reports that he first noticed a gradual decline in sexual function 12 months ago after he was diagnosed with diabetes. K.B. reports that he is no longer able to achieve a full erection and cannot maintain his partial erection for intercourse. He states that he is very frustrated by his inability to perform sexually and stated that he no longer feels like a good husband. His wife is beginning to feel that his inability to perform is directly related to her, and they are experiencing problems in their relationship. He states that he no longer experiences nocturnal erections and has noticed his libido is "not as good as it used to be." K.B.'s PMH is positive for HTN (hypertension), hyperlipidemia, and diabetes. He is currently taking fosinopril (Monopril) 20 mg qd, atorvastatin (Lipitor) 20 mg, and metformin (Glucophage) 1000 mg bid. He is sedentary and does not exercise regularly. He is requesting treatment for his erectile dysfunction.

1. What is erectile dysfunction?

2. Why is it important to diagnose men with ED?

3. Identify at least 10 disease states that are known to cause ED.

4. What is the most likely cause of K.B.'s ED?

You are the RN working in the ED clinic. It is your responsibility to complete the intake interview, order the standard lab work, and complete a physical exam.

5. What information would you include?

6. You order a CBC, BMP, LFT (liver function tests), lipids, testosterone, prolactin, lutenizing hormone, TSH, PSA, UA according to the clinic protocol. Give your rationale for ordering each of these tests.

7. K.B. asks you what treatments are available. Identify three different treatments and list the pros and cons of each.

8. You documented "small, soft testicles" on your assessment. What screening labs are particularly important in light of your assessment findings?

9. From what other intervention would K.B. and his wife benefit?

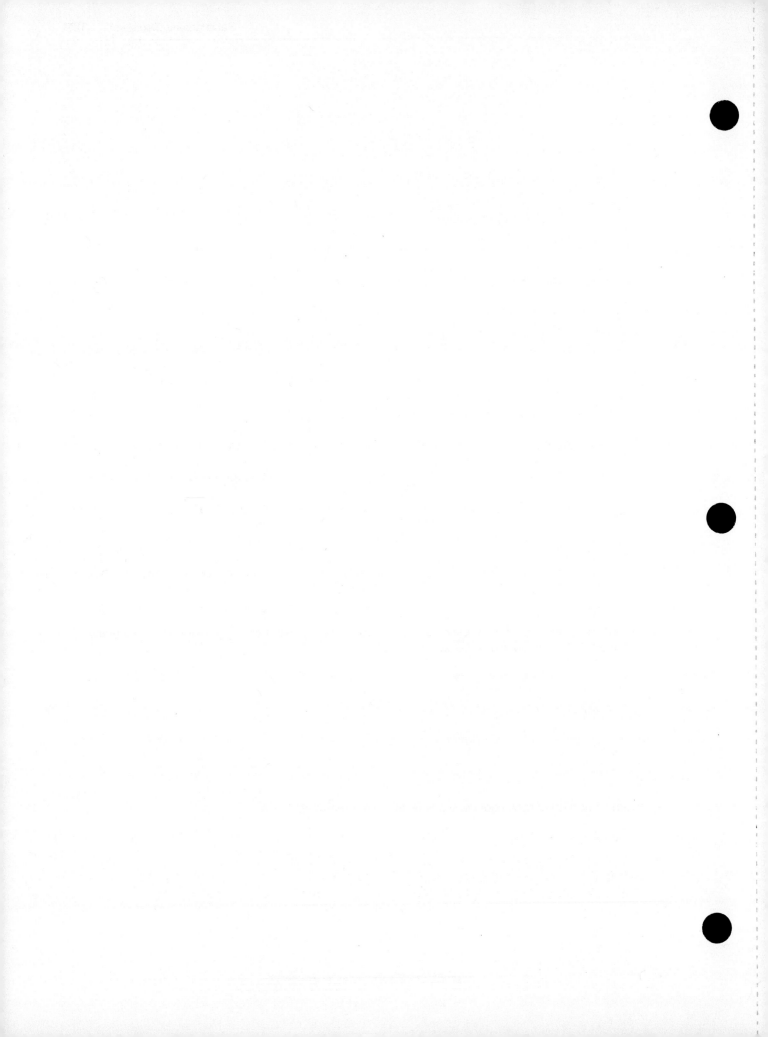

Case Study 10

Name ____________________ Class/Group __________ Date __________

Group Members ____

INSTRUCTIONS: All questions apply to this case study. Your responses should be brief and to the point. Adequate space has been provided for answers. When asked to provide several answers, they should be listed in order of priority or significance. Do not asume information that is not provided. Please print or write clearly. If your response is not legible, it will be marked as ? and you will need to rewrite it.

Scenario

F.F., a 58-year-old man with type 2 DM (non-insulin-dependent diabetes mellitus), presents at the ED with severe R flank and abdominal pain, and N/V. The abdomen is soft and without tenderness. The right flank is extremely tender to touch and palpation. VS are 142/80, 88, 20, 99.0° F; urinalysis shows hematuria; an IV of .9 NS is started and is to infuse at 125 mL/h. An IVP (intravenous pyelogram) confirms the diagnosis of a staghorn-type stone in the R renal pelvis. The R kidney looks enlarged. F.F. states that he did not sleep well last night and has not eaten much today. He is obviously very fatigued. His laboratory results are as follows: Na 144 mmol/L, K 4.0 mmol/L, Cl 101 mmol/L, CO_2 26 mmol/L, BUN 30 mg/dL, creatinine 3.6 mg/dL, glucose 260 mg/dL, uric acid 5.0 mg/dL, Ca 9.0 mg/dL, phos 2.6 mg/dL, total protein 7.8 g/dL, albumin 4.0 g/dL, total bilirubin 0.3 mg/dL, direct bilirubin 0.1 mg/dL, chol 200 mg/dL, alk phos 61 U/L, LDH total 100 U/L, AST (SGOT) 13 U/L, ALT (SGPT) 13 U/L, GGTP 40 U/L, amylase 98 U/L.

1. F.F.'s pain is treated with IV morphine. It is late afternoon before he is admitted to your unit, and he is scheduled for lithotripsy in the morning. What specific priorities do you identify for F.F.?

2. The physician has prescribed gentamicin 80 mg IVPB q8h. You question the physician about giving this large of a dose of gentamicin to F.F. You are met with angry and belittling statements. Articulate why you should question this specific order for F.F.

3. How should you handle the situation with the physician in order to protect the patient and promote a collegial relationship?

4. A staghorn stone can cause chronic infection and renal pelvis obstruction that may result in the need for nephrectomy. What may be the impact of this problem on his long-term kidney function?

5. Analyze the relationship between creatinine and GFR and predicting kidney function.

6. Later, as you walk past his bed, you notice F.F. crawling off the end of the bed. What are you going to do?

F.F. is going to be admitted. You call the unit nurse to give the report. You tell her he's been up all night with pain that has just been relieved by IV morphine. You don't know whether he's going to have lithotripsy or surgery; surgery is unlikely because the stone is so large.

7. You tell F.F. he is going to be admitted and will probably need surgery for his kidney stone. He looks at you, panicked, and says, "I can't do that. I don't have any insurance. This is costing me a wad already." How are you going to respond?

Case Study 11

Name ______________________ Class/Group __________ Date __________

Group Members ____

INSTRUCTIONS: All questions apply to this case study. Your responses should be brief and to the point. Adequate space has been provided for answers. When asked to provide several answers, they should be listed in order of priority or significance. Do not asume information that is not provided. Please print or write clearly. If your response is not legible, it will be marked as ? and you will need to rewrite it.

Scenario

You are working in the ICU of an acute care hospital and assume the care of E.B., a 78-year-old woman who is 3 days post inferior wall MI. E.B. had been healthy before admission except for a longstanding history of osteoarthritis treated with rofecoxib (Vioxx) 50 mg daily and longstanding hypertension treated with atenolol (Tenormin) 50 mg daily. On presentation to the ED, E.B. had severe hypertension (210/122 mm Hg); therefore, thrombolytics were contraindicated. An IV was started with D_5W at KOR and she was taken directly to the cardiac catheterization lab for acute PTCA (percutaneous transluminal coronary angioplasty). Her angioplasty was successful, and she has been pain-free since the PTCA. You are reviewing E.B.'s lab work and note the following values: Na 142 mmol/L, K 4.6 mmol/L, Cl 100 mmol/L, CO_2 26 mmol/L, BUN 60 mg/dL, creatinine 3.8 mg/dL, glucose 158 mg/dL.

Keep Open Rate (KVO)

1. What abnormalities are there in E.B.'s lab work?

   BUN and creatinine

2. What are possible causes for these abnormalities?

   Severe hypertensive, MI, nephrotoxic drugs.

3. Describe prerenal, intrarenal, and postrenal causes of acute renal failure (ARF). Given the potential causes of E.B.'s elevated BUN and creatinine, how would they be categorized?

Prerenal - MI, hypotensive
Intrarenal - Vioxx
Postrenal - obstruction, artherosclerosis, PTCA (use of dyes)

You are given the results of E.B.'s lab work from today. The results are Na 140 mmol/L, K 5.0 mmol/L, Cl 104 mmol/L, CO_2 24 mmol/L, BUN 68 mg/dL, creatinine 4.0 mg/dL, glucose 104 mg/dL. You have also noted her urine output for the past 8 hours is 160 mL.

4. Based on these values, what is your next action going to be?

Call the doctor!

5. Define *oliguria* and *anuria*. Which term best describes E.B.'s renal function?

Oliguria — < 400cc /day
Anuria — <100 cc/ day.
She is oliguric.

6. In reviewing E.B.'s VS, you cannot identify any episodes of hypotension since her admission. What might be a possible explanation for her increase in BUN and creatinine?

- Chronic nephrotoxic use.
- Hypertension Hx
- Contrast dye

7. What are your interventions and priorities for a patient in ARF?

Fluid volume levels (I&O, labs, resp/cardiac symptoms)
Monitor K^+ (EKG)

8. E.B. has been very quiet. Suddenly she asks you, "Am I going to die?" How will you respond?

9. You talk to her about the possibility of dialysis, which may be a treatment option for her. She responds, "You know, I'm 78 years old. I've had a pretty good life, and I don't want to be hooked to a machine." What will you say?

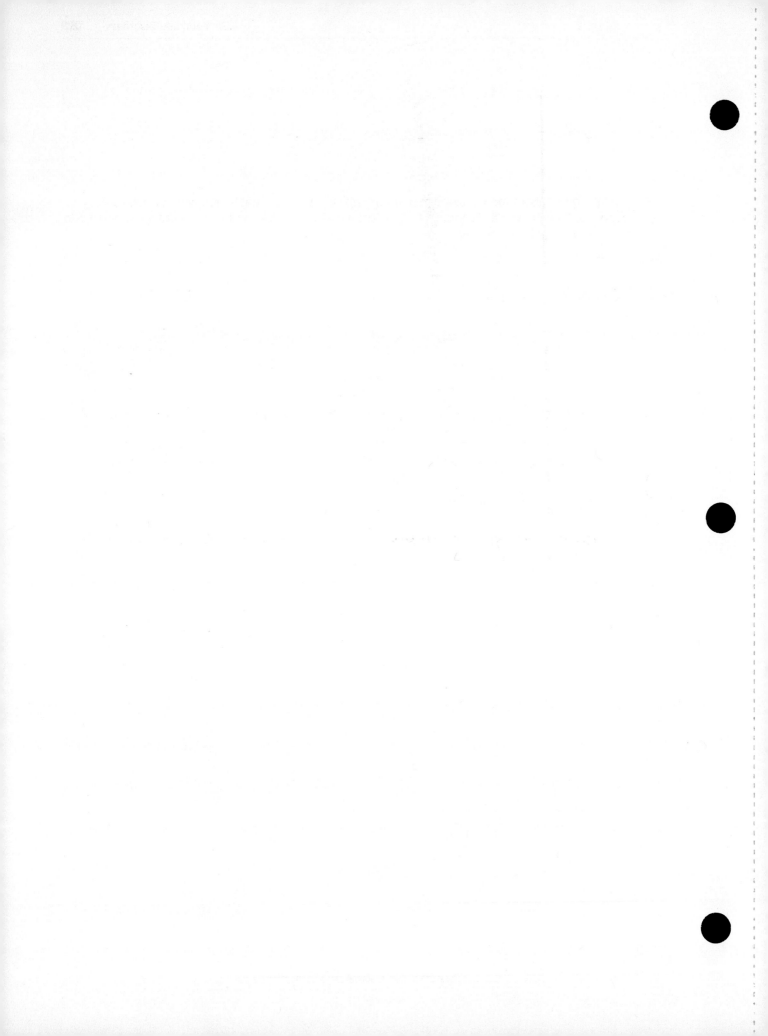

Case Study 12

Name ______________________ Class/Group __________ Date __________

Group Members ____

INSTRUCTIONS: All questions apply to this case study. Your responses should be brief and to the point. Adequate space has been provided for answers. When asked to provide several answers, they should be listed in order of priority or significance. Do not asume information that is not provided. Please print or write clearly. If your response is not legible, it will be marked as ? and you will need to rewrite it.

Scenario

N.H., an 89-year-old widow, recently experienced a left cerebrovascular accident (CVA). She has R-sided weakness and expressive aphasia with minimal swallowing difficulty. N.H. has a PMH of L CVA 2.5 years ago, chronic atrial flutter, and HTN. She has a negative psychiatric history and has lived with her daughter's family in a rural town since her previous stroke. Since admission to an acute care facility 5 days ago, N.H. has gained some strength, has become oriented to person and place, and is anxious to begin her rehabilitation program. She is transferred for rehabilitation to your skilled nursing facility with the following orders: hydrochlorothiazide 25 mg PO qd, digoxin 0.125 mg PO qd, aspirin 81 mg PO qd, warfarin (Coumadin) 5 mg PO qd, acetaminophen (Tylenol) 325 mg q6h prn for pain, zolpidem 5 mg PO hs PRN for sleep. Diet: mechanical soft, low Na with ground meat. Other strategies: maintain Foley to DD and then follow up with bladder training; facilitate referrals for speech, OT, and PT to evaluate and treat swallowing, communication, and functional abilities.

1. What lab orders would you anticipate as a result of this specific list of orders? With each response, describe your rationale.

2. At the interdisciplinary care conferences, you report that bladder training is progressing and recommend removing the catheter if N.H.'s mobility and communication abilities have progressed sufficiently. The group and N.H. agree that she is ready for the Foley catheter to be removed. Identify three problems that N.H. is at risk for developing following catheter removal. Describe specific interventions for each problem.

3. Two days after the Foley is removed, you observe that N.H.'s urine is cloudy and concentrated and has a strong odor. What are your immediate actions?

4. N.H. is started on sulfamethoxazole 400 mg/trimethoprim 160 mg (Bactrim DS) 1 tab PO bid × 10 days. However, 2 days later N.H. is in the bathroom, and she is very upset. There is blood on the toilet, and the water is bright red with blood. You help the CNA clean N.H. and help her into bed. Describe your assessment steps. What complications do you anticipate?

5. You complete your assessment and report your findings to the physician. You obtain an order for a straight catheterized urine specimen for C&S. Identify at least two potential causes for N.H.'s hematuria.

6. N.H.'s UTI is responding to antibiotics, and you want to prepare her and her daughter for eventual discharge. What specific issues must be considered in the teaching/discharge planning to prevent a recurrence of infection?

7. You talk with N.H.'s daughter about her understanding of caregiving responsibilities for her mother. What kind of questions are you going to ask to assess if she is capable of taking on this additional burden?

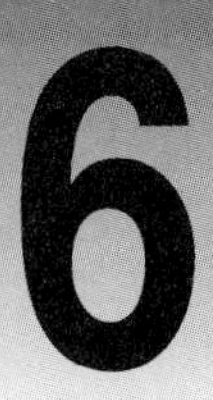

Neurologic Disorders

Case Study 1

Name ______________________ Class/Group __________ Date __________

Group Members ____

INSTRUCTIONS: All questions apply to this case study. Your responses should be brief and to the point. Adequate space has been provided for answers. When asked to provide several answers, they should be listed in order of priority or significance. Do not asume information that is not provided. Please print or write clearly. If your response is not legible, it will be marked as ? and you will need to rewrite it.

Scenario

M.E. is a 62-year-old woman who has a 5-year history of progressive forgetfulness. She is no longer able to care for herself, has become increasingly depressed and paranoid, and recently started a fire in the kitchen. After extensive neurologic evaluation, M.E. is diagnosed as having Alzheimer's disease. Her husband and children have come to the Alzheimer's unit at your ECF (extended-care facility) for information about this disease and to discuss the possibility of placement for M.E. You reassure the family that you have experience dealing with the questions and concerns of most people in their situation.

1. How would you explain Alzheimer's disease to the family?

2. The husband asks, "How did she get Alzheimer's? We don't know anyone else who has it." How would you respond?

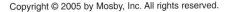

3. After asking the family to describe M.E.'s behavior, you determine that she is in stage two of Alzheimer's three stages. Describe common S/S for each stage of the disease.

4. The daughter expresses frustration at the number of tests M.E. had to undergo and the length of time it took for someone to diagnosis M.E.'s problem. What tests are likely to be performed and how is Alzheimer's disease diagnosed?

The husband states, "How are you going to take care of her? She wanders around all night long. She can't find her way to the bathroom in a house she's lived in for 43 years. She can't be trusted to be alone any more; she almost burnt the house down. We're all exhausted; there are three of us, and we can't keep up with her." You acknowledge how exhausted they must be from trying to keep her safe. You tell the family that there is no known treatment but Alzheimer's units have been created to provide a structured, safe environment for each person.

5. Describe the Alzheimer's-related nursing interventions R/T (related to) each of the following nursing care problems: self-care deficits, disturbed sleep pattern, impaired verbal communication, impaired cognitive function, risk for injury, and agitation.

6. M.E.'s son asks what different medications might be prescribed for M.E. How would you describe the purpose of antiseizure, cognitive, antipsychotic, antidepressive, or sedative medications for a patient like M.E.?

You try to comfort the family by telling them that the problems they are experiencing are very common. You explain that family support is a major focus of your program.

7. List four ways that M.E.'s family might receive the support they need.

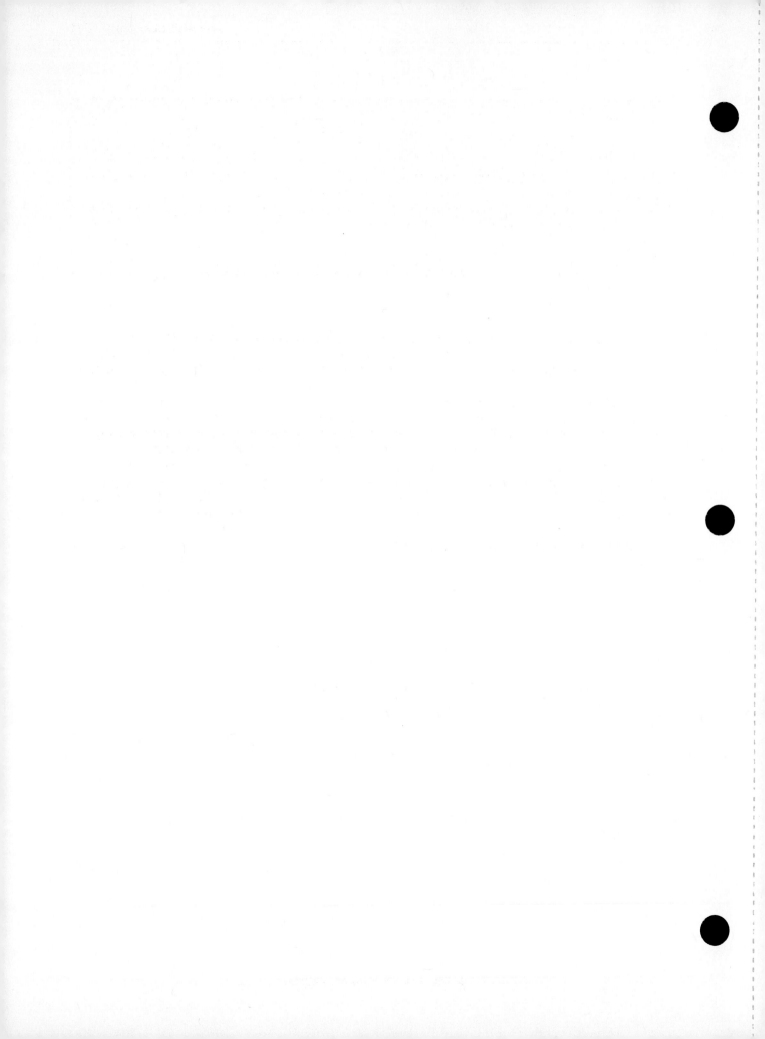

Case Study 2

Name ______________________ Class/Group __________ Date __________

Group Members ____

INSTRUCTIONS: All questions apply to this case study. Your responses should be brief and to the point. Adequate space has been provided for answers. When asked to provide several answers, they should be listed in order of priority or significance. Do not asume information that is not provided. Please print or write clearly. If your response is not legible, it will be marked as ? and you will need to rewrite it.

Scenario

C.B. is a 58-year-old male with Guillain-Barré syndrome (GBS). He was transferred to a skilled nursing facility that cares for patients requiring mechanical ventilation 2 days ago. C.B. is a single, self-supporting man from a small town. He presented to his family physician with symptoms of fatigue, mylagias, fever, and chills, which were accompanied by a hacking cough in early January. He was diagnosed with viral influenza. Three weeks later he developed bilateral weakness, numbness and tingling of his lower extremities, which rapidly progressed into his upper body. He was brought to the ED (Emergency Department) after his brother recognized the seriousness of his condition. Shortly after arrival he became totally paralyzed and required endotracheal intubation and mechanical ventilation. He was then admitted to the Neurologic Critical Care Unit, where he spent 1 month. He underwent a tracheotomy before being transferred to a medical floor where he spent several weeks. He was treated for pneumonia while hospitalized in the medical floor. His pneumonia resolved prior to transfer to a skilled care facility for further rehabilitation and continued ventilatory support.

1. What is the etiology of Guillain-Barré syndrome?

2. What type of individual is likely diagnosed with Gullian-Barré syndrome?

3. What are the clinical manifestations of GBS?

4. Is C.B.'s case typical?

5. How is GBS diagnosed?

6. Why does life-threatening respiratory dysfunction occur?

7. How are C.B.'s nutritional needs being maintained?

8. What interventions can you implement to decrease C.B.'s fear and anxiety?

9. What is the medical management for GBS?

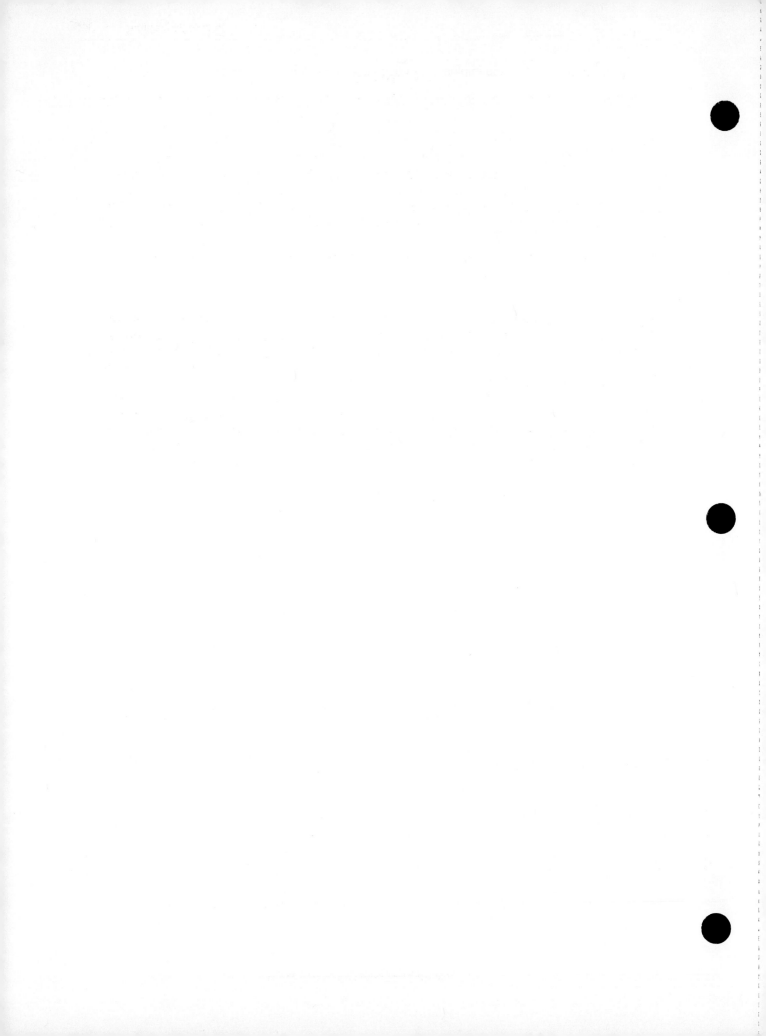

Case Study 3

Name ______________________________ Class/Group __________ Date __________

Group Members ____

INSTRUCTIONS: All questions apply to this case study. Your responses should be brief and to the point. Adequate space has been provided for answers. When asked to provide several answers, they should be listed in order of priority or significance. Do not asume information that is not provided. Please print or write clearly. If your response is not legible, it will be marked as ? and you will need to rewrite it.

Scenario

L.C. is a 78-year-old white male with a 4-year history of Parkinson's disease (PD). He is a retired engineer, married, and lives with his wife in a small farming community. He has four adult children who live close by. He is on carbidopa/levodopa, pergolide, and amantadine. L.C. reports that overall he is doing "about the same" as he was at his last clinic visit 6 months ago. He reports that his tremor is about the same, his gait is perhaps a little more unsteady, and his fatigue is slightly more noticeable. L.C. is also concerned about increased drooling. The patient and his wife report that he is taking carbidopa/levodopa 25/100 mg, two tablets qd and carbidopa/levodopa SA 50/200 mg, one tablet at bedtime. On the previous visit they were encouraged to try taking the carbidopa/levodopa CR more times throughout the day, but they report that he became very somnolent with that dosing regimen. He also reports that his dykinetic movements appear to be worse just after taking his carbidopa/levodopa.

1. What is parkinsonism?

2. What is Parkinson's disease?

3. What are the clinical manifestations of Parkinson's disease? Place a star next to the symptoms L.C. has mentioned.

4. L.C.'s wife asks you, "How do the doctors know L.C. has Parkinson's disease? They never did a lot of tests on him." How is the diagnosis of PD made?

5. L.C.'s wife comments "I don't even know which one of his medicines he takes for his Parkinson's." What medications are used for PD?

6. L.C. asks, "If I don't have enough dopamine, then why don't they give me a dopamine pill?" Why can't oral dopamine be given as replacement therapy?

7. Levodopa is always given in combination with carbidopa. Why?

8. What is the current recommended nutritional management for Parkinson's?

9. L.C.'s wife is getting their belongings together to leave when she asks, "They can do surgery for everything else, why can't they do surgery to fix Parkinson's?" What types of surgical treatments are available for patients with PD?

10. What are 3 interventions that should be implemented in caring for L.C.?

11. You are a Case Manager. Identify six things that you would assess to determine if L.C. could be cared for in his home.

Case Study 4

Name ____________________ Class/Group __________ Date __________

Group Members ____

INSTRUCTIONS: All questions apply to this case study. Your responses should be brief and to the point. Adequate space has been provided for answers. When asked to provide several answers, they should be listed in order of priority or significance. Do not asume information that is not provided. Please print or write clearly. If your response is not legible, it will be marked as ? and you will need to rewrite it.

Scenario

It is early morning and N.T., a 79-year-old woman, is getting out of bed. She has a mild headache over the right temple, is fatigued, and feels slightly weak. She calls for her husband to let him know she will be going back to bed for a while. When her husband comes in to check her he finds that she is having trouble saying words and has a slight left-sided facial droop. When he helps her up from the bedside, he notices weakness in her left hand and convinces her to go to the local ED (Emergency Department). Her first CT (computed tomography) scan was negative for CVA (cerebrovascular accident); however, the second CT scan (18 hours later) reveals a small CVA in the right hemisphere. She is still experiencing expressive aphasia, left facial droop, left-sided hemiparesis, and what is presumed to be symptoms of mild dysphagia. Her PMH (past medical history) includes paroxysmal A-fib (atrial fibrillation), HTN (hypertension), hyperlipidemia, and a remote Hx (history) of DVT (deep vein thrombosis). A recent cardiac stress test was normal and her blood pressure has been well controlled. She admits to being under recent stress with the death of her husband's adult son. She is hospitalized for 4 days and discharged with orders for outpatient rehabilitation for speech and physical therapy. Medications prior to CVA were flecanide, HRT (hormone replacement therapy), amlodipine (Norvasc), aspirin, simvastatin (Zocor), and trandolopril (Mavik). She is discharged on flecanide, amlodipine, clopidogrel (Plavix), aspirin, simvastatin, and trandolopril.

1. What other information would be necessary for evaluating the *cause* for the CVA?

2. If her deficits are temporary, how long might it take before they are completely reversed?

3. Why was N.T. placed on clopidogrel post-CVA?

4. Why was the initial CT scan negative for stroke?

5. N.T. is not on HRT (hormone replacement therapy) post-CVA, why would this medication be discontinued?

6. Is there any benefit from continuing simvastatin after her CVA?

7. Is there treatment that can be initiated in the ED to stop a CVA from progressing?

8. Your coworker states, "I always heard that paroxysmal atrial fibrillation is a precursor to stroke." Is this statement true or false?

9. Which of the following is *not* a symptom of CVA:
   A. Headache
   B. Lethargy
   C. Lumbar pain
   D. Blurred vision

10. As you walk into the nurses' station, the charge nurse is talking to N.T.'s doctor. She ordered a modified barium swallow study and referral for speech-language pathologist, OT (occupational therapist) and RD (registered dietitian). Give the rationale for these orders.

11. What lab test may be abnormal during CVA?

12. N.T's blood pressure should be well controlled. What BP (blood pressure) level should be considered normal for her based on the Seventh Report of the Joint National Committee on Prevention, Detection, Evaluation, and Treatment of High Blood Pressure (JNC 7)?

Case Study 5

Name ______________________ Class/Group __________ Date __________

Group Members ____

INSTRUCTIONS: All questions apply to this case study. Your responses should be brief and to the point. Adequate space has been provided for answers. When asked to provide several answers, they should be listed in order of priority or significance. Do not asume information that is not provided. Please print or write clearly. If your response is not legible, it will be marked as ? and you will need to rewrite it.

Scenario

T.H. is a 55-year-old male with an 8 month Hx of progressive muscle weakness. Initially, he tripped over things and seemed to drop everything. He never wanted to do anything because he was always exhausted. He sought medical assistance when his speech became slurred and he started to drool. During his initial evaluation the MD noted frequent, severe muscle cramps, muscle twitching, and inappropriate and uncontrollable periods of laughter. After a lengthy period of diagnostic tests, T.H. received the diagnosis of ALS (amyotrophic lateral sclerosis). He is very upset and bewildered about this disease that he's "never even heard of." You are a home health nurse who is seeing T.H. for the first time.

1. How would you explain ALS to T.H.?

2. Who gets ALS?

3. How common is ALS?

4. P.C. has many questions. P.C. asks you, "How long can I expect to live?" How should you respond?

5. P.C. asks, "Will I slowly lose my mind?"

6. P.C. then asks, "Are there any treatments?"

ALS is a very difficult disease to diagnose. No one test or procedure can definitively establish the diagnosis of ALS. Often the diagnosis is made after ruling out other diseases that mimic ALS.

7. What diagnostic tests can be done to make the diagnosis of ALS?

8. Because ALS affects so many body systems, you will be working with many disciplines. For each discipline, define the role these workers would play in P.C.'s treatment.

9. You hold a family meeting to recruit adequate help for the caregiver (usually patient's spouse or child). Why is this important?

10. P.C. asks you, "How will the end probably come for me?" What should you tell him?

11. How can you advise him to prepare for possible pneumonia or respiratory failure?

Case Study 6

Name ______________________ Class/Group __________ Date __________

Group Members ____

INSTRUCTIONS: All questions apply to this case study. Your responses should be brief and to the point. Adequate space has been provided for answers. When asked to provide several answers, they should be listed in order of priority or significance. Do not asume information that is not provided. Please print or write clearly. If your response is not legible, it will be marked as ? and you will need to rewrite it.

Scenario

J.B. is a 58-year-old retired postal worker who has been on your floor for several days receiving plasmapheresis qod for myasthenia gravis (MG). Before this admission, he had been relatively healthy. His medical Hx includes HTN controlled with verapamil and glaucoma treated with timolol (ophthalmic preparation). About a year ago, J.B. started experiencing difficulty chewing and swallowing, diplopia, and slurring of speech, at which time he was placed on pyridostigmine (Mestinon). Recently J.B. was diagnosed with a sinus infection and treated with ciprofloxacin. On admission, J.B. was unable to bear any weight or take fluids through a straw. There have been periods of exacerbation and remission since admission.

1. J.B.'s wife asks you, "What may have caused my husband to get worse?" What explanation should you give her?

2. You are visiting with J.B.'s wife, who tells you she doesn't have a lot of information about MG and she would like to know more about it so that she will feel more comfortable talking to her husband. What should you tell her?

3. The wife asks you to explain what to look for in MG. What should you tell her?

4. J.B.'s wife asks how this disease is diagnosed. "How do they know that my husband has myasthenia gravis?" What should you tell her?

5. J.B.'s wife asks, "What are some options for treatment of MG?" How should you explain the different treatments?

6. List four factors that could predispose J.B. to an exacerbation of his illness.

7. J.B.'s wife asks what the doctors and nurses watch for while her husband is in the hospital. How should you explain these activities?

8. J.B.'s wife wants to know when he will be able to go home. How should you respond?

9. J.B.'s wife asks you what information she will need before taking her husband home. How should you explain this to her?

10. J.B.'s wife asks you, "What is the difference between cholinergic crisis and myasthenic crisis?" What explanation should you give her?

11. What supportive measures can you suggest to J.B.'s wife that she can undertake or arrange on behalf of her husband?

Bonus Question: Which institute under the National Institutes of Health (NIH) is primarily responsible for MG information and research?

Note: Another excellent source of information is:
Myasthenia Gravis Foundation of America
123 W. Madison Street
Suite 800
Chicago, IL 60602
Telephone: (800) 541-5454 Fax: (312) 853-0523
E-mail: *info-request@myasthenia.org*

Case Study 7

Name ________________ Class/Group ________ Date ________

Group Members ________________________________

INSTRUCTIONS: All questions apply to this case study. Your responses should be brief and to the point. Adequate space has been provided for answers. When asked to provide several answers, they should be listed in order of priority or significance. Do not asume information that is not provided. Please print or write clearly. If your response is not legible, it will be marked as ? and you will need to rewrite it.

Scenario

You have been asked to see D.V. in the neurologic clinic. D.V. has been referred by his internist, who thinks his patient is having symptoms of multiple sclerosis (MS). D.V. is a 25-year-old man who has experienced increasing urinary frequency and urgency over the past 2 months. Because his female partner was treated for an STD (sexually transmitted disease), D.V. also underwent treatment, but the symptoms did not resolve. D.V. has also recently had two brief episodes of eye "fuzziness" associated with diplopia and brightness. He has noticed ascending numbness and weakness of the R arm with inability to hold objects over the past few days. Now he reports rapid progression of weakness in his legs.

1. MS is an inflammatory disorder of the nervous system causing scattered, patchy demyelinization of the CNS (central nervous system). What does myelin do? What is demyelinization?

2. MS is characterized by remissions and exacerbations. What happens to the myelin during each of these phases?

3. Isn't D.V. too young to get MS? What is the etiology?

4. What assessment data from the case study caused the physician to suspect a possible diagnosis of MS?

Diagnostic tests are often done to R/O other disorders with similar symptoms. A diagnosis will be made when other disorders have been R/O, when the patient has two or more exacerbations, when there is slow, steady progression, and when the patient has two or more areas of demyelinization or plaque formation.

5. What are four common diagnostic tests you can begin to teach D.V. about?

6. D.V. asks you, "If this turns out to be MS, what is the treatment?"

7. As part of your teaching plan, you want D.V. to be aware of situations or factors that are known to cause an exacerbation of symptoms. List four.

8. The National Multiple Sclerosis Society (800-344-4867), http://www.nmss.org, Third Ave, 6th Floor, New York, NY 10017-3288, and the Multiple Sclerosis Association of America (800-833-4MSA), *http://www.msaa.com*, are great resources for D.V. List several resources available in the community that D.V. may find helpful.

D.V. confides in you that he has been very depressed since his parent's divorce and the onset of these symptoms. He tells you that he knows his girlfriend hasn't been faithful, but he's afraid of living alone. He's afraid if he tells her about his M.S. diagnosis, she'll leave him.

9. What are you going to do with this information?

10. In view of his personal history and current diagnosis, what two critical psychosocial issues are you going to monitor in his follow-up visits?

D.V. takes advantage of his time with the psychiatric nurse specialist, joins a local MS support group, and tells his girlfriend to move out. He later marries a woman from the support group.

Case Study 8

Name ________________ Class/Group ________ Date ________

Group Members ________________

INSTRUCTIONS: All questions apply to this case study. Your responses should be brief and to the point. Adequate space has been provided for answers. When asked to provide several answers, they should be listed in order of priority or significance. Do not asume information that is not provided. Please print or write clearly. If your response is not legible, it will be marked as ? and you will need to rewrite it.

Scenario

J.G. is a 34-year-old P1G1 (para 1, gravida 1) woman who underwent an emergency cesarean delivery after a prolonged labor, during which she exhibited a sudden change in neurologic functioning and started seizing. Since that time, she has experienced three tonic-clonic (grand mal) seizures. She was diagnosed as having a basal ganglion hematoma with infarct and was started on phenytoin. Postdelivery, J.G. demonstrated dyskinesia, resulting in frequent falls during ambulation. Once the seizure disorder appeared to be under control, she was transferred to a rehabilitation facility for evaluation, and 2 weeks of intensive PT (physical therapy). She is now home, where she is doing quite well but still has occasional falls and is receiving PT 3 times a week in her home. She remains on phenytoin and has had no seizures since her release from the rehabilitation facility. As case manager for J.G.'s HMO, you make a home visit with her and her family for evaluation of long-term, follow-up care.

1. A seizure is not a disease in itself but a symptom of a disease. What is the term for chronically recurring seizures?

2. Does J.G. have epilepsy?

3. The three main phases of a seizure are the preictal, ictal, and postictal. Differentiate between the three phases, and list clinical symptoms you may observe when a patient is having a seizure.

4. What is the pathophysiology of a seizure?

5. J.G. had grand mal, or tonic-clonic, seizures. Describe this type of seizure. List five other types of seizures.

6. Some patients know they are about to have a seizure. What is this preseizure warning called, and what form does it take?

7. Besides the brain injury, what are some other possible conditions that could be contributing to J.G's lowered seizure threshold?

8. List five different classifications of antiseizure medications.

9. J.G.'s husband comes to visit and asks you what he should do if she has a seizure at home. What do you tell him?

10. Her husband states that he is afraid for J.G. to take care of the baby. What would you say to him?

11. J.G.'s husband tells you that his wife is not good at remembering to take medication. What are some strategies that you should review with J.G. and her husband to increase the likelihood of compliance?

12. J.G. asks, "If I get my blood level under control, will it stay at the same level as long as I take my medicine?" How would you answer her question?

13. J.G.'s husband asks whether the drugs could harm his wife in any way. What general information would you give them about anticonvulsants?

14. J.G.'s husband says, "I was watching *ER* last night, and they showed this guy who just kept on having a seizure. That doctor had to give him lots of medicine before he came out of it." How would you explain status epilepticus and why is it a medical emergency?

Optional Project: Look up the Medic-Alert website, and plan a 10-minute presentation for patients/consumers/families on the importance of people with seizure disorders wearing standardized identification. Include instructions on cost, benefits, and how they can get Medic-Alert identification.

For additional information contact:

Medic-Alert
2323 Colorado Avenue
Turlock, CA 95382
Telephone: (800) 432-5378
Website: http://www.medicalert.org

Case Study 9

Name ______________________ Class/Group __________ Date __________

Group Members ____

INSTRUCTIONS: All questions apply to this case study. Your responses should be brief and to the point. Adequate space has been provided for answers. When asked to provide several answers, they should be listed in order of priority or significance. Do not asume information that is not provided. Please print or write clearly. If your response is not legible, it will be marked as ? and you will need to rewrite it.

Scenario

You are assigned to take care of M.X. on this evening's shift. In report you are told that she is a 40-year-old obese (112 kg) woman who arose from a sitting position and experienced acute and severe low back pain 3 weeks ago. She was diagnosed with herniated disks L4-L5 and L5-S1. Dr. W., who performed a lumbar laminectomy 3 days ago, is concerned because her WBC count has gone from 8100/cmm to 19,600/cmm.

1. What is meant by the term *herniated disk (herniated nucleus pulposus)*?

2. What tests may be performed to detect and diagnose the herniation?

3. What is a laminectomy?

4. Identify two general objectives of postoperative nursing care of M.X.?

5. What is meant by "log-rolling"?

6. You ask four coworkers to help you log-roll M.X. As one nurse enters the room she makes a statement about breaking her back trying to move M.X. You are a little overweight yourself and watch M.X.'s face when she hears the remark. How would you handle the situation?

7. Patients who have undergone a lumbar laminectomy frequently experience paralytic ileus and urinary retention. Why?

8. What are two possible sources of infection that may account for M.X.'s elevated WBC count?

9. M.X. asks you how you would know if her wound were infected. Differentiate between signs and symptoms of wound infection for M.X.

10. Discharge planning should begin the day M.X. is admitted to your unit. What factors should discharge planning include?

11. List seven written home care instructions that should be reviewed and given to M.X. before discharge.

M.X. is treated with aggressive antibiotic therapy for a UTI (urinary tract infection). With the help and support of her family, she is discharged home where she makes a complete recovery. After referral for consultation with a medical nutritionist, M.X. starts on a healthy low-fat diet and loses 21 lb over the next 9 months. When you were arranging her discharge papers, you discovered that M.X. was a scriptwriter for soap operas. Six months after her discharge, she calls to meet you for coffee. She asks whether you would like to supplement your income by consulting with her on realistically presenting the role of nurses in soap operas. She said it was your professionalism that gave her this idea.

Case Study 10

Name ________________________ Class/Group __________ Date __________

Group Members ____

INSTRUCTIONS: All questions apply to this case study. Your responses should be brief and to the point. Adequate space has been provided for answers. When asked to provide several answers, they should be listed in order of priority or significance. Do not asume information that is not provided. Please print or write clearly. If your response is not legible, it will be marked as ? and you will need to rewrite it.

Scenario

F.N. is a 57-year-old housewife, happily married with grown children, and two new grandchildren. F.N. made an appointment with her optometrist to explore a progressive OS (L eye) visual loss over a 9-month period. Her eye exam was essentially normal, and the optometrist referred her to a neurologist. After work-up, a 2.5-cm brain mass was found, and surgery was scheduled. Her only PMH (past medical history) is hypertension, for which she takes long-acting nifedipine (Procardia XL) 60 mg qd. Her PSH (past surgical history) includes T&A (tonsilectomy and adnoidectomy) as a child, cholecystectomy, and a TAH (total abdominal hysterectomy) at age 42. She also takes a conjugated estrogen (Premarin) 0.625 mg qd.

1. Name four tests that can be done to evaluate for brain tumor.

There is no standardized, universally accepted system of classifying brain tumors. They can be classified according to histologic basis, intraaxial vs. extraaxial, or malignant vs. benign.

2. Using the term *benign* when discussing brain tumors is somewhat misleading. Why?

3. Onset of neurologic symptoms is usually insidious, and they exhibit symptoms in relation to the area of the brain where the tumor is located. List six general symptoms associated with many brain tumors.

4. Dexamethasone (Decadron) is commonly prescribed when a tumor is diagnosed and the presence of IICP is demonstrated. It is administered preoperatively and postoperatively, and in conjunction with radiation and chemotherapy. Why is dexamethasone prescribed, and why should it not be abruptly stopped?

5. Other common supportive medications include antiseizure, diuretics, H_2 blockers, analgesics, antiemetics, antidepressants, and osmotic diuretic. Indicate why each is used.

6. Once the diagnosis is made, the patient and family must be involved in the plan for treatment. Treatment depends on the type and location of the tumor and can include surgery, radiation, chemotherapy, or any combination of these. The patient also has the right to refuse treatment. Identify four other considerations the medical team, patient, and family will consider in devising a treatment plan.

7. Describe common responses to a diagnosis of a brain tumor.

8. F.N. draws up a living will and health care power of attorney after she hears the diagnosis. She also sits down with her family and makes her wishes known. Why is this important for F.N. in particular and for everyone in general?

9. You enter F.N.'s room to take VS and she says, "What if I come out of surgery and I'm different? Or what if I die? My grandbabies will never know me." You hear the concern in her voice. Suggest several ways that F.N. can communicate with her loved ones in the event that her surgery is unsuccessful.

11. F.N. has the surgery and is admitted to ICU (intensive care unit) postoperatively. She does very well and remains neurologically intact (qh neurologic checks). Her BP is slightly elevated (147/68); the rest of her VS are normal; she has two peripheral IVs, TED hose, O_2 at 4 L/NC (nasal cannula), and a Foley. Postoperatively, F.N.'s K level drops to 2.7 mmol/L, and glucose is 202 mg/dL. Describe possible reasons why these two laboratory values are abnormal, and identify what treatment will be ordered to correct each.

F.N. did suffer mild neurologic damage as a result of the surgery. She was discharged to a rehabilitation facility, and eventually recovered most of her lost function. She continues to enjoy an active life and has become involved in helping others facing similar experiences.

For additional information contact:

The Brain Injury Association Inc.
105 North Alfred Street
Alexandria, VA 22314
Telephone: (703) 236-6000

Case Study 11

Name ______________________ Class/Group __________ Date __________

Group Members ____

INSTRUCTIONS: All questions apply to this case study. Your responses should be brief and to the point. Adequate space has been provided for answers. When asked to provide several answers, they should be listed in order of priority or significance. Do not asume information that is not provided. Please print or write clearly. If your response is not legible, it will be marked as ? and you will need to rewrite it.

Scenario

T.W. is a 22-year-old man who fell 50 ft from a chairlift while skiing and landed on hard-packed snow. He was found to have a T10-T11 fracture with paraplegia. He was initially admitted to the SICU (Surgical Intensive Care Unit) and placed on high-dose steroids for 24 hours. He was taken to surgery 48 hours post accident for spinal stabilization. He spent 2 additional days in the SICU, 5 days on the neurologic unit, and now is ready to be transferred to your rehab unit. He continues to have no movement of his lower extremities.

1. The goal of treatment in the acute phase of spinal cord injury (SCI) is to help T.W. survive the injury and maintain physiologic stability through the period of spinal shock. Once the acute phase is over, T.W. moves into the postacute and early rehabilitation phases. What are the treatment goals for T.W. in these phases?

2. Considering a hierarchy of rehabilitative needs for patients like T.W., number the following from highest (1) to lowest (5) priority.
   __ Community integration and employment
   __ Accomplishment of self-care and ADLs
   __ Self-actualization
   __ Stabilization of the physiologic systems
   __ Adjustment to living at home

3. T.W. receives high-dose steroid therapy every 24 hours; then he is placed on a smaller maintenance dose. What effect will steroids have on T.W.?

4. List three critical potential infections that T.W. should be monitored for throughout his hospitalization.

A person with an SCI at the T10-12 level should be independent in a wheelchair and able to manage ADLs, including bowel and bladder care.

5. T.W. is taking vitamin C 250 mg PO bid. What is the purpose of this?

You request a consultation with an RD (registered dietitian) because you realize that T.W. needs proteins for healing; however, too much protein can stress his kidneys. The RD will adjust his diet to ensure adequate amount of protein, carbohydrates, calcium, magnesium, and zinc.

6. Rehabilitation teaching includes teaching T.W. how to manage his urinary drainage system. What would this teaching include?

7. What is the usual amount of time for the return of reflex function of the bladder?

8. The large bowel musculature has its own neural center that can directly respond to distention caused by fecal material. This is what allows most SCI patients to regain bowel control. What dietary instructions are important for T.W.?

9. T.W. should also be taught bowel training techniques. What would this teaching include?

10. What medications can assist with a bowel program?

11. Describe digital stimulation.

12. T.W. asks you whether he'll ever be able to have sex again. What do you tell him, and what are some possible referrals?

For patients with lesions at T6 or above, there is the potential for AD (autonomic dysreflexia). Noxious stimulus below the level of injury triggers the sympathetic nervous system, causing massive release of catecholamines producing vasoconstriction. The patient develops severe hypertension (as high as 240–300/150 mm Hg), pounding headache, bradycardia, blurred vision, nausea, nasal congestion, and flushing and sweating above the level of the injury and goose bumps or pallor below the level of the injury. Potential causes include bladder distention, obstruction, infection, spasms, catheterization, and bladder irrigations done too fast or with cold fluid; bowel constipation, impaction, or rectal stimulation; and alterations in skin integrity including pressure, infection, injury, and cold or hot. AD can cause retinal hemorrhage, CVA, and seizure activity.

13. What are interventions R/T AD?

For additional information, contact:

National Spinal Cord Injury Association
Telephone: (800) 962-9629
E-mail: *resource@spinalcord.org*

Case Study 12

Name ________________ Class/Group ________ Date ________

Group Members ________________________________

INSTRUCTIONS: All questions apply to this case study. Your responses should be brief and to the point. Adequate space has been provided for answers. When asked to provide several answers, they should be listed in order of priority or significance. Do not asume information that is not provided. Please print or write clearly. If your response is not legible, it will be marked as ? and you will need to rewrite it.

Scenario

G.B.'s family reports that he has had progressive back pain since his decompression laminectomy 4 months ago and is now unable to walk. He has become increasingly confused over the past 2 weeks, has occasional SOB (shortness of breath), and is now unable to care for himself. He looks dehydrated and possibly septic. G.B. is very angry at being brought to the hospital and states, "I had this back worked on 4 months ago and I don't intend to have it done again!" G.B. is 72 years old and has had multiple health problems including GI hemorrhages, hypertension (HTN), elevated glucose, chronic lymphocytic leukemia (CLL), a remote history of kidney stones, an appendectomy, shrapnel from the Korean war, and a fracture (fx) of the R femur from a mining accident. His family reports that G.B. was allergic to penicillin as a child but cannot remember what reaction he experienced.

1. Based on the previous information, review the following list of admission orders. Place an "I" by each inappropriate order and state why it is inappropriate.

 ___ Routine VS
 ___ Routine neurologic checks
 ___ Up ad lib
 ___ CBC with diff, BMP (basic metabolic panel), UA (urinalysis), ABG, PT/INR and PTT
 ___ O_2 to keep Sao_2 greater than 90%
 ___ IV D_5½NS with 20 mEq of KCl/L at 100 mL/h
 ___ NPO
 ___ Cefazolin (Kefzol, Ancef) 1 g IV q8h
 ___ Ranitidine (Zantac) 50 mg IV q8h
 ___ Codeine 30 mg IM q4–6h prn for pain
 ___ Droperidol (Inapsine) 0.25 mL IV q8h prn for nausea
 ___ Acetaminophen (Tylenol) 650 mg PO q4–6h prn for fever

2. Admission VS are 165/85, 76, 20, 36.7°C. Do any of the VS concern you? Explain.

3. You get the following lab results: Na 132 mmol/L, K 3.7 mmol/L, Cl 98 mmol/L, CO_2 27 mmol/L, BUN 13 mg/dL, creatinine 0.6 mg/dL, glucose 138 mg/dL, WBC 36,000/cmm, Hgb 10.8 g/dL, Hct 31.3%, platelets 130,000/cmm. You call the physician to report them. What orders do you anticipate in regard to a change in IV solution?

4. What part of G.B.'s PMH is consistent with the CBC results?

5. What noninvasive diagnostic test might be done to determine G.B.'s problem?

6. Why would an MRI be contraindicated in G.B.'s case?

7. G.B.'s family had to leave the hospital for a short time. When you enter his room, you find him trying to climb over the side rails. What should you consider before applying a vest (Posey) or wrist restraints?

8. As the afternoon progresses, G.B.'s oxygen saturation decreases from 92% on 2 L O_2/NC to 82%. The physician orders oxygen by mask at 6 L. Name at least three interventions that can help improve his oxygenation status?

9. Diagnostic tests reveal that G.B. has an epidural abscess near his laminectomy incision, and he is scheduled for surgery. G.B. has already stated he does not plan to have any more surgery. Do you feel he is competent to make the decision? How would you proceed with obtaining consent?

The family tells the surgeon to go ahead with the surgery, against G.B.'s wishes. It was decided that he is not competent to make the decision for himself at this time.

10. What are considerations for discharge planning?

Case Study 13

Name ______________________ Class/Group __________ Date __________

Group Members ____

INSTRUCTIONS: All questions apply to this case study. Your responses should be brief and to the point. Adequate space has been provided for answers. When asked to provide several answers, they should be listed in order of priority or significance. Do not asume information that is not provided. Please print or write clearly. If your response is not legible, it will be marked as ? and you will need to rewrite it.

Scenario

Y.W. is a 23-year-old male student from Thailand studying electrical engineering at the university. He was ejected from a moving vehicle, which was traveling 70 mph. His injuries included a severe closed head injury with an occipital hematoma, bilateral wrist fractures, and a R pneumothorax. During his NICU (Neurological Intensive Care Unit) stay, Y.W. was intubated and placed on mechanical ventilation, had a feeding tube inserted and was placed on tube feedings, had a Foley catheter to down drain, and had multiple IVs inserted. He developed pneumonia 1 month after admission.

1. Describe the term *primary head injury.*

2. Describe secondary head injury.

3. Why is IICP so clinically important, and what are five S/S?

4. List four medication classifications and eight nursing measures that the ICU nurses could use to control or decrease the ICP.

5. Y.W.'s medication list includes clindamycin 150 mg per feeding tube q6h, ranitidine (Zantac elixir) 150 mg per feeding tube bid, and phenytoin (Dilantin) 100 mg IVPB (intravenous piggy back) tid. Indicate the reasons for each.

6. A stat portable CXR is ordered after each CVC (central venous catheter) is inserted. According to hospital protocol, no one is permitted to infuse anything through the catheter until the CXR has been read by the physician or radiologist. What is the purpose of the CXR, and why isn't fluid infused through the catheter until after the CXR is read?

Y.W. spent 2 months in acute care and is now on your rehabilitation unit. He follows commands but tends to get very agitated with too much stimulation. His tracheostomy site is well healed, and the pneumonia is finally resolving. He is still receiving supplemental tube feeding and has some continued incontinence of both bowel and bladder. Y.W. has a very supportive group of friends who are students at the university; several of them are also from Thailand.

7. Y.W.'s latest lab results are as follows: Na 149 mmol/L, K 4.2 mmol/L, Cl 119 mmol/L, CO_2 21 mmol/L, BUN 12 mg/dL, creatinine 1.2 mg/dL, glucose 123 mg/dL, WBC 15,400/cmm, Hgb 14.9 g/dL, Hct 36.4%, platelets 140,000/cmm. Are any of these of concern to you, and what would you suggest to correct them?

8. Are you surprised by Y.W.'s agitated behavior? Explain.

9. Outline a general rehabilitation plan for Y.W. based on the above data.

10. Y.W.'s mother has just arrived in the United States and speaks no English. What measures can be taken to facilitate communication between medical personnel and the mother?

11. Y.W.'s mother will need a place to stay while in the United States. What can you do to facilitate the initial contact with the Thai community?

12. What special discharge planning considerations are there in this case?

Case Study 14

Name ______________________ Class/Group __________ Date __________

Group Members ____

INSTRUCTIONS: All questions apply to this case study. Your responses should be brief and to the point. Adequate space has been provided for answers. When asked to provide several answers, they should be listed in order of priority or significance. Do not asume information that is not provided. Please print or write clearly. If your response is not legible, it will be marked as ? and you will need to rewrite it.

Scenario

K.B. is a 21-year-old male, with a PMH of seizure disorder controlled with carbamazepine (Tegretol), was accidentally struck in the head by a pitched baseball while batting in a baseball game. He was unconscious momentarily, about 5 seconds, then awakened and was alert and responsive. After a few hours, K.B. returned home with complaints of a "splitting" headache, drowsiness, slight confusion, and some nausea. K.B. was taken to the local hospital ED (emergency department), where a CT scan revealed a left subdural hematoma. He has been transferred to your medical center, which has a neurosurgeon on call.

1. The ED RN gives you the above information during a phoned report. What other information do you need to prepare for this patient?

2. Because you occasionally have trouble remembering the layers of the brain and different hematomas, you look up subdural hematoma before S.B. arrives. What do you find?

3. K.B.'s subdural hematoma is considered acute because symptoms appeared within 24–48 hours of injury. What are the other classifications of subdural hematomas?

4. What are common S/S of an acute subdural hematoma?

5. Why are the elderly and alcoholics at risk for chronic subdural hematomas?

6. What neurologic changes and indicators would you monitor in K.B. for IICP?

7. Why is it especially important to make sure K.B. is taking his carbamazepine and has a therapeutic serum level?

8. The decision was made, in K.B.'s case, not to do a craniotomy. When would a neurosurgeon decide to treat medically vs. perform surgery?

9. Burr holes usually are effective in treating acute subdural hematomas, while a craniotomy is often performed for subacute and chronic subdural hematomas. Why?

10. Why would hypotonic IV solutions such as D_5W be avoided in K.B.?

11. How would you position K.B. in bed in order to help control ICP?

12. What other interventions would be appropriate to implement in the care of K.B.?

Goal: All therapies are directed toward decreasing ICP and preventing deterioration of neurologic status.

13. K.B.'s LOC started to decrease. What information would you provide to the neurosurgeon when you call?

14. How would you provide support to the family?

15. The neurosurgeon has ordered codeine IV as a pain medication. Why did he order codeine instead of another narcotic?

Case Study 15

Name ______________________ Class/Group __________ Date __________

Group Members ____

INSTRUCTIONS: All questions apply to this case study. Your responses should be brief and to the point. Adequate space has been provided for answers. When asked to provide several answers, they should be listed in order of priority or significance. Do not asume information that is not provided. Please print or write clearly. If your response is not legible, it will be marked as ? and you will need to rewrite it.

Scenario

C.J. is a 22-year-old concert pianist and is scheduled to perform tonight. Before her performance, she told a friend that she was experiencing what she called "the worst headache I've ever had." She decides that she must perform despite the pain and she takes 2 ES (extra strength) Tylenol. During her performance, she stops playing, reaches up to grasp her head, then she falls unconscious. When the paramedics arrive, she is intubated, an IV is started with NS, and her ECG reveals a sinus tachycardia.

Upon arrival to the ED, she has a Glascow Coma Scale score of 3. Her husband reports a history of hypertension but states she recently quit taking her medication because it made her feel tired. She is trying to quit smoking; she has cut down to ½ PPD (pack per day), and has a remote history of cocaine use. He says that she has complained of worsening, intermittent headaches for the past few weeks.

1. What is the Glasgow Coma Scale?

2. What is a subarachnoid hemorrhage (SAH)?

3. What are the causes of a SAH?

4. How is the diagnosis of SAH made?

5. How are SAHs graded?

6. What kinds of aneurysms cause SAH?

Once the CT scan is done on C.J., the diagnosis of SAH is made and she is transported to the ICU and closely monitored.

7. What are two main problems closely associated with SAH?

8. Identify the treatment given after SAH.

9. What is the recommended treatment for SAH?

10. What considerations should be made for patients with SAH?

Case Study 16

Name ________________________ Class/Group __________ Date __________

Group Members ____

INSTRUCTIONS: All questions apply to this case study. Your responses should be brief and to the point. Adequate space has been provided for answers. When asked to provide several answers, they should be listed in order of priority or significance. Do not asume information that is not provided. Please print or write clearly. If your response is not legible, it will be marked as ? and you will need to rewrite it.

Scenario

D.H., a 54-year-old resort owner, has multiple chronic medical problems including type 2 DM for 25 years, which has progressed to insulin-dependent DM for the past 10 years; a renal transplant 5 years ago with no signs of rejection at last biopsy; HTN; and remote peptic ulcer disease (PUD). His medications include insulin, immunosuppressive agents, and two antihypertensive drugs. He visited his local physician with C/O L ear, mastoid, and sinus pain. He was diagnosed with sinusitis and *Candida albicans* infection (thrush); cephalexin and nystatin were prescribed. Later that evening he developed N/V, hematemesis, and weakness, and he was taken to the ED. He was admitted and started on IV antibiotics, but his condition worsened throughout the night; his dyspnea increased and he developed difficulty speaking. He was flown to your tertiary referral center and was intubated en route. On arrival, D.H. had decreased LOC with periods of total unresponsiveness, weakness, and cranial nerve deficits. His diagnosis is meningitis complicated by an aspiration pneumonia and atrial fibrillation. D.H. has continued fever and leukocytosis despite aggressive antibiotic therapy.

1. Why is D.H. at particular risk for infection?

2. Describe bacterial meningitis.

3. What is the probable route of entry of bacteria into D.H.'s brain?

4. How do you think D.H. might have developed an aspiration pneumonia?

5. What factors influenced the physicians' decision to transport D.H. from a smaller hospital to a tertiary referral center?

6. Name four tests that could be used in the diagnosis of meningitis.

7. D.H. is taking the following medications: NPH insulin and sliding-scale regular insulin, sucralfate, azathioprine, imipenem methylprednisolone, digoxin, and metronidazole. Indicate why he is receiving each medication.

8. The lab just called you with a glucose result of 350 mg/dL. Identify three factors that could contribute to D.H.'s elevated glucose level.

9. List seven interventions for management of D.H.'s current problems.

10. List six interventions given to prevent complications.

11. D.H.'s family is staying at a nearby motel. His adult son brings his mother to the hospital. Mrs. H. says she just wants to stay with her husband around the clock. She states, "I took care of him for 35 years now, and I'm not going to abandon him now when he needs me the most." How would you respond?

Note: These are stressful times for all individuals involved. Anything nurses can do to help alleviate the stress contributes to the well-being of patients and families. In these situations, you might consider asking if the family would like to talk with a spiritual counselor.

D.H.'s infection destroyed his cadaver kidney. He developed MSOF (multiple system organ failure) and died 7 weeks later.

Case Study 17

Name ______________________ Class/Group ___________ Date ___________

Group Members ____

INSTRUCTIONS: All questions apply to this case study. Your responses should be brief and to the point. Adequate space has been provided for answers. When asked to provide several answers, they should be listed in order of priority or significance. Do not asume information that is not provided. Please print or write clearly. If your response is not legible, it will be marked as ? and you will need to rewrite it.

Scenario

S.B. is a 17-year-old male who lost control of his SUV (sport utility vehicle) and struck a tree. Witnesses reported he was not restrained and his face hit the windshield on impact. When paramedics arrived S.B. was responsive but confused, had significant facial swelling, and C/O pain in his right wrist and left forearm. The paramedics initiated C-spine precautions, strapped him to a backboard, started O_2 @ 15 L/min via a nonrebreather mask, and started a 16-gauge IV with 0.9% NS. VS: 120/75, 125, 36, Sao_2 94%. On arrival to the local ED 5 minutes later his VS were 110/62, 110, R 28–32 and shallow, 99%. An additional 16-gauge IV was inserted and the following labs were drawn: CBC, type and screen, CMP, PT/PTT INR, and ETOH level. The trauma physician completed a head to toe assessment and found the following: Obeys commands, responds to voice but not oriented to time or place. Generalized facial edema with full-thickness 2-cm cheek laceration and bilateral mandibular depressed fractures. Blood behind L TM (tympanic membrane), edema with slight discoloration over L mastoid process. Mid to upper chest contusions W/O crepitus, breath sounds clear. Abdomen slightly firm, nontender. Catheterized for 500 mL clear yellow urine, Neg for blood, glucose, ketones. Positive deformity of R wrist and diffuse tenderness L lower forearm.

1. S.B.'s skull x-ray was negative for basilar skull fracture. How significant is this finding?

2. On arrival, S.B. had slight discoloration over L mastoid process, and blood behind the L tympanic membrane. What is the significance of this finding?

3. Why did S.B. have edema with slight discoloration and not ecchymosis over the mastoid process?

4. Identify two complications associated with basilar skull fracture?

5. Why is a dural tear likely to produce a CSF leak?

6. The term “raccoon eyes” is frequently used when describing someone who has a BSF. Explain the term “raccoon eyes.”

7. What is the most reliable diagnostic indicator for basilar skull fracture?

8. How would you test S.B. for evidence of CSF leakage?

9. Identify the most serious complication of basilar skull fracture?

10. What are the symptoms of an anterior fossa fracture (fracture of the paranasal sinuses)?

11. What are the symptoms of a posterior fossa fracture (fracture of temporal petrous bone)?

12. S.B. is suspected of having a BSF. Why don't you want to place an NGT (nasogastric tube) in S.B.?

13. What is the treatment strategy for a BSF with a *limited* CSF leak?

14. Acetazolamide (Diamox) is a medication often prescribed with those requiring continued observation after BSF. Why is this medication prescribed?

15. Which cranial nerves are most likely to be affected by a BSF?

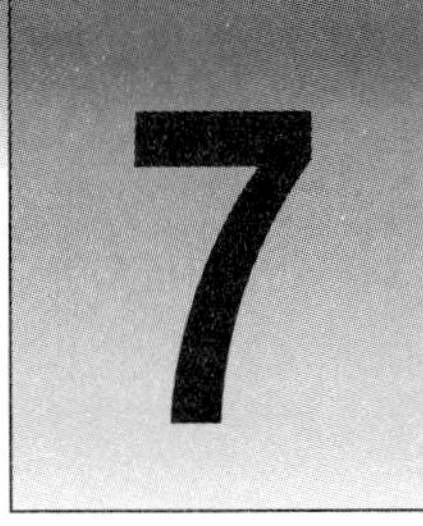

Endocrine Disorders

Case Study 1

Name ________________ Class/Group ________ Date ________

Group Members ________________

INSTRUCTIONS: All questions apply to this case study. Your responses should be brief and to the point. Adequate space has been provided for answers. When asked to provide several answers, they should be listed in order of priority or significance. Do not asume information that is not provided. Please print or write clearly. If your response is not legible, it will be marked as ? and you will need to rewrite it.

Scenario

E.H. is a 60-year-old woman who has rheumatoid arthritis. For the past 12 years, she has been taking prednisone 40 mg daily, and NSAIDs (nonsteroidal antiinflammatory drugs) to control her disease and symptoms. As a result of her autoimmune disorder and long-term steroid use, E.H. has adrenal insufficiency and osteoporosis. The physician adjusts her steroid dosage for replacement therapy. You are asked to conduct educational sessions designed to teach E.H. about her condition and the treatment she needs.

1. E.H. states she doesn't understand how her taking steroids has caused her body to lose its ability to produce the "the real thing." How would you explain this paradox in terms she can understand?

2. People receiving steroid replacement should be taught S/S that signal the dosage is too low. What are the S/S of inadequate steroid replacement?

3. What would the RD (registered dietitian) teach someone like E.H. about the nutritional implications of adrenal insufficiency?

4. E.H. confides in you that she is afraid of taking steroids any longer because she has read about the deleterious effects of steroid abuse by athletes. How would you counter this misconception and alleviate E.H.'s concern?

5. How would teaching differ for this patient (on replacement therapy) as compared with teaching required for the patient taking therapeutic doses of glucocorticoids?

6. The patient states she is under a lot of stress because of her son's recent diagnosis of cancer and her husband's upcoming retirement. What are the teaching implications of this information?

7. You realize that taking exogenous cortisol can result in a variety of pathophysiologic alterations often described as Cushing's syndrome. Because E.H. will be taking lifelong steroids, would you expect to see the S/S associated with Cushing's syndrome in this individual? Explain your answer.

8. What S/S should you teach E.H. to monitor that would indicate excessive cortisol therapy?

9. You instruct E.H. on administration of a parenteral form of hydrocortisone. Under what circumstances should she take the parenteral form of the drug?

10. What measures should E.H. take to prevent an acute episode of adrenal insufficiency?

11. E.H. tells you she never used to take pills at all. She says she hates to be "addicted to a drug." What will you tell her?

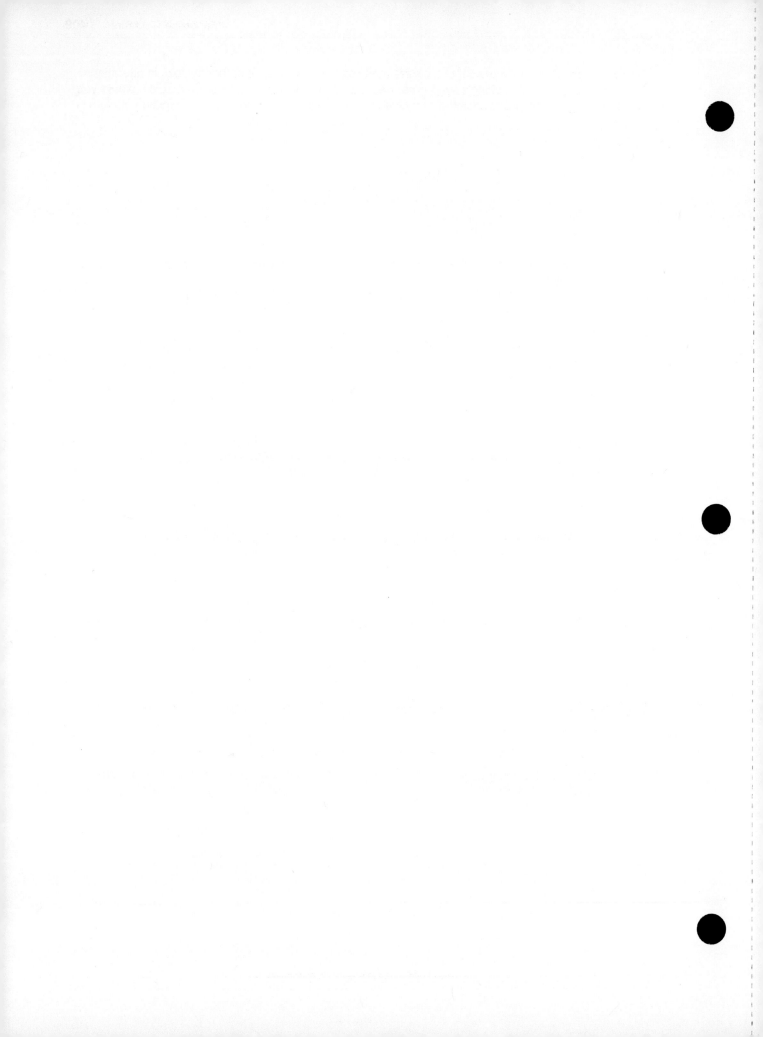

Case Study 2

Name ______________________________ Class/Group __________ Date __________

Group Members ____

INSTRUCTIONS: All questions apply to this case study. Your responses should be brief and to the point. Adequate space has been provided for answers. When asked to provide several answers, they should be listed in order of priority or significance. Do not asume information that is not provided. Please print or write clearly. If your response is not legible, it will be marked as ? and you will need to rewrite it.

Scenario

You are working as a RN in a large women's clinic. A 24-year-old Asian female arrives for her regularly scheduled obstetric appointment. She is in her 26th week of pregnancy and is a primigravida. After examining the patient, the nurse midwife tells you to schedule Y.L. for a 50-g glucose challenge. You review Y.L.'s chart and note she is 5′3″, weighs 143 lb, and her BMI (body mass index) is 25. Her father has type 2 diabetes, and both paternal grandparents had type 2 diabetes. You enter the room to talk to Y.L.

1. You instruct Y.L. to drink a 50-g solution of glucose and have her blood drawn 1 hour after ingesting the solution. What is the purpose of a 50-g glucose challenge?

2. The results came back from the lab. Y.L.'s blood sugar was 151 mg/dL. What does this mean?

Based on the elevated screening test, Y.L. was scheduled for a 100-g glucose load. The lab results are as follows:

Time of Test	Patient Value	Normal Value
Fasting:	101 mg/dL	<95 mg/dL
1 hour	193 mg/dL	<180 mg/dL
2 hour	132 mg/dL	<155 mg/dL
3 hour	111 mg/dL	<140 mg/dL

3. Y.L. had an elevated fasting and 1-hour test and was diagnosed with GDM (gestational diabetes mellitus). What is GDM?

4. List five risk factors for GDM. Place a star next to those risk factors that Y.L. has.

You schedule Y.L. with the dietitian later that same day because MNT (medical nutrition therapy) is the primary treatment for the management of GDM. She is also scheduled to meet with other members of the diabetes management team later in the week.

5. During the appointment with the dietitian, Y.L. gives a diet history that is high in noodles and rice with very little protein. She informs the dietitian she is lactose-intolerant but can have dairy products occasionally in small portions. Why is it important that Y.L. take a calcium supplement along with her prenatal vitamins?

6. What is the goal of MNT?

7. Why is the MNT for a person with GDM higher in fat and protein?

8. Everyone's body metabolizes foods in different ways; however, no woman with GDM can metabolize concentrated simple sugars without a sharp rise in blood glucose. Name five examples of simple sugars.

9. Complex carbohydrates do not cause a rapid rise in blood sugar when eaten in small amounts. Identify five foods from this group.

10. Y.L. was instructed to monitor her fasting blood glucose first thing in the morning and 2 hours after every meal. What is the significance of this request?

11. Y.L. was instructed to complete ketone testing using the first-voided urine in the morning. What is the rationale for this request?

Case Study 3

Name ______________________ Class/Group __________ Date __________

Group Members ____

INSTRUCTIONS: All questions apply to this case study. Your responses should be brief and to the point. Adequate space has been provided for answers. When asked to provide several answers, they should be listed in order of priority or significance. Do not asume information that is not provided. Please print or write clearly. If your response is not legible, it will be marked as ? and you will need to rewrite it.

Scenario

This scenario continues Case Study 2.

Y.L. continues to work with the diabetes team over the next few weeks, attending classes for gestational mothers. She received information on perinatal implications, maternal risks, and long-term implications of GDM. The dietary goal was to provide adequate protein and fewer carbohydrates in Y.L.'s diet. The importance of eating three meals and three snacks/day were stressed. Y.L.'s bedtime snack was increased because she had periodic trace to mild ketones. She started walking 30 to 60 minutes every day. At Y.L.'s 30th week appointment her diary indicates mild and occasional moderate ketones every morning for the past week and fasting blood sugars between 103 and 112 mg/dL. All other readings were within normal range. The patient reports that she never missed her bedtime snack. The diabetes team agrees that Y.L. should be started on a small dose of NPH insulin at bedtime.

1. Y.L. expresses concern regarding insulin injections and asks why she can't take oral insulin like other people she knows. How should you respond to this question?

2. What is the purpose of bedtime administration of NPH insulin?

3. How did the diabetes team establish that Y.L. was insulin-insufficient and not having starvation ketosis?

4. You are responsible for Y.L.'s insulin training. Identify five points that you will discuss with her.

5. List six signs and symptoms of hypoglycemia.

6. Y.L. began to report elevated blood sugars 2 hours after breakfast. She was started on R (regular) insulin 30 min (before meals) AC qam (every morning). She was instructed not to exercise during the time the insulin is peaking. What is the rationale for this recommendation?

7. Y.L. learned that there can be fetal complications associated with GDM. List three perinatal concerns?

8. Maternal complications are also seen when women develop GDM. Identify three complications.

9. You inform Y.L. about the long-term implications of having GDM and stress eating sensibly, exercising, and losing any additional weight after delivery. Most women return to a normal glucose state after delivery. It is recommended that glucose tolerance be evaluated 6 to 12 weeks postpartum. What are Y.L.'s chances of developing diabetes later in life?

Case Study 4

Name ______________________ Class/Group __________ Date __________

Group Members ____

INSTRUCTIONS: All questions apply to this case study. Your responses should be brief and to the point. Adequate space has been provided for answers. When asked to provide several answers, they should be listed in order of priority or significance. Do not asume information that is not provided. Please print or write clearly. If your response is not legible, it will be marked as ? and you will need to rewrite it.

Scenario

Y.L. makes an appointment to come to the clinic where you are employed. She has been complaining of chronic fatigue, increased thirst, constantly being hungry, and frequent urination. She denies any pain, burning, or low back pain on urination. She tells you she has a vaginal yeast infection that she has treated numerous times with OTC (over-the-counter) medication. She admits to starting smoking since going back to work full time as a clerk in a loan company. She also complains of having difficulty reading numbers and reports making frequent mistakes. She says by the time she gets home and makes supper for her family, then puts her child to bed, she is too tired to exercise. She reports her feet hurt; they often "burn or feel like there are pins in them." She reports that after her delivery, she went back to her traditional eating pattern, which you know is high in carbohydrates.

In reviewing Y.L.'s chart, you notice she has not been seen since the delivery of her child 6 years ago. She has gained a considerable amount of weight; her current weight is 173 lb. Today her BP is 152/97 mm Hg and her plasma glucose is 291 mg/dL. The PCP (primary care provider) orders the following labs: UA, HbA1c (hemoglobin A1c), fasting CMP, CBC, fasting lipid profile, and a baseline 24-hour urine collection to assess creatinine clearance. The lab values are as follows: fasting glucose 184 mg/dL, A1c 10.4, UA +glucose, –ketones, cholesterol 256 mg/dL, triglycerides 346 mg/dL, LDL (low-density lipids) 155 mg/dL, HDL (high-density lipids) 32 mg/dL, ratio 8.0. Y.L. is diagnosed with type 2 diabetes.

After meeting with Y.L. and discussing management therapies, the PCP decides to start MDI (multiple dose injection) insulin therapy and have the patient count carbohydrates. Y.L. is scheduled for education classes and is to work with the diabetes team to get her blood sugar under control.

1. Identify the three methods used to diagnose DM.

2. Identify three functions of insulin.

3. Insulin's main action is to lower blood sugar levels. Several hormones produced in the body inhibit the effects of insulin. Identify three.

4. Y.L. was started on lispro (Humalog) and glargine (Lantus) insulin with carbohydrate counting. What is the most important point to make when teaching the patient about glargine?

5. Because Y.L. has been on regular insulin in the past, you want to make sure she understands the difference between regular and lispro. What is the most significant difference between these two insulins?

6. What is the peak time and duration for lispro insulin?

7. Y.L. wants to know why she can't take NPH and regular insulin. She is more familiar with them and has taken them in the past. Explain why the provider chose lispro and glargine insulin over NPH and regular insulin?

8. Y.L.'s culture prefers foods high in carbohydrates. What is carbohydrate counting and why would this method work well for Y.L.?

9. What symptoms did Y.L. report today that led you to believe she has some form of neuropathy?

10. What findings in Y.L.'s history place her at increased risk for the development of other forms of neuropathy?

11. What are some changes that Y.L. can make to reduce the risk or slow the progression of both macrovascular and microvascular disease?

12. Y.L. is enrolled in a smoking cessation class. Why is it so important that she stop smoking?

Case Study 5

Name ______________________ Class/Group __________ Date __________

Group Members ____

INSTRUCTIONS: All questions apply to this case study. Your responses should be brief and to the point. Adequate space has been provided for answers. When asked to provide several answers, they should be listed in order of priority or significance. Do not asume information that is not provided. Please print or write clearly. If your response is not legible, it will be marked as ? and you will need to rewrite it.

Scenario

You work in a diabetes treatment center located in a large teaching hospital. The first patient you meet is K.W., a 35-year-old female, who presented 2 years ago with symptoms of severe fatigue and blurred vision. She thought this was due to long hours of working at a computer. The doctor who examined her told her she had "borderline diabetes," gave her a 1200 calorie ADA (American Diabetes Association) diet, and told her to lose weight. Her medical record from that visit indicates the following information: Wt 190 lb, Ht 5′4″, BP 140/90, urine normal, random blood glucose 155 mg/dL.

1. The correct term for "borderline diabetes" is impaired glucose tolerance. How would you have explained this term to K.W.?

2. What are the criteria for the diagnosis of IGT?

3. What laboratory value indicated that K.W. had impaired glucose tolerance?

4. What recommendations would you have made to K.W. to minimize her risk of developing DM? Identify two factors.

K.W. did not think she had a problem and ignored the doctor's advice. Three days ago K.W. went to see the doctor after a 1 month Hx of severe fatigue, HA (headaches), nocturia, thirst, and some burning and tingling in her feet. She smokes and does not exercise. She states she does not have time to cook, so most of her meals are at fast-food restaurants. Family Hx: father died of a MI in his early 40s, her mother is alive and has DM and HTN.

Her doctor ran a number of tests; the results are as follows: random glucose 205 mg/dL, next day fasting glucose 140 mg/dL, HbA1c 9.5%, chol 310 mg/dL, trig 700 mg/dL, HDL 30 mg/dL, LDL 140 mg/dL, ratio 10.3, Cr 0.9 mg/dL, wt 204 lb, BMI 35, BP 160/96. She is diagnosed with type 2 DM and is started on metformin for her diabetes and lisinopril for her HTN. She is referred to the diabetes treatment center for comprehensive education.

4. What laboratory values are now diagnostic for type 2 diabetes?

Your educational materials are divided into three basic areas: medical nutrition therapy, exercise, and pharmacotherapy.

5. Identify important content to be included under medical nutrition therapy.

6. Identify important content to be included under exercise. Address potential benefits, precautions and recommendations.

7. Identify important content to be included under pharmacologic therapy.

K.W. expresses concern over the burning and tingling in her feet. She comments, "I've heard many people with diabetes lose their toes." You take this opportunity to teach K.W. about neuropathy and foot care.

8. How would you educate K.W. about neuropathy?

9. No diabetic education program would be complete without addressing good foot care. Identify 7 points you would include when teaching K.W. about proper diabetic foot care.

10. Given all the information in the foregoing scenario, what diabetes-related complication do you believe K.W. is most at risk for and why?

11. List at least three interventions for reducing K.W.'s risk for macrovascular disease.

12. K.W. states she and her husband were planning on having another child in a year to two. She wants to know how her having diabetes will affect this. Pregnancy and diabetes is a very complex issue. What basic information can you share with K.W. today without overwhelming her?

Case Study 6

Name ______________________ Class/Group ____________ Date ____________

Group Members ____

INSTRUCTIONS: All questions apply to this case study. Your responses should be brief and to the point. Adequate space has been provided for answers. When asked to provide several answers, they should be listed in order of priority or significance. Do not asume information that is not provided. Please print or write clearly. If your response is not legible, it will be marked as ? and you will need to rewrite it.

Scenario

You are working as a nurse at the Veterans Administration Medical Center. Early in the day you meet C.R., a 38-year-old African-American male whose chief complaint is thirst and polydipsia. C.R. tells you he has always enjoyed good health, but 2 weeks ago he developed symptoms of dry mouth, urinary frequency, and polydipsia. At that time he was working on a job clearing asbestos from a building. Because he was dressed in an air-supplied protective suit, he assumed his symptoms were due to dehydration and overheating. When the project ended his symptoms persisted and he noticed a 20 lb weight loss. He also reports blurred vision and some mild cramping in both lower extremities. He states his grandmother developed diabetes in her 50s. VS: 139/90, 90, 99.4° F, 92%, Ht 5′8″, wt 230 lb, BMI 35. Lab results: glucose 917 mg/dL, HbA1c 12.5%, chol 283 mg/dL, trig 721 mg/dL, C-peptide 2.4, urine glucose >1000, urine protein neg, ketones trace. An IV was started and 1 L NS with 5 U of regular insulin is infused over 1 hour. C.R.'s glucose decreases to the 300 mg/dL range, and he is admitted to your floor.

1. List the major risk factors for diabetes mellitus (DM). Place a star next to the risk factors that C.R. has.

2. List the major signs and symptoms of DM. Place a star next to the signs and symptoms C.R. presents with.

The next day you are assigned to work on the acute medicine floor. One of your patients is C.R., whom you met yesterday. C.R. had a fasting glucose this morning of 160 mg/dL and has been Dx (diagnosed) as having type 2 DM. He is to be discharged tomorrow on 15 U NPH + 7 U regular insulin bid. He will meet with the RD (registered dietitian) later today, is scheduled to attend the diabetes class next week, and will be seen by the CDE (certified diabetes educator) a week after the class for individualized teaching and insulin titration. C.R. also has an appointment with an endocrinologist in 1 month to decide if he is to remain on insulin or be switched to oral agents.

3. You know there is much C.R. needs to learn about diabetes, but time is limited. What “survival skills” for diabetes management does he need to learn before he can go home safely? List your ideas according to monitoring, medication, and acute complications.

4. The RD receives an emergency telephone call and must leave the hospital. The job of teaching the basics of nutrition becomes your responsibility. What should you teach C.R.?

5. C.R. has a 20-year-old friend who is on insulin and has type 1 diabetes. C.R. is on insulin and thinks he must have type 1 as well, but his doctor told him he has type 2 diabetes. He asks you to explain the difference. How should you respond?

6. C.R. is type 2 because his C-peptide lab test shows that he is still producing endogenous insulin. What is a C-peptide?

7. C.R. expressed concern over his blurred vision. He reports "My vision was just fine before all this started." He is worried because he has heard that "people with diabetes go blind." What would you tell C.R.?

8. Identify two ocular complications of DM.

9. While you are teaching C.R. to use his glucometer, he asks, "The doctor said something about my A1c being too high. What does that mean?" How would you explain this to him?

The American Association of Clinical Endocrinologists (AACE) recommends an HbA1c level of 6.5% or less. The American Diabetes Association still recommends 7.0% or less.

Case Study 7

Name ______________________________ Class/Group __________ Date __________

Group Members ____

INSTRUCTIONS: All questions apply to this case study. Your responses should be brief and to the point. Adequate space has been provided for answers. When asked to provide several answers, they should be listed in order of priority or significance. Do not asume information that is not provided. Please print or write clearly. If your response is not legible, it will be marked as ? and you will need to rewrite it.

Scenario

You graduated 3 months ago and are working with a home care agency. Included in your caseload is J.S., a 60-year-old man suffering from chronic obstructive pulmonary disease (COPD) R/T cigarette smoking. He has been on home oxygen, 2 L O_2/NC, for several years. Approximately 10 months ago, he was started on chronic oral steroid therapy. Medications include ipratropium (Atrovent) inhaler, salmeterol (Serevent) inhaler, dexamethasone, digoxin, and furosemide (Lasix). On the way to J.S.'s home, you make mental note to check him for S/S of Cushing's syndrome.

1. Differentiate between Cushing's syndrome and Cushing's disease.

2. Your assessment includes the following findings. Determine if the findings are attributable to J.S.'s COPD or possible Cushing's syndrome. Place an L beside the symptoms consistent with lung disease and a C next to those consistent with Cushing's syndrome.

    ______ Barrel chest
    ______ Full-looking face ("moon facies")
    ______ BP 180/94 mm Hg
    ______ Pursed-lip breathing, especially when patient is stressed
    ______ Striae over trunk and thighs
    ______ Bruising on both arms
    ______ Acne
    ______ Diminished breath sounds throughout lungs
    ______ Truncal obesity with supraclavicular and posterior upper back fat

3. You inform the physician of the patient's S/S. The physician believes J.S. has developed Cushing's syndrome and decides to change his prescription from dexamethasone to prednisone given on alternate days. Explain the rationale for this change.

4. Identify possible consequences of suddenly stopping the dexamethasone (Decadron) therapy.

5. Cushing's syndrome can affect memory. It will be easy to forget what medications have been taken, especially when there are several different drugs and some are taken on alternating days. List at least three ways you can help J.S. remember to take his pills as prescribed.

6. J.S. states that his appetite has increased but he is losing weight. He reports trying to eat but he gets SOB and cannot eat any more. How would you address this problem? How might his diet be modified?

7. You advise J.S. to take his prednisone in the morning with food. You ask him a series of questions R/T his vision and joint pain. Discuss the rationale for your line of questioning.

8. Differentiate between the glucocorticoid and mineralocorticoid effects of prednisone.

9. How would your assessment change if J.S. were taking a glucocorticoid that also has significant mineralocorticoid activity?

10. Review J.S.'s list of medications. Based on what you know about the side effects of loop diuretics and steroids, discuss the potential problem of administering these in combination with digoxin.

11. Realizing that patients like J.S. are susceptible to all types of infections, you write guidelines to prevent infection. Identify four major points that these guidelines will include.

Case Study 10

Name ______________________ Class/Group __________ Date __________

Group Members ____

INSTRUCTIONS: All questions apply to this case study. Your responses should be brief and to the point. Adequate space has been provided for answers. When asked to provide several answers, they should be listed in order of priority or significance. Do not asume information that is not provided. Please print or write clearly. If your response is not legible, it will be marked as ? and you will need to rewrite it.

Scenario

You are working on an oncology unit and will be receiving a patient from the recovery room. The PACU (postanesthesia care unit) nurse calls and gives the following report: C.P., a 50-year-old woman with a subtotal thyroidectomy for multinodular goiter and left superior and right inferior parathyroidectomy because of adenoma. The EBL (estimated blood loss) was 25 mL. VS are 130/82, 80-90, 20, 94% on RA (room air). She has a peripheral IV of D_5½NS with 20 mEq KCl and 10 mEq calcium gluconate infusing at 100 mL/h. She has received a total of 50 mg meperidine IVP, and she remains AAO (awake, alert, oriented). C.P.'s PMH includes TAH (total abdominal hysterectomy) for fibroids and low-level radiation treatments to the neck 38 years ago for eczema. Her medications include estradiol, lovastatin, and levothyroxine. Both parents are living; her father had an MI at 70 years old, her mother has hypothyroidism but never had thyroid tumors. Preoperative laboratory findings: Ca 11.2 mg/dL, phosphorus 2.4 mg/dL, Cl 106 mmol/L, alkaline phosphatase 112 U/L, elevated parahormone and TSH (thyroid-stimulating hormone) levels, Cr 1.4 mg/dL.

1. What additional data should you obtain from the recovery room nurse?

2. What preparations will you make before C.P. arrives?

3. You receive C.P. from the recovery room. How will you focus your initial assessment, and why?

4. During your initial assessment, you document negative Chvostek's and Trousseau's signs. Describe data that would support this conclusion.

5. Identify the m... risk factor that may have contributed to the development of parathyroid adenoma in C.P.

6. Identify four issues R/T C

7. Identify four actions you should include in the postoperative care of C.P.

8. Identify measures that reduce the risk for postoperative swelling.

9. After surgery, C.P.'s thyroid hormone levels were elevated and the doctor ordered propranolol 80 mg ER (extended release) tabs for "surgically induced thyrotoxicosis." Is this reaction expected following parathyroid surgery or did something go wrong during surgery? Explain.

10. 18 hours after surgery, C.P. calls you into her room C/O numbness around her mouth and tingling at the tips of her fingers. She appears restless but is AAO. Realizing that C.P. may be experiencing hypocalcemia, you notify the physician. What should you do in the interim before the physician returns your call?

11. What emergency equipment should you gather?

C.P. is given supplemental calcium gluconate and recovers without further complications. C.P. is started on calcium carbonate bid, given a F/U (follow-up) appointment in 3 weeks, and is discharged 24 hours postoperatively.

Case Study 11

Name ______________________________ Class/Group __________ Date __________

Group Members ____

INSTRUCTIONS: All questions apply to this case study. Your responses should be brief and to the point. Adequate space has been provided for answers. When asked to provide several answers, they should be listed in order of priority or significance. Do not asume information that is not provided. Please print or write clearly. If your response is not legible, it will be marked as ? and you will need to rewrite it.

Scenario

W.V., a 40-year-old woman, has been referred to the endocrine clinic of a large metropolitan medical center by her primary care physician. She presents with a history of bilateral hemianopsia, headaches, amenorrhea, dyspareunia, and lethargy. An extensive history reveals polyuria and polydipsia. Her family physician suspects an anterior pituitary tumor. GH, prolactin, TSH, LH, and FSH levels are unremarkable. A dexamethasone suppression test (or cortisol/ACTH challenge test) and 24-hour urine for 17-hydroxysteroids (17-OHCS) are planned.

1. W.V. is aware of the high probability of a pituitary tumor, but she doesn't understand why the physician wants to test her kidneys. How would you explain the relationship between the pituitary and adrenal glands and the need for adrenal function studies to her?

2. Identify four problems R/T W.V.'s care.

The dexamethasone suppression test is normal, but the 24-hour urine collection indicates 17-OHCS is elevated. An MRI is ordered.

3. The MRI confirms a macroadenoma of the anterior pituitary. The physician advises a transsphenoidal hypophysectomy. What questions would you anticipate W.V. might have?

4. While W.V.'s physician arranges for her admission to the hospital and schedules her transsphenoidal hypophysectomy, you enter her examining room to conduct preoperative teaching. You find W.V. crying. She says she is embarrassed by the hormonal changes and states, "I'm afraid my husband won't love me anymore." What approaches would be appropriate for addressing the patient's fear?

5. During preoperative teaching, W.V. states she is fearful of the procedure. She says she doesn't understand how a tumor in the brain can be removed through the nose. How would you explain the procedure to minimize her fear?

6. Identify two major teaching needs for postop care based on the transsphenoidal approach. Outline important educational points for each area to address during preop teaching with W.V.

7. W.V. is admitted and undergoes a successful transsphenoidal hypophysectomy. Ten hours postop, W.V. calls her nurse into her room C/O postnasal drip. She is frequently swallowing. What five actions should the nurse take? Include your rationales.

8. The nurse notes the following assessment findings: VS 100/66, 98, 16; W.V. C/O thirst; her skin is flushed; her urine output 300 mL/h with a specific gravity of 1.003, and she is flaccid (no muscle tone). What additional information should you gather before calling the physician?

9. The nurse suspects fluid volume deficit R/T inadequate release of ADH. While waiting for the surgeon to return her call, what should the nurse's priority intervention(s) be?

10. The surgeon orders a serum and urine osmolality and electrolytes. The labratory reports a urine osmolality of 95 mosm/kg, serum osmolality of 315 mosm/kg, and sodium level of 146 mmol/L. Discuss the significance of each.

11. Replacement therapy for diabetes insipidus includes administration of desmopressin. What is this drug and how is it given?

12. How will the nurse evaluate the effectiveness of drug and fluid therapy?

Case Study 12

Name ______________________ Class/Group __________ Date __________

Group Members ____

INSTRUCTIONS: All questions apply to this case study. Your responses should be brief and to the point. Adequate space has been provided for answers. When asked to provide several answers, they should be listed in order of priority or significance. Do not asume information that is not provided. Please print or write clearly. If your response is not legible, it will be marked as ? and you will need to rewrite it.

Scenario

You are a nurse on a medical unit. One of your patients, T.L., a 40-year-old man who works as a communications supervisor, is being evaluated for uncontrolled HTN. He C/O frequent episodes of chest pain and palpitations, diaphoresis, job stress, nervousness, epigastric distress after eating, and pounding migraine headaches that leave him exhausted. He states that these episodes have increased in frequency and duration; he now experiences several episodes a week, and each episode lasts 1 to 3 days. He has taken a variety of antihypertensive medications, none of which has successfully controlled his HTN. His BP is labile; sometimes it is normal, and other times it is 220/120 mm Hg. Cardiac work-up reveals no significant cardiovascular abnormalities. He has a 27-pack-year smoking history. T.L.'s 24-hour urine analysis reveals vanillylmandelic acid (VMA) 12 mg/24 h; epinephrine 45 ng/24 h, and norepinephrine 100 ng/24 h; CT scan reveals a single adrenomedullary tumor. T.L. is diagnosed with pheochromocytoma and scheduled for an adrenalectomy.

1. The physician informs T.L. that an adrenal tumor is causing his symptoms. T.L. is obviously upset with his diagnosis. He states he doesn't understand how a tumor on top of his kidney can cause high BP. He asks whether this means he has cancer. How would you respond?

2. The physician advises T.L. to undergo an adrenalectomy. He is immediately started on phenoxybenzamine (Dibenzyline) 10 mg PO q12h. This medication is titrated upward q3d until T.L.'s supine BP is below 160/90 mmHg and his standing BP is above 85/40. Propranolol (Inderal) 20 mg PO qid is added to control his tachyarrhythmia. What is the connection between these two drugs and the diagnosis?

3. Some people experience paroxysmal, or sudden, periodic attacks of HTN that correspond to the release of epinephrine and/or norepinephrine. Under what circumstances would T.L. most likely experience a paroxysmal hypertensive event?

4. What measures to prevent a paroxysmal hypertensive event should you teach T.L.?

5. Following the surgery, T.L. is taken directly to the ICU. The anesthesiologist gives the admitting nurse the following report: the surgery went well, and T.L. should wake up shortly; his VS have been running 180/90, 88, 16, 96.1° F; he's got a left subclavian Swan-Ganz catheter and two large-bore peripheral IVs with D_5W running at a total of 125 mL/h; urine output during OR was 200 mL. What additional data should the ICU nurse elicit from the anesthesiologist?

6. Identify three postoperative issues R/T T.L.'s care.

7. For each issue identified in question 6, outline two to three interventions/measures.

8. During shift assessment (second postoperative day), the nurse notes that T.L. seems less alert, his grip strength is markedly weaker than yesterday, and his mucous membranes are dry. The previous nurse reported that he had vomited twice in the last hour. The cardiac monitor shows peaked T waves and a widened QRS complex. VS are 120/72, 94, 14, 101° F. What conclusions can you draw from the foregoing data?

All these findings suggest adrenal insufficiency.

9. Based on the nurses' assessment findings, what general treatment measures would you anticipate?

10. Outline four measures that are critical during this period.

11. T.L. is stabilized and is scheduled to be discharged home. During discharge teaching, T.L. asks whether he will require medication for the rest of his life. How should you respond to T.L.?

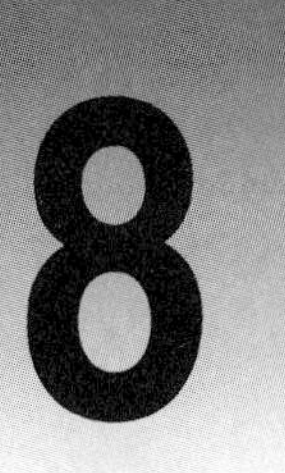

Immunologic Disorders

Case Study 1

Name ______________________ Class/Group __________ Date __________

Group Members ______________________________________

INSTRUCTIONS: All questions apply to this case study. Your responses should be brief and to the point. Adequate space has been provided for answers. When asked to provide several answers, they should be listed in order of priority or significance. Do not asume information that is not provided. Please print or write clearly. If your response is not legible, it will be marked as ? and you will need to rewrite it.

Scenario

You are a nurse at a local health clinic. T.Q. comes in to your clinic and informs you of his immunodeficiency problem. He has just moved here to go to school. He gives you a letter from his attending physician, a vial of gamma globulin, and asks you to give him his "shot." The letter, written by T.Q.'s physician, states that he was diagnosed with primary immunodeficiency disease 18 years ago. He has an adequate number of B cells but they fail to mature properly and become plasma cells or immunoglobulin. T.Q. states he has a history of chronic respiratory and gastrointestinal (GI) infections. He is maintained on 0.66 ml/kg gamma globulin IM every 3 weeks, and has tolerated this well. He has no known drug allergies (NKDA). His vital signs (VS) are stable.

1. Can you honor this patient's prescription? Why or why not? How could you provide him with his injection?

2. What should you do while the physician is verifying information?

3. Once the clinic physician receives confirmation from T.Q.'S physician, he will order the gamma globulin. What questions would you ask T.Q. that would reassure you that the medication he brought was safe to administer?

4. Briefly describe the maturation cycle of the B cell.

5. What immunoglobulin deficiency does T.Q. have?

6. Before T.Q. leaves what should you assess?

7. You note on T.Q.'s health record that he has not received his polio, measles, mumps, or rubella vaccines. What explanation can be given for the lack of these vaccinations?

T.Q. returns in 3 weeks with complaints of (C/O) a stuffy nose.

8. What will you assess to further evaluate his stuffy nose?

9. If T.Q. is developing a sinus infection, what signs are you likely to encounter upon examining him?

T.Q.'s nares do not appear swollen or red, although he does have some clear mucus drainage. His temperature is normal at 98.4° F. T.Q. is due for his next injection of gamma globulin.

10. Should you give the medication or ask him to return when he is no longer having nasal stuffiness? Why or why not?

11. How do primary immunodeficiencies differ from secondary immunodeficiencies?

12. What is the most common primary immunodeficiency?

13. Explain why T.Q. is at greater risk for the development of infections than his classmates.

Case Study 3

Name ______________________ Class/Group __________ Date __________

Group Members ____

INSTRUCTIONS: All questions apply to this case study. Your responses should be brief and to the point. Adequate space has been provided for answers. When asked to provide several answers, they should be listed in order of priority or significance. Do not asume information that is not provided. Please print or write clearly. If your response is not legible, it will be marked as ? and you will need to rewrite it.

Scenario

J.P., a 56-year-old man, developed a severe viral infection and suffered fatigue, fever, and myalgia. Although he recovered from the acute episode, J.P. never quite regained normal activity level. Six months later, J.P. continues to find it difficult to work a 10-hour day as a brick mason, so he returns to his physician. Diagnostic studies reveal congestive heart failure (CHF) R/T postviral cardiomyopathy. Following medical management with digoxin (Lanoxin) and furosemide (Lasix), his condition stabilizes and he returns to work, but his attendance is erratic. J.P.'s condition gradually deteriorates, and he is readmitted to the hospital 16 months later with C/O dyspnea with minimal exertion, fatigue, orthopnea, chest pain, anorexia, and feelings of abdominal fullness. He has 1+ peripheral edema and is diaphoretic. Further studies reveal that J.P. has cardiac dilation, moderate to gross ventricular hypertrophy, and poor systolic ejection fraction, consistent with severe congestive cardiomyopathy. Because J.P.'s only other health problem is mild hypertension, heart transplant evaluation is recommended. J.P. and his wife discuss his prognosis and he agrees to an evaluation for possible heart transplantation.

1. If J.P. is accepted for cardiac transplantation, what data will be collected in addition to his PMH, current diagnostic findings, and cardiac evaluation?

2. What criteria for heart transplantation does J.P. meet that will make him eligible for cardiac transplantation?

3. Cite five contraindications for cardiac transplant.

4. J.P. is accepted for cardiac transplant and placed on the waiting list. What fears or concerns may J.P. experience during this waiting period?

J.P. receives a phone call to report to the hospital immediately because a donor heart has become available.

5. What compatibility tests are performed to determine eligibility for transplantation and to ensure as close a match as possible?

6. As the nurse on the transplant unit, how can you best help J.P. prepare for his heart transplant?

J.P.'s surgery and recovery are uncomplicated and he is sent home and referred to cardiac rehabilitation after adjustment of his immunosuppression therapy and appropriate teaching. J.P. is readmitted for low-grade fever and dyspnea 6 weeks after surgery. Cardiac biopsies demonstrate moderate acute rejection.

7. What is the etiology of acute rejection, and how does it differ from chronic rejection?

8. The nurse can anticipate that prompt immunosuppressive therapy will be instituted using what drug? How does this drug alter the rejection process?

9. What is the most important intervention for J.P. at this time, and why?

J.P. responds positively to steroid therapy and is released to home after 5 days. J.P. is again admitted to the hospital with renewed C/O of dyspnea, low-grade fever, and ankle swelling 7 months later. Both J.P. and his wife are anxious and fearful.

10. Explain what may be happening to J.P. physiologically.

11. How will treatment for this episode of graft rejection differ from treatment for his earlier episode of rejection?

12. J.P.'s prognosis for the future will depend on what factors?

Case Study 4

Name ______________________ Class/Group __________ Date __________

Group Members ____

INSTRUCTIONS: All questions apply to this case study. Your responses should be brief and to the point. Adequate space has been provided for answers. When asked to provide several answers, they should be listed in order of priority or significance. Do not asume information that is not provided. Please print or write clearly. If your response is not legible, it will be marked as ? and you will need to rewrite it.

Scenario

W.V. is a 57-year-old man who lives with his wife and two teenage sons. W.V. developed chronic renal failure 20 years ago after acute renal failure due to phenacetin use. (W.V. took phenacetin since his early 20s for migraine headaches. Large doses of phenacetin over the years can cause analgesic-induced nephropathy. This drug has subsequently been removed from the market.) W.V. was initially placed on hemodialysis but was switched to peritoneal dialysis so he could remain employed as an auto mechanic. Three months ago W.V. received a cadaveric transplant, or cadaver kidney. He recovered without complications and his serum laboratory values returned to normal. He was placed on immunosuppressive therapy, including cyclosporine and prednisone and was discharged to home. W.V. returned to work 3 weeks later.

Today W.V. reports to his physician for routine follow-up. His VS are 148/92, 88, 24, 99.2° F. His lab data reveal the following: serum creatinine 1.2 mg/dl, BUN 22 mg/dl, normal serum electrolytes. W.V. has gained 5 pounds since discharge from the hospital.

1. What histocompatibility studies are generally performed before renal transplant, and why are they important?

2. By what criteria is W.V. considered a good candidate for renal transplantation?

3. If W.V.'s kidney is producing sufficient urine and he is feeling well, why is it necessary to monitor his laboratory data?

4. What is the possible significance of W.V.'s current blood pressure (BP)?

5. How does the drug cyclosporine protect W.V.'s kidney from rejection, and what are the most important side effects of this drug that W.V. must be taught to monitor?

6. How will W.V. know whether he is experiencing organ rejection?

7. If W.V. begins to reject his kidney, how would the rejection be classified, and what S/S would most likely be present?

8. Identify at least four ways that W.V. might experience difficulty adjusting to his organ transplant.

9. How can you best support W.V. and his family?

10. Why is it necessary for W.V. to be concerned about infection?

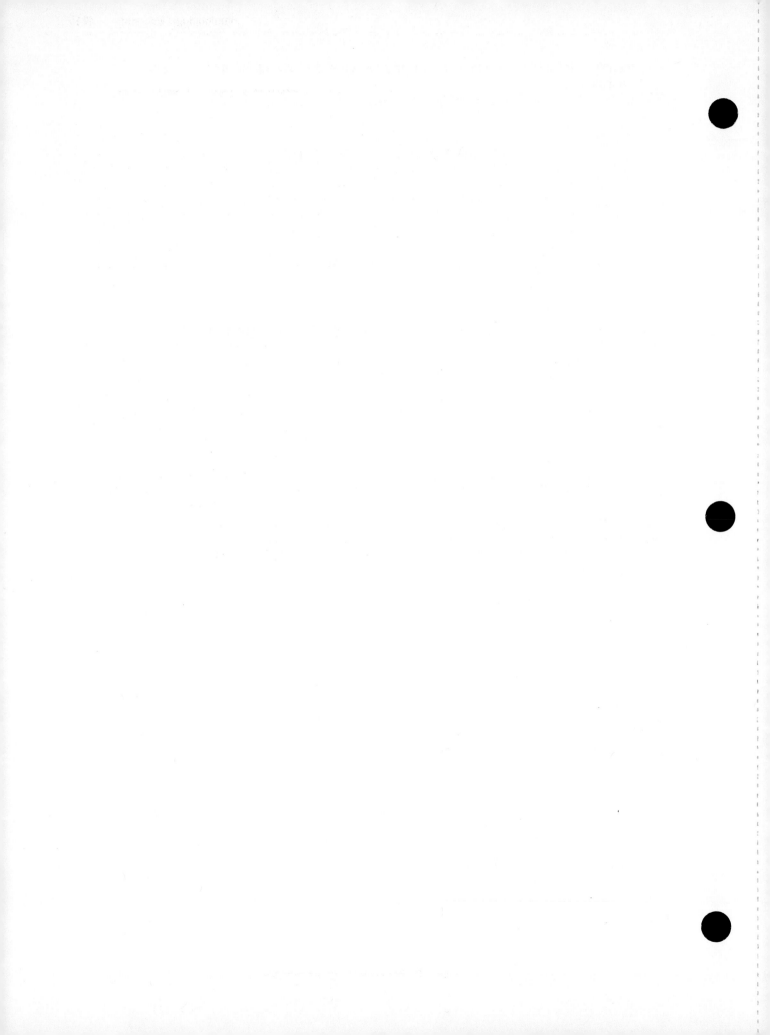

11. What laboratory data will most likely be monitored on K.D. in the future?

12. List at least five other opportunistic infections that K.D. is at risk for developing.

For additional information, check the following resources.
National Institute of Allergy and Infectious Diseases: www.niaid.nih.gov/ and www.niaid.nih.gov/publications/hivaids/hivaids.htm
Another comprehensive source of information: www.thebody.com

Case Study 6

Name ______________________ Class/Group __________ Date __________

Group Members ____

INSTRUCTIONS: All questions apply to this case study. Your responses should be brief and to the point. Adequate space has been provided for answers. When asked to provide several answers, they should be listed in order of priority or significance. Do not asume information that is not provided. Please print or write clearly. If your response is not legible, it will be marked as ? and you will need to rewrite it.

Scenario

D.W. is a 23-year-old married woman with three children less than the age of 5. She presented to her physician 2 years ago with vague C/O intermittent fatigue, joint pain, and low-grade fever. Her physician noted small patchy areas of vitiligo and a scaly rash across her nose, cheeks, back, and chest at that time. Laboratory studies revealed that D.W. had a positive antinuclear antibody titer, positive lupus erythematosus (dsDNA), positive Anti-Sm (antismooth muscle antibody), elevated C-reactive protein and erythrocyte sedimentation rate (ESR), and decreased C3 and C4 serum complement. Joint x-rays demonstrated joint swelling without joint erosion. D.W. was subsequently diagnosed with SLE. She was initially treated with sulindac 200 mg PO bid and prednisone 20 mg PO qd, bed rest, and ice packs. She was counseled regarding her condition, advised to balance rest and activity, eat a well-balanced diet, use strategies to reduce stress, and avoid direct sunlight. D.W. responded well to treatment and was eventually told she could report for follow-up every 6 months unless her symptoms became acute. D.W. resumed her job in environmental services at a large geriatric facility.

1. What is the significance of each of D.W.'s laboratory findings?

2. Given that most tests are nonspecific, how is SLE diagnosed?

3. What priority problems need to be addressed with D.W.?

Eighteen months after diagnosis, D.W. seeks out her physician because of puffy hands and feet and increased fatigue. D.W. reports that she has been working longer hours because of the absence of two of her fellow workers. Diagnostic evaluation reveals that her BUN and serum creatinine are slightly elevated and that she has 2+ protein and 1+ red blood cells (RBCs) in her urine.

4. Of what significance are these findings, and what is the relationship of such findings to D.W.'s diagnosis of SLE?

5. How will D.W.'s treatment and care plan likely change?

D.W. is seen in the immunology clinic twice monthly during the next 3 months. Although her condition does not worsen, her BUN and serum creatinine remain elevated. While at work one afternoon, D.W. begins to feel dizzy and develops a severe headache. She reports to her supervisor, who has her lie down. When D.W. starts to become disoriented, her supervisor calls 911, and D.W. is taken to the hospital. D.W. is admitted for probable lupus cerebritis R/T acute exacerbation of her disease.

6. What preventive measures should be instituted to protect D.W. at this time?

7. What additional problems indicative of CNS involvement R/T SLE should D.W. be assessed for?

D.W.'s dose of methylprednisolone is increased and she is started on plasmapheresis.

8. What major complications associated with immunosuppression therapy will D.W. have to be monitored for?

9. What does plasmapheresis do, and why might it reduce the S/S associated with SLE?

10. What data would support the assumption that D.W.'s condition is stabilizing?

11. Identify at least five topics that D.W. must be taught before she is discharged that may help her lead as normal a life as possible.

12. You note that D.W.'s husband is visiting her this afternoon. You enter the room to ask whether they have any questions. D.W.'s husband states, "I have tried to tell her that she cannot go back to work. Sure, we need the money, but the kids and I need her more. I'm afraid that this lupus has weakened her whole body and it will kill her if she goes back to work. Is that right?" How would you respond to his concerns?

Additional information on SLE can be found through the following resources:

www.nlm.nih.gov/medlineplus/lupus.html *or*

www.nih.gov/niams/ (National Institute of Arthritis and Musculoskeletal and Skin Diseases)

Bonus Project: Locate and print a patient education handout on SLE in both English and Spanish. Attach it to this assignment.

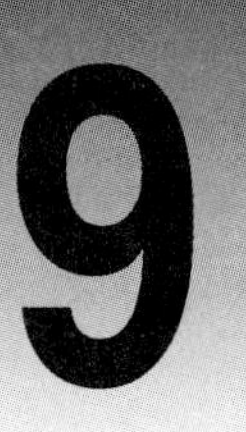

Oncologic and Hematologic Disorders

Case Study 1

Name ______________________ Class/Group __________ Date __________

Group Members ______________________________________

INSTRUCTIONS: All questions apply to this case study. Your responses should be brief and to the point. Adequate space has been provided for answers. When asked to provide several answers, they should be listed in order of priority or significance. Do not asume information that is not provided. Please print or write clearly. If your response is not legible, it will be marked as ? and you will need to rewrite it.

Scenario

You are a home health nurse who has been seeing P.C., who has a diagnosis of lung cancer for approximately 1 year. Her provider recently informed her that her cancer is no longer treatable; the focus of her treatment will change from curative measures to symptom relief. She is confused and somewhat angry with her provider. She vaguely remembers the term "palliative treatment" when discussing her situation with her provider but doesn't know what it means.

1. How would you describe palliative treatment?

P.C. confides that she always felt that she may not survive her illness, but has never formally written down her wishes concerning what types of treatment she would or would not want. You advise her to complete an advance directive and/or living will.

2. What is the purpose of these two documents?

3. Why should these be completed?

4. What health care decisions are considered in these documents?

5. How are advance directives and living wills formalized?

6. P.C. states she is confused and has mixed feelings about her health care wishes right now. She asks, “If I fill out this form, can I change my mind down the road?” How should you answer this question?

7. You inform P.C. that you will help with symptomatic control of her illness. What types of things will you focus on?

8. As P.C. becomes more frail and incoherent, what treatment will be given?

Case Study 2

Name ______________________ Class/Group __________ Date __________

Group Members ____

INSTRUCTIONS: All questions apply to this case study. Your responses should be brief and to the point. Adequate space has been provided for answers. When asked to provide several answers, they should be listed in order of priority or significance. Do not asume information that is not provided. Please print or write clearly. If your response is not legible, it will be marked as ? and you will need to rewrite it.

Scenario

B.B., a 53-year-old divorced professional woman, was diagnosed with stage T1 N0 M0 infiltrating ductal breast cancer on her right side based on a lumpectomy and axillary lymph node dissection more than a year ago. After her radiation therapy (daily treatments for 6 weeks) was completed, she was placed on tamoxifen (to be taken for 5 years). She has been coming to the clinic every 3 months for her checkup in the year since her treatment was completed. In addition to working at the clinic, you are a volunteer consultant to the Encore-YWCA support group for women who have had breast cancer, where B.B. regularly attends. The group has invited you to present "Breast Cancer: Prevention, Screening, and Detection Guidelines" at their next meeting.

1. What is tamoxifen? Why are women placed on long-term tamoxifen therapy as a treatment for breast cancer?

2. What is an axillary lymph node dissection? Why did B.B. have an axillary lymph node dissection with her lumpectomy?

3. B.B. was diagnosed with stage T1 N0 M0 breast cancer. What does that mean?

4. What risk factors for breast cancer will you include in your group presentation?

5. What will you teach the group about early detection of breast cancer?

6. What educational equipment can help women learn how to perform BSE correctly and how to detect lumps?

7. Describe the technique for performing BSE correctly.

8. One of the women in the group shows you how the arm on the side that had the breast cancer is more swollen than the other arm. She said she is having a lot of trouble with this. What do you think is happening? How will you explain this to her? What will you advise her?

9. B.B. raises her hand and tells you she heard she should never have her blood pressure (BP) taken in her affected arm (the right arm in her case). You remember that you told her this in the office, but you realize she was probably too anxious or tired to remember exactly what you said. What will you advise her and the other women present?

10. B.B. also says she was told to watch for infection in her affected arm. She asks why that's important. What will you tell her?

11. What are some other things breast cancer survivors can do to manage or prevent lymphedema? (List four.)

For more information on risk factors, consult the following resources:

The Department of Defense Breast Cancer Decision Guide
www.bcdg.org/

American Cancer Society
1599 Clifton Road, NE
Atlanta, GA 30329-4251
800-ACS-2345
www.cancer.org

National Cancer Institute (NCI)
Building 31, Room 10A03
31 Center Drive, MSC 2580
Bethesda, MD 20892-2580
www.nci.nih.gov

National Cancer Information Service
800-4-CANCER

Case Study 3

Name ______________________ Class/Group __________ Date __________

Group Members ____

INSTRUCTIONS: All questions apply to this case study. Your responses should be brief and to the point. Adequate space has been provided for answers. When asked to provide several answers, they should be listed in order of priority or significance. Do not asume information that is not provided. Please print or write clearly. If your response is not legible, it will be marked as ? and you will need to rewrite it.

Scenario

C.W. is a 42-year-old divorced woman with adenocarcinoma (cancer) of the lung with metastasis (spread) to the brain and liver. She is the single parent of a 17-year-old son, has experienced episodic health care, is currently unemployed because of poor health, and has no health insurance. She has smoked one to two packs per day for 20 years. Past medical history (PMH) includes cholecystectomy, hysterectomy, and breast augmentation. In May of last year she developed scapular and arm pain on her right side, was diagnosed with adenocarcinoma of the lung, and underwent a wedge resection of the upper right lobe of the lung. Because she had no insurance, she did not receive follow-up care (e.g., radiation therapy and/or chemotherapy).

C.W. developed pain in her right temple 48 hours ago and was seen in the emergency department (ED), where she was given cephradine (Velosef). C.W. had a seizure 24 hours later, was transported to the ED, and was diagnosed as having an allergic reaction to the cephradine. She was instructed to call her family doctor. C.W.'s doctor was unavailable for 48 hours. After suffering a tonic-clonic (grand mal) seizure at home, she was admitted to a rural hospital. A computed tomography (CT) scan revealed a large mass in the right frontal area of her brain. Dexamethasone (Decadron) was given IV, and an oncologist in the metropolitan area was consulted. C.W. was transferred to your oncology unit postseizure with slightly slurred speech and intermittent bone pain. She has lost 22 pounds in the past year. She is receiving hydrocodone/acetaminophen (Lortab) one or two 5 mg tablets every 3 to 4 hours, as needed. C.W.'s record lists codeine and milk allergies.

1. Identify the usual location, growth rate, and likelihood of metastasis of adenocarcinoma of the lung.

2. Is the presence of bone pain and weight loss significant?

3. What tests are likely to be performed to determine whether C.W.'s adenocarcinoma has metastasized?

4. The tests are performed, and C.W. is diagnosed with adenocarcinoma of the lung with metastasis to lymph nodes, liver, and brain. She is scheduled to receive 10 radiation therapy treatments to the whole brain (3 as an inpatient, 7 as an outpatient). Identify five needs that you will address with C.W. and her son.

After her third radiation treatment, C.W. is discharged on the following medications: dexamethasone 4 mg PO q8h; propoxyphene/acetaminophen (Darvocet-N) 100 mg PO (orally) q4h prn (as needed); prochlorperazine maleate (Compazine Spansules) 15 mg PO q12h prn; temazepam 30 mg PO prn.

5. What is the rationale for C.W. receiving each medication?

Two months' posthospital discharge and follow-up therapy, C.W. continues to have increasing symptoms of pain, anorexia, weight loss, edema in extremities, and insomnia. Her son accompanied her to the physician's office. While his mother is having her blood drawn, he asks the nurse what is going to happen to his mother.

6. How would you respond to him?

7. He asks what he can do to help his mother. What information could you give him?

8. As C.W.'s disease progresses, what signs and symptoms (S/S) can be anticipated, and what kind of relief can be provided?

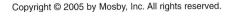

9. C.W.'s son says he's never been around someone who is dying before. He expresses fear he won't know what to do. How can you help him?

Case Study 4

Name ______________________ Class/Group __________ Date __________

Group Members ______________________________

INSTRUCTIONS: All questions apply to this case study. Your responses should be brief and to the point. Adequate space has been provided for answers. When asked to provide several answers, they should be listed in order of priority or significance. Do not asume information that is not provided. Please print or write clearly. If your response is not legible, it will be marked as ? and you will need to rewrite it.

Scenario

A.T. is a 21-year-old college student. He works part-time as a manual laborer, uses half a can of smokeless tobacco each week, and drinks a six-pack of beer on the weekend. A year ago in September, he discovered a small, painless lump in his lower left neck. Over the quarter, he experienced increasing fatigue and a 10-pound weight loss that he attributed to "working and studying too hard." In the spring he saw a nurse practitioner at the student health center who immediately referred him to an oncologist. A lymph node biopsy revealed Hodgkin's disease. The gallium scan, bone scan, and CT scan of the chest, abdomen, and pelvis all came back negative. A staging laparotomy was conducted a month later to confirm the diagnosis. His diagnosis was Hodgkin's disease, stage IA, mixed cellularity. You are a staff nurse in the outpatient oncology services when A.T. comes in.

1. A.T. wants to know what Hodgkin's disease is and how he "caught" it. What will you tell him?

2. A.T. wants to know what "stage IA" means; he also wants to know the significance of the test results. What are you going to tell him?

A few days later you see A.T. in the oncologist's office during his appointment to discuss the treatment regimen for radiation therapy. His prescribed radiation treatment regimen (outpatient) includes Monday through Friday with treatments scheduled for approximately 6 to 10 weeks. Admission assessment findings on his first visit to the outpatient oncology clinic at the end of January are weight 193 pounds, height 78 inches. Vital signs (VS) 124/66, 60, 16, 98.0° F (oral). Cardiovascular: heart rate regular. Respiratory: clear to auscultation. Neuromuscular/skeletal, GI, and genitourinary (GU): negative. Integumentary/oral: incision from staging laparotomy well approximated without erythema, edema, pain, or drainage. Incision from lymph node dissection healing well, oral mucosa pink and moist, no palpable adenopathy.

3. What abnormal assessment findings do you recognize in the previous information?

4. A.T. jokes with you that he's "going to get nuked and glow." What information would you include in your teaching to prepare him for radiation treatments?

5. You have developed a good relationship with A.T. during the multiple visits required for his radiation therapy. He shares some futuristic goals and says, "What are the chances that I will beat this cancer?" Respond to A.T.'s request.

Other kinds of cancer may occur many years later as a result of the toxic effects of earlier treatment. This is one reason why cancer specialists are reluctant to use the word "cured."

6. What other issues of survivorship may affect patients like A.T. (e.g., insurance, employability)?

7. How and what are you going to counsel and teach A.J. about potential sterility/infertility side effects of treatment?

8. Six weeks into therapy A.T. drags himself into the clinic one Friday, drops into a chair, and wearily states, “I’m quitting. If this is what life is like, it’s not worth living.” How would you respond to him?

9. When A.T. checks in this week, he weighs 177 pounds. When you express concern, he tells you he just doesn’t have any appetite. How are you going to respond? List at least four interventions.

10. At his final appointment, A.T.'s laboratory values are white blood count (WBC) 3.3 thou/cmm, hemoglobin (Hgb) 14 g/dl, hematocrit (Hct) 41%, and platelets 369 thou/cmm. His VS are 120/76, 84, 20, 98.0° F (oral). Weight 175 pounds. Do any of these values concern you? Explain.

A.T. is discharged from radiation and scheduled to see an oncologist every 3 months for follow-up care.

Case Study 5

Name ______________________ Class/Group __________ Date __________

Group Members ____

INSTRUCTIONS: All questions apply to this case study. Your responses should be brief and to the point. Adequate space has been provided for answers. When asked to provide several answers, they should be listed in order of priority or significance. Do not asume information that is not provided. Please print or write clearly. If your response is not legible, it will be marked as ? and you will need to rewrite it.

Scenario

V.M. is a 39-year-old African-American man who has SCD, sometimes called sickle cell anemia, marked by frequent episodes of severe pain. His anemia has been managed with multiple transfusions, and he shows signs of chronic renal failure. He is a nonsmoker, nondrinker, and is on Social Security disability. His regular medications are pentoxifylline (Trental), oxycodone/acetaminophen, and folic acid. In hematology clinic this morning, V.M.'s Hgb measured 6.7 g/dl. He received 2 units packed red cells (PRC) over 3 hours and then went home. He developed dyspnea and SOB approximately one to 1½ hours later, and his wife called 911. The emergency medical system (EMS) crew initiated oxygen and transported V.M. to the ED.

1. What is sickle cell disease, and how is it R/T (related to) race?

2. The stiff, sickled RBCc tend to cause vascular occlusions with subsequent local infarction. As a rule, the spleen suffers so many vaso-occlusive/infarction episodes that it is greatly reduced in size and is rendered nonfunctional by the time the individual is 6 years of age. What are the implications of having a nonfunctioning spleen?

3. Identify two mechanisms that contribute to anemia in patients with SCD.

4. On arrival to the ED, the physician asks V.M. if he is in pain and if he needs meperidine (Demerol). V.M. answers no to both questions. Why did the physician ask these two questions?

5. V.M.'s arterial blood gases (ABGs) on 9 L O_2/simple face mask show Pao_2 (partial pressure of oxygen in arterial blood) 74 mm Hg, Is V.M. being adequately oxygenated?

6. V.M. complains of (C/O) being SOB. Do you believe his low Hgb level is responsible for his complaints?

You perform a quick assessment and note a systolic murmur and crackles in V.M.'s bases bilaterally. VS are 176/102, 94, 28, 97° F (oral). As you start an IV, you draw blood for CBC with differential, basic metabolic panel, calcium, and phosphorus and send it for analysis.

7. Your assessment findings are consistent with fluid overload. What four findings led you to that conclusion?

8. What action would you expect the physician to take next, and why?

The lab values return: Na 137 mmol/L, K 4.9 mmol/L, Cl 110 mmol/L, CO_2 16 mmol/L, BUN 27 mg/dl, CR 2.7 mg/dl, Ca 8.2 mg/dl, Po_4 4.7 mg/dl, WBC 4.3 thou/cmm, Hgb 7.8 g/dl, Hct 20.9%, platelets 208 thou/cmm.

9. What is the significance of the lab results, and why?

The physician prescribes furosemide (Lasix) 20 mg IVP now, methylprednisolone (Solu-Medrol) 125 mg IVP, and ceftriaxone (Rocephin) 1 g intravenous piggyback (IVPB) after the furosemide.

10. Explain the significance of using each of these drugs.

11. Why is it difficult to crossmatch blood to transfuse V.M.?

As V.M.'s SOB is relieved, he shakes the physician's hand and thanks him for asking about the presence of pain and the need for pain medication. V.M. states, "One of my biggest fears is that I'll come here in crisis and the doctor won't treat my pain aggressively enough. I don't want to be labeled as a drug seeker or an emergency room abuser."

12. Why would V.M. be concerned about obtaining adequate pain control in the ED?

V.M. voids 1900 ml within 2 hours of the furosemide administration. On repeat assessment, the systolic murmur is audible, but all lung fields are clear. Repeat VS are 160/94, 82, 20, 98° F (oral). V.M. is discharged to home on his previous medications.

13. What issues would you address with V.M. before he is discharged?

For more information contact:
Comprehensive Sickle Cell Centers
www.rhofed.com/sickle/

Case Study 6

Name ______________________ Class/Group __________ Date __________

Group Members ____

INSTRUCTIONS: All questions apply to this case study. Your responses should be brief and to the point. Adequate space has been provided for answers. When asked to provide several answers, they should be listed in order of priority or significance. Do not asume information that is not provided. Please print or write clearly. If your response is not legible, it will be marked as ? and you will need to rewrite it.

Scenario

D.M. is a married 36-year-old woman with four children who works part-time as a clerk. She is 5′8″ tall and weighs 135 pounds. She has insurance through her husband's employer. She has never smoked and has an occasional social drink. She has PMH of plastic surgery for breast implants in August of last year. When she returned for her breast implant check-up 10 months later, a 2.2 cm lump was discovered in her right breast. When a biopsy indicated the lump was malignant, she elected to have a lumpectomy and axillary lymph node dissection. The pathology report indicated that 3 of 14 lymph nodes were positive. Her CT scan and bone scans were negative. You are a staff nurse at the group oncology clinic where she was referred to receive chemotherapy. After she completes chemotherapy she is scheduled to receive radiation therapy. Admitting diagnosis: infiltrating ductal carcinoma, stage T2 N1 M0, premenopausal, estrogen receptor (ER) 3+, progesterone receptor (PR) negative, and Her2-neu 3+. (Note: Her2-neu is also known as C-ErbB-2.)

1. D.M. wants you to explain exactly what stage T2 N1 M0 means. What will you tell her?

2. Next, D.M. wants to know what the ER, PR, and Her2-neu values mean.

3. She asks you to explain what her chances of survival are. How will you explain this to her?

4. D.M. will be receiving six cycles of combination chemotherapy, consisting of doxorubicin (Adriamycin), and cyclophosphamide (Cytoxan). What are the major side effects you want to prepare her for?

5. Elaborate on issues R/T head/hair care.

6. What is a major complication in patients receiving a high amount of doxorubicin?

7. Explain to D.M. in lay terms what she needs to know about immunosuppression.

D.M. completes her chemotherapy. She lost most of her hair and has been wearing a scarf but now her hair is beginning to grow back. She is being transferred to the radiation therapy department for treatment and is scheduled to begin radiation therapy.

You perform an admission assessment. Findings are as follows: weight 148 pounds; VS 104/70, 80, 20, 98.0° F (oral). Cardiovascular: S_1 S_2 without murmurs or rubs. Respiratory: clear to auscultation throughout. Neuromuscular/skeletal: negative, patient C/O of fatigue, no C/O bone pain. GI: without hepatosplenomegaly or masses. GU: negative. Integumentary/oral: hair growth ¼ inch over entire head, oral mucosa reddened, and patient C/O soreness. Lymph node: no palpable adenopathy in the cervical, supraclavicular, axillary, or inguinal nodes. Extremities: no peripheral edema, all peripheral pulses palpable.

8. What areas of the above assessment concern you? Explain.

D.M. receives 6 weeks of daily (weekdays) radiation therapy treatments with a total dose of 6400 cGy. She has a terrible time with fatigue, and at one point tells you, "When I lie down, I can't become enough of the bed!" You helped her develop an activity-rest plan and support her in obtaining outside help with housework. At her last visit, she tells you, "Now I hope I can see my kids grow up." She is scheduled to return to the oncologist every 3 months for follow-up care and monitoring.

9. D.M. comes to her scheduled follow-up appointment. She appears very anxious. When questioned, she tells you, "I've been worried about my daughters. What if they get breast cancer? What can I do to help them?" What is your response?

10. You ask her whether she has other questions. She tells you she is worried about the breast cancer coming back and wants to know whether she would have to go through the chemotherapy and radiation therapy all over again. What can you do, and what will you tell her?

D.M. seems to do fine for a while. On her 9-month follow-up visit, she tells you she has been having headaches for the past few weeks. Her magnetic resonance image (MRI) indicates she has metastases to the brain. She undergoes a bone marrow transplant; unfortunately, it fails to stop her cancer. She dies at the age of 38, leaving behind four children, ages 4 through 14.

Case Study 7

Name ______________________ Class/Group __________ Date __________

Group Members ____

INSTRUCTIONS: All questions apply to this case study. Your responses should be brief and to the point. Adequate space has been provided for answers. When asked to provide several answers, they should be listed in order of priority or significance. Do not asume information that is not provided. Please print or write clearly. If your response is not legible, it will be marked as ? and you will need to rewrite it.

Scenario

A.V. is a 37-year-old married housewife with a 35-pack-year history of smoking. She says she "just can't quit." She denies alcohol (ETOH) use. Height is 5′7″; weight, 115 pounds. Her PMH includes C-sections for all three children ages 6, 14, and 18. She does not have insurance. She noticed a "canker sore" on the anterior lateral aspect of her left tongue several months ago. Over time, she developed a sore throat and ear pain. The family nurse practitioner at the low-income clinic sent her to a specialist, who performed a biopsy of her anterior tongue. The diagnosis was squamous cell carcinoma poorly differentiated T2 N0. Before her surgery she had complete panoramic views of her mandible; fluoride trays were made followed by a partial glossectomy and excision of the floor of her mouth. Three weeks after surgery, multiple teeth are scheduled to be extracted. Afterward she will be scheduled for 8 weeks of radiation therapy in your outpatient clinic.

1. Describe the rationale for this prophylactic treatment: teeth extraction, panoramic views, fluoride trays.

2. Identify and describe preoperative care for partial glossectomy.

3. Identify and describe potential postoperative care for partial glossectomy.

4. Identify and describe potential postoperative complications resulting from a partial glossectomy. Plan appropriate interventions and patient teaching strategies to manage these complications.

5. When she returns for her first postop visit to your clinic, she appears to be quite distressed to hear about the radiation therapy. Although she still has considerable trouble speaking, she explains she really didn't think much about it before surgery. She seems quite embarrassed as she tells you her family has no insurance, and they were barely making it earlier. Now she says she is getting "nasty letters" from the hospital demanding payment. What can you do?

6. As she sits by you, she keeps her hand over her mouth and jaw. She is wearing her hair so that it hangs down over her face. Her jaw and neck still are swollen from the surgery and tooth extraction. She avoids eye contact with you. How will you respond?

Case Study 8

Name ______________________ Class/Group __________ Date __________

Group Members ____

INSTRUCTIONS: All questions apply to this case study. Your responses should be brief and to the point. Adequate space has been provided for answers. When asked to provide several answers, they should be listed in order of priority or significance. Do not asume information that is not provided. Please print or write clearly. If your response is not legible, it will be marked as ? and you will need to rewrite it.

Scenario

D.L., a 21-year-old single man who works as a plumber's assistant, developed low back pain "from a work injury" 2 weeks ago. He had no PMH and is a lifetime nonsmoker, nondrinker. He is instructed to take diclofenac (Voltaren) 50 mg PO tid for 6 weeks and cyclobenzaprine (Flexeril) 10 mg PO tid for 6 weeks. Within 2 to 3 days, he develops a fever (101.6° F, oral), and a rash develops over his entire body. He shows dramatic bruising; he also develops a decreased appetite and a sore mouth. He is taken to the ED at a rural hospital when he starts vomiting blood. His labs are WBC 31.7 thou/cmm, Hgb 10.1 g/dl, Hct 29%, and platelets 16 thou/cmm. Arrangements are made to transfer him to the regional medical center (where you work on the hematology/oncology unit) to see an oncologist for a workup and to be admitted to the hospital for therapy. A bone marrow biopsy confirms the diagnosis of ALL (acute lymphoblastic leukemia).

1. What is ALL, and what are other names for this same condition?

2. You are the leukemia support and education group leader for your hospital. Patients attending your sessions have acute/chronic lymphocytic leukemia, acute/chronic myelogenous leukemia, myelodysplastic syndrome, and multiple myeloma. Your topic for discussion today is the etiology of these oncologic/hematologic disorders. D.L.'s older brother, T.L., is a nursing student, and he wants to know how many kinds of leukemia there are and if they are caused by the same thing. List the related diseases in the leukemia family and what is thought to cause each.

   For more information on ALL see www.leukemia.org.

- Chronic lymphocytic leukemia (CLL): Appears to be R/T autoimmune disorders such as lupus and hemolytic anemia. There is a higher incidence of CLL in the elderly and older individuals diagnosed with CLL tend to have a better prognosis.
- Chronic myelogenous leukemia (CML): The incidence of CML increases with exposure to radiation, benzene, and alkylating drugs used in the treatment of cancer.
- Myelodysplastic syndrome: associated with exposure to benzene products, radiation, and alkylating chemotherapy agents (e.g., busulfan, carboplatin, chlorambucil, cisplatin, cyclophosphamide, ifosfamide, nitrogen mustard, and thiotepa).
- Multiple myeloma: chromosome abnormalities, host genetic factors, chronic antigenic stimulation, and viruses are thought to contribute to the development of plasma cell dyscrasias.

3. D.L. asks you what the chances are for someone, like him, with ALL. What can you tell him?

D.L. is scheduled to receive the initial induction combination chemotherapy by IV and intrathecal (IT) routes. He will be receiving doxorubicin, vincristine, and cyclophosphamide IVP, methotrexate IT, and prednisone PO. He will be hospitalized about 3 weeks. He will be scheduled for intense consolidation courses, and then maintenance therapy for 1 year. The induction and consolidation courses are intense drug therapies, requiring multiple blood product infusions and antibiotic therapy to aid recovery. Because of his projected required course of therapy, he will be unable to work and will probably lose his insurance.

D.L.'s admission assessments are as follows: VS 140/74, 90, 24, 103.3° F (oral). Weight is 150 pounds. Cardiovascular: normal sinus rhythm, no S_3, S_4, rubs, or murmurs, all peripheral pulses present. Respiratory: clear to auscultation. Neuromuscular/skeletal: grossly intact. Motor and sensory examination normal. GI: spleen about five fingerbreadths below the right costal margin—tender; liver is not enlarged; no ascites or intraabdominal mass or CVA tenderness. GU: rectal not done. Integumentary/oral: HEENT, nomocephalic, pupils level, round, reactive to light in accommodation; no sclera icterus; conjunctivae very pale; funduscopic examination benign; oropharynx has some gingival lesions; mucous membranes moist and pale; tympanic membranes normal; neck supple; trachea midline; thyroid normal; no murmurs or JVD. To facilitate D.L.'s chemotherapy and blood product infusion, a triple-lumen subclavian catheter is inserted.

4. Describe potential effects the acute leukemia, treatment, and rehabilitation have on the socioeconomic status and family relationships of people like D.L.

5. During the next 14 days, D.L. receives irradiated platelets and leukoreduced ("filtered" irradiated) RBCs. What is the rationale for using irradiated, leukoreduced blood products? Describe the administration/monitoring procedure for these products.

6. D.L. will continue to receive intense combination chemotherapy for several more weeks. Because of limited finances, his hospitalization stay will be cut short. What are the major self-care management issues for home care that need to be reinforced?

7. D.L. is going to be staying with his parents. T.L. has promised to help with D.L.'s care. In addition, a home care nurse will visit him twice weekly. You are going to teach D.L. and his brother, T.L., to care for and use his triple-lumen subclavian catheter. What will you tell them?

Before he leaves, T.L. says, "You know, I've been studying about some of this stuff in my medical-surgical class, but I had no idea how bad it feels to go through this. I hope this makes me a better, more sensitive nurse."

Case Study 9

Name ______________________ Class/Group __________ Date __________

Group Members ____

INSTRUCTIONS: All questions apply to this case study. Your responses should be brief and to the point. Adequate space has been provided for answers. When asked to provide several answers, they should be listed in order of priority or significance. Do not asume information that is not provided. Please print or write clearly. If your response is not legible, it will be marked as ? and you will need to rewrite it.

Scenario

C.P. is a 71-year-old married farmer, with a PMH of hernia surgery in 1965 and prostate surgery in 1992 for benign prostatic hyperplasia (BPH). C.P. does not drink but he has smoked for 40 years; the past 3 years he has smoked 2-3 PPD. He has NKDA. Six months ago C.P. visited the local rural health clinic with C/O progressive cough and chest congestion. Despite a week of antibiotic therapy, C.P. continued to worsen; he experienced progressive dyspnea and productive cough, and he began to have night sweats. C.P. refuses to be admitted to the hospital ("There's no one to look after the cows") but agrees to go for a chest x-ray (CXR). His insurance company also insists on this being done on an outpatient basis. The radiologist reads C.P.'s CXR as left hilar lung mass, probable lung cancer. C.P. is scheduled for a diagnostic fiberoptic bronchoscopy with endobronchial lung biopsy as an outpatient to confirm the diagnosis.

1. What is fiberoptic bronchoscopy? What information will a fiberoptic bronchoscopy with endobronchial lung biopsy provide?

2. As the nurse who works with the pulmonologist, it is your responsibility to prepare C.P. for the fiberoptic bronchoscopy procedure. What would you include in your teaching plan?

3. What is your responsibility during and immediately after the bronchoscopy?

4. C.P. tolerates the procedure well. He returns to the office in 4 days to learn the results of his test. The pulmonologist tells C.P. and his wife that he has oat cell lung cancer and explains that it is a very fast-growing cancer with a poor prognosis. This kind of lung cancer is directly R/T C.P.'s history of smoking. What is your role at this time?

C.P. is scheduled to begin combination chemotherapy with cisplatin (Platinol) and etoposide (VePesid). He plans to continue to work the farm as long as possible; his brother-in-law has promised to help him.

5. How would you explain combination chemotherapy and how it works to C.P. and his wife?

6. C.P.'s wife tells you she's heard that chemotherapy makes you really sick. How would you explain chemotherapy side effects?

7. What are the most common side effects of cisplatin and etoposide?

8. Based on your knowledge of the most common side effects, list at least seven interventions that should be incorporated into his plan of care.

9. C.P. needs to have a working understanding of how to balance his treatments with his work. You sit down with C.P. to plan a daily work/activity/rest schedule to accommodate his treatments and side effects. List at least four concepts you would emphasize.

10. C.P. receives cisplatin 60 mg in 100 ml normal saline (NS) IV over 1 to 2 hours daily, the first 3 days of each month for 6 months, and etoposide 200 mg in 250 ml NS IV over 1 to 2 hours daily, the first 3 days of each month for 6 months. What is the nadir for each drug, and what implications does the nadir have for C.P.?

A month later, when C.P. returns for his second round of chemotherapy, he C/O SOB, chest tightness, and palpitations. He looks exhausted. Electrocardiogram (ECG) and CXR reveal A-fib and LLL (left lower lobe) pneumonia with left pleural effusion. C.P. is admitted to the hospital with the following laboratory values: WBC 2.5 thou/cmm, RBC 5.6 thou/cmm, Hgb 17.7 g/dl, Hct 51.7%, platelets 252.0 thou/cmm, Na 131 mmol/L, K 4.2 mmol/L, Cl 90 mmol/L, CO_2 25 mEq/L, BUN 13 mg/dl, creatinine 0.8 mg/dl, glucose 105 mg/dl.

11. What do these lab values indicate?

12. The pulmonologist performs a thoracentesis and prescribes cefotaxime 1 g IV and q8h erythromycin 500 mg IV q6h. What factor in C.P.'s background will complicate his diagnosis of pneumonia?

13. C.P.'s condition continues to deteriorate. He tells you he doesn't want to live like this, but the doctor wants to continue with aggressive therapy. Discuss the pros and cons of continued therapy and what role you can play in helping him.

C.P. refuses the second round of chemotherapy and is discharged to home. He receives no further treatment and dies 2 weeks later.

Case Study 10

Name ______________________________ Class/Group __________ Date __________

Group Members ____

INSTRUCTIONS: All questions apply to this case study. Your responses should be brief and to the point. Adequate space has been provided for answers. When asked to provide several answers, they should be listed in order of priority or significance. Do not asume information that is not provided. Please print or write clearly. If your response is not legible, it will be marked as ? and you will need to rewrite it.

Scenario

You are caring for J.B., a 56-year-old woman with colon cancer. PMH includes colon resection followed by combined chemotherapy approximately 18 months ago; recently diagnosed with recurrence of colon cancer; chemotherapy was administered for five of the eight scheduled cycles; previous significant weight loss (current height, 67″; weight, 105 pounds); 50-pack-year (2 PPD × 25 yr) smoking history. J.B. is admitted for acute N/V and dehydration. She is nutritionally depleted. Her physician determines that diagnostic evaluation requires exploratory laparotomy. VS 150/90, 124, 26, 100° F.

1. List at least five major risks and potential complications for J.B.

2. The physician performs an exploratory laparotomy for lysis of adhesions, small bowel resection, colectomy, and colostomy with Hartmann's pouch. After surgery J.B. is admitted to the SICU (surgical intensive care unit) with a large abdominal dressing. You roll J.B. side-to-side to remove the soiled surgical linen, and the dressing becomes saturated with a large amount of serosanguineous drainage. Would the drainage be expected after abdominal surgery? Explain.

3. Traditionally the physician performs the first dressing change. Why is this done?

4. The physician removes the surgical dressing. The wound edges are well approximated, the suture line is edematous, the staples are intact, the transverse colostomy rosebud looks pink in the middle and dark around the edges, and there are two Jackson-Pratt drains in the right abdomen. Do any of these findings concern you, and why?

The physician prescribes the following total parenteral nutrition (TPN) orders: amino acids 10% 100 ml; dextrose 70%, 1000 ml; water for injection 1000 ml; sodium acetate 20 mEq; sodium phosphate 20 mEq; potassium acetate 20 mEq; KCl 90 mEq; calcium gluconate 20 mEq; magnesium sulfate 10 mEq; regular insulin 10 units; multivitamins 1 amp; heparin 1200 units. Infuse 3000 ml volume over 24 hours daily.

5. List and explain at least five management activities you should provide to minimize the potential side effects of the TPN for J.B.

6. The TPN infusion is complete, the alarm is sounding, and the pharmacy has not delivered the next bottle of TPN. What action should you take, and why?

7. Within minutes of sitting in the chair, you note that J.B. is becoming increasingly pale and diaphoretic. Her pulse is rapid and irregular and she C/O being nauseated and dizzy. What actions should you take next?

8. J.B. looks at you and tells you that she knows she is never going to leave the hospital alive. She says she has a lot of regrets. She confides that she used to drink a lot and wasn't a good mother to her three children; her son hasn't spoken to her in 15 years. How should you respond?

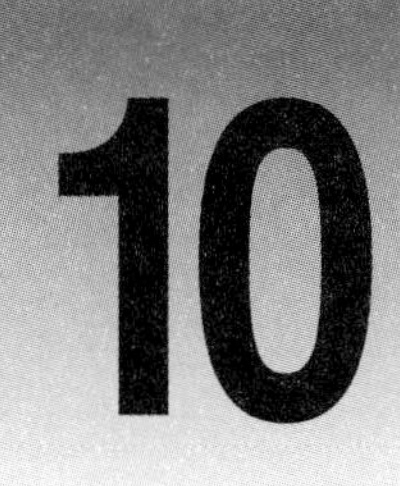

Women's Health Disorders

Case Study 1

Name ______________________ Class/Group __________ Date __________

Group Members ____

INSTRUCTIONS: All questions apply to this case study. Your responses should be brief and to the point. Adequate space has been provided for answers. When asked to provide several answers, they should be listed in order of priority or significance. Do not asume information that is not provided. Please print or write clearly. If your response is not legible, it will be marked as ? and you will need to rewrite it.

Scenario

K.W. is an 18-year-old who comes to Planned Parenthood for a pregnancy test because a condom had broken during intercourse the night before. Her last menstrual period (LMP) was 13 days ago and was normal. She always has a monthly menstrual cycle. She is extremely nervous about pregnancy because she is beginning college on a scholarship soon. She states there have been no other acts of unprotected intercourse since her LMP. She did take oral contraceptives briefly in the past but discontinued use due to weight gain and mood swings.

1. As the RN working in the clinic, should you run a pregnancy test?

2. K.W. asks if she is at risk for pregnancy. How should you respond?

3. She asks what contraceptive options are available to her at this point. How should you answer?

4. K.W. says, "Are you talking about having an abortion?" Formulate a response.

There are three EC options: contraceptive pills containing estrogen and progesterone, progesterone only pills, and the copper intrauterine device (IUD).

5. She asks you to explain the differences among the various options. What would you tell her?

6. She asks you about side effects. What would you tell her?

7. Which of the above methods of EC would you offer this patient?

8. How would you counsel this patient?

Case Study 2

Name ______________________ Class/Group __________ Date __________

Group Members ____

INSTRUCTIONS: All questions apply to this case study. Your responses should be brief and to the point. Adequate space has been provided for answers. When asked to provide several answers, they should be listed in order of priority or significance. Do not asume information that is not provided. Please print or write clearly. If your response is not legible, it will be marked as ? and you will need to rewrite it.

Scenario

L.W., a 20-year-old college student, comes to the clinic for a pregnancy test. She has been sexually active with her boyfriend of 6 months and her menstrual period is now 2 weeks late. The pregnancy test is positive. The patient begins to cry saying, "I don't know what to do."

1. How would you begin to counsel L.W.?

2. What options does a woman experiencing an unplanned pregnancy have?

3. If your role is to assist her in making the choice, what information would you want L.W. to identify?

4. What are the nurse's moral and ethical obligations in this situation?

5. L.W. wants to know when she has to decide.

6. L.W. asks you if there are any things she should be doing now to take care of herself. You would tell her:

7. L.W. asks you to tell her about abortion. What should you tell her?

8. L.W. wants you to explain the difference between vacuum aspiration and medical abortion. How would you explain this to her?

9. She tells you that she has heard that if a woman has an abortion she may not be able to get pregnant again. How would you counsel her?

10. What type of emotional reactions do women experience following an abortion?

11. What factors affect carrying a pregnancy to term? L.W. asks you about the importance of prenatal care. Explain.

12. Finally, L.W. wants to know about adoption. What should you tell her?

Case Study 3

Name ______________________ Class/Group __________ Date __________

Group Members ____

INSTRUCTIONS: All questions apply to this case study. Your responses should be brief and to the point. Adequate space has been provided for answers. When asked to provide several answers, they should be listed in order of priority or significance. Do not asume information that is not provided. Please print or write clearly. If your response is not legible, it will be marked as ? and you will need to rewrite it.

Scenario

You are working in a busy OB/GYN office and the last patient of the day is P.B., a 36-year-old, who is planning on getting married soon. She wants to use birth control, but is not sure what to choose. Her fiancé is in law school and they do not have health insurance so she is anxious not to get pregnant yet. She asks you to review the various methods and help her explore what is best for her.

1. What past medical information will you need to ask P.B. about?

2. Are there any other conditions that would influence the choice of a contraceptive method?

3. Is P.B. at risk for sexually transmitted infections?

4. What lifestyle information will help you assist P.B. in choosing an appropriate method for her?

5. P.B. asks you about the effectiveness rating of available birth control methods. Categorize your response according to the follow efficacy ratings: most effective (more than 99%), highly effective (97%-99%), and moderately effective (less than 90%).

6. P.B. asks you to explain the main advantages and disadvantages of the most effective methods.

7. What are the main advantages and disadvantages of the contraceptive methods in the highly effective category?

8. What about the moderately effective birth control methods? What are the main advantages and disadvantages?

9. She wants to know about cost with each method because she will be on a tight budget, with limited insurance coverage.

10. She asks you which method you would pick. What do you tell her?

Case Study 4

Name ______________________ Class/Group __________ Date __________

Group Members ____

INSTRUCTIONS: All questions apply to this case study. Your responses should be brief and to the point. Adequate space has been provided for answers. When asked to provide several answers, they should be listed in order of priority or significance. Do not asume information that is not provided. Please print or write clearly. If your response is not legible, it will be marked as ? and you will need to rewrite it.

Scenario

You are working as the triage nurse in the emergency department (ED) at a busy tertiary care center. A woman comes in complaining of (C/O) very heavy vaginal bleeding and extreme pain. S.K. is single, 47 years of age, and has been bleeding for 24 hours, soaking a pad an hour. She thinks her LMP was 2 months ago, but they have been irregular, and she isn't sure. She has had some spotting during the past 6 months, and is very afraid of the amount of bleeding in the past 24 hours. She works in a law firm as a paralegal and was very embarrassed yesterday when she leaked around her pad and stained a chair in the conference room. She has two sexual partners currently and has two children from a previous marriage.

1. Identify three conditions that would require emergency care and could prove life threatening.

You determine that S.K. is stable at the present level of bleeding; her VS are 110/68, 88, 22. She is not diaphoretic or pale. Her blood loss, although significant, does not present as hemorrhage with imminent hypovolemic shock.

2. She looks horrified and asks you, "Could I be pregnant?" How should you respond?

3. S.K. reports she hasn't been using birth control because she has sex so rarely. She wants to know if a urine pregnancy test would tell her whether she is pregnant. Provide information about a urine pregnancy test.

You go on to explain that there are other concerns with her heavy bleeding, so an ultrasound will be done to determine if she is pregnant and to exclude some of the most serious possible causes of her bleeding. You ask her how she would feel if she were pregnant and she says, "It would ruin my life." She states she is a single mother with two children in junior high school.

4. What can you tell her to help her with her obvious distress?

You inform her that you have counselors if she needs to talk to someone. "Everything we do here today or talk about is confidential."

During her ultrasound her BP drops to 90/42 and she C/O considerable cramping. The physician asks you to start an IV and infuse 1 L of D5LR to replace the volume lost during the last 24 hours and writes a prescription for meperidine (Demerol) 25 mg IV.

5. Before administering the meperidine, what should you ask her?

Her ultrasound is negative for pregnancy; she does not have an ectopic or intrauterine pregnancy. The ultrasound shows a very thick endometrial lining, even after 24 hours of bleeding.

6. S.K. is obviously relieved about the pregnancy, but while the physician is out of the cubicle writing discharge orders, she expresses fear that this could be cancer. What should you tell her to reassure her?

7. S.K. asks what she can do to keep this from happening again. Please respond.

8. What risk factors should you ask her about before discussing birth control pills as a treatment option?

9. If S.K. is prescribed birth control pills for the treatment of her bleeding problem, what other risks should she be aware of if she is using the pills for birth control?

S.K. is more comfortable now. The physician suggests birth control pills to control her bleeding. He tells her to take two pills a day for 2 or 3 days until her bleeding stops, then continue with one pill/day for the rest of the cycle.

10. What warning signs and symptoms do you want to tell her about as she starts her contraceptive pills?

You give her the telephone number of her OB/GYN and suggest she make the appointment right away. Reinforce that an endometrial biopsy to see if she has any abnormal cells with her heavy bleeding would be a good idea. Again, you stress she should go to her OB/GYN right away if the bleeding increases or the birth control pills do not stop her bleeding. She states that she understands.

Case Study 5

Name ______________________________ Class/Group __________ Date __________

Group Members ____

INSTRUCTIONS: All questions apply to this case study. Your responses should be brief and to the point. Adequate space has been provided for answers. When asked to provide several answers, they should be listed in order of priority or significance. Do not asume information that is not provided. Please print or write clearly. If your response is not legible, it will be marked as ? and you will need to rewrite it.

Scenario

You are the nurse in a walk-in clinic. A.P. is being seen this morning for a 2-day history of diffuse but severe abdominal pain. She has C/O nausea without vomiting but denies vaginal bleeding or discharge. A.P. claims to have had unprotected sex with several partners, some of whom have penile discharge. Her LMP ended 3 days ago. She has no known drug allergies (NKDA) and denies previous medical or psychiatric problems. VS are 108/60, 110, 20, 100.6° F (tympanic).

Physical examination finds her abdomen is very tender. The slightest touch of her abdomen causes her to wince with pain. Bowel sounds are normal. Pelvic examination finds purulent material pooled in the vaginal vault, which appears to be coming from the cervix. A sample of the vaginal drainage is obtained and sent for culture.

1. What medical interventions can you anticipate?

2. Based on A.P.'s stated history and the results of the vaginal examination, the physician treats her also for *Chlamydia* infection. Formulate a care plan for A.P. that can be shared with the community agency for follow-up.

3. Based on the previous question, identify the potential issues for noncompliance and what other action might encourage successful compliance.

The physician has the option of treating A.P. by one of two different methods. First, the physician could prescribe treatment over a period of 1 week; A.P. would be given the first dose of doxycycline (Monodox) 100 mg PO, then would be given a prescription for the same to be taken PO bid for 7 days. Second, the physician could prescribe a one-time dose of azithromycin (Zithromax) 1 g PO, which could be administered in the clinic.

4. A one-time dose of azithromycin 1 g PO is ordered for A.P. Why is this a good choice for her?

5. *Chlamydia* infection is considered a STD that is mandated to be reported to the public health department (PHD). Why?

6. You ask if someone has talked with A.P. about "safe sex." She laughs and tells you there is nothing safe about sex. Undaunted, you ask if she would be willing for you to discuss the use of condoms with her sexual partners. She tells you that she's already careful; if she doesn't know the guy, she uses condoms every time. How are you going to respond?

7. You ask A.P. if she has been tested for HIV. She says no, she doesn't know anyone with acquired immunodeficiency syndrome (AIDS), and she doesn't do sex with gay men. Now what are you going to say?

Case Study 6

Name ____________________ Class/Group __________ Date __________

Group Members ____

INSTRUCTIONS: All questions apply to this case study. Your responses should be brief and to the point. Adequate space has been provided for answers. When asked to provide several answers, they should be listed in order of priority or significance. Do not asume information that is not provided. Please print or write clearly. If your response is not legible, it will be marked as ? and you will need to rewrite it.

Scenario

T.C. is a 30-year-old woman who 3 weeks ago underwent a vaginal hysterectomy and right salpingo-oophorectomy for abdominal pain, and endometriosis. Postoperatively she experienced an intraabdominal hemorrhage, and her hematocrit (Hct) dropped from 40.5% to 21%. She was transfused with three units of packed red blood cells (PRBCs). Following discharge she continued to have abdominal pain, chills, and fever and was subsequently readmitted twice: once for treatment of postoperative infection and the second time for evacuation of a pelvic hematoma. Despite treatment, T.C. continued to have abdominal pain, chills, fever, and nausea and vomiting (N/V).

T.C. has now been admitted to your unit following an exploratory laparotomy. VS are 130/70, 94, 16, 37.6° F (tympanic). She is easily aroused and oriented to place and person. She dozes between verbal requests. She has a low-midline abdominal dressing that is dry and intact and a Jackson-Pratt (JP) drain that is fully compressed and contains a scant amount of bright red blood. Her Foley to down drain has clear yellow urine. She has an IV of 1000 ml D_5½NS infusing at 100 ml/hr in her left forearm, with no swelling or redness. T.C. is receiving IV morphine sulfate for pain control through a patient-controlled analgesia (PCA) pump. The settings are dose 2 mg, lock-out interval 15 min, 4-hour maximum dose of 30 mg. When aroused, she states that her pain is an 8 on a scale of 1 to 10. She also has 2 L O_2/NC, and her Sao_2 by pulse oximeter is 93%.

1. During your assessment you note that T.C.'s R is 16 and shallow. Articulate your plan for a more complete assessment of T.C.s' condition. Include factors to be considered, the supporting rationale, and your actions.

The unit is very busy when T.C. is returned from the postanesthesia care unit (PACU). Staffing is minimal. You are concerned about monitoring T.C. carefully enough. Your present patient load is six; of these, two patients are newly postop and one is getting ready for discharge. You have a nursing assistant who helps you and another R.N. You are most concerned with T.C.'s respiratory status and the possibility that she may, in her drowsy state, self-administer a dose of narcotic that would further reduce her respiratory status despite the lock-out time.

2. Formulate a plan, given the resources mentioned previously.

3. Pain control using the PCA can be very tricky. Throughout the first postop day, it has been difficult to juggle T.C.'s need for pain medication and depression of her respiratory status. Discuss the concepts of controlling pain with IV narcotics and factors that may be adjusted to better control her pain.

4. T.C. is beginning to withdraw from conversations with you and the other staff. She sleeps most of the day and is not eating. At times she is tearful and is irritable with her husband. You believe that she is showing signs of depression. What actions should you take to help her?

5. T.C. and her husband are talking one evening, and you overhear that they are very dissatisfied with the care provided by the physician. They believe that he has mismanaged T.C.'s care. They are discussing getting an attorney. They ask you what you think. What do you do?

6. You state, "Tell me what's going on with you right now. Maybe I can help you be more comfortable." What would be the benefit of taking this approach?

7. Mr. C. says, "No one is telling us anything. My wife came in here for a simple hysterectomy. She ends up with four surgeries. She still has pain, and she's worse off than when she started. Somebody has screwed up big time. Then they have the nerve to send me a bill. This morning they demanded $185,000. I'm not paying a dime until she gets better." How are you going to respond?

8. You ask her if she would like to be tested for HIV. It won't cost her anything, and no one will know the results but her; it's completely confidential. She agrees to the test and it comes back positive. What is her prognosis?

Case Study 7

Name ______________________ Class/Group __________ Date __________

Group Members ____

INSTRUCTIONS: All questions apply to this case study. Your responses should be brief and to the point. Adequate space has been provided for answers. When asked to provide several answers, they should be listed in order of priority or significance. Do not asume information that is not provided. Please print or write clearly. If your response is not legible, it will be marked as ? and you will need to rewrite it.

Scenario

P.T. is a married 30-year-old gravida 4 para 1203 (1 full-term pregnancy, 2 premature births, 0 abortions, 3 living children) at 28 weeks' gestation, arriving in the labor and delivery unit at a level two hospital complaining of lower back pain and frequency of urination. She states that she feels occasional uterine cramping and believes that her membranes have not ruptured.

1. You are the charge nurse and admit P.T. What other information do you need from P.T. to determine what you will do next?

2. P.T.'s prenatal chart is not in the labor and delivery unit because she is so early in the pregnancy. What additional obstetric information do you need to ask her at this time?

3. How will you assess this patient, before calling her physician? Identify seven factors you should address.

4. What other problems could be going on with P.T. that you should consider?

P.T.'s history reveals that she had one preterm delivery 4 years ago at 31 weeks' gestation. The infant girl was in the neonatal intensive care unit (NICU) for 3 weeks and discharged without sequela. The second preterm infant boy was delivered 2 years ago at 35 weeks' gestation and spent 4 days in the hospital before discharge. She has no other risk factors for preterm labor. VS are normal. Her vaginal examination was essentially within normal limits: cervix long, closed and thick, membranes intact. Abdominal examination: nontender, with fundal height at 29 cm, fetus in a vertex presentation.

5. While you are waiting for laboratory results, what therapeutic measures are there to consider?

Two hours later the laboratory results indicate a UTI, white blood cells (WBC) are within normal limits (WNL) and fetal fibronectin was negative. The contraction monitor indicates only occasional mild contractions. Her physician discharges her to home on an antibiotic for the UTI.

6. What follow-up measures should be considered?

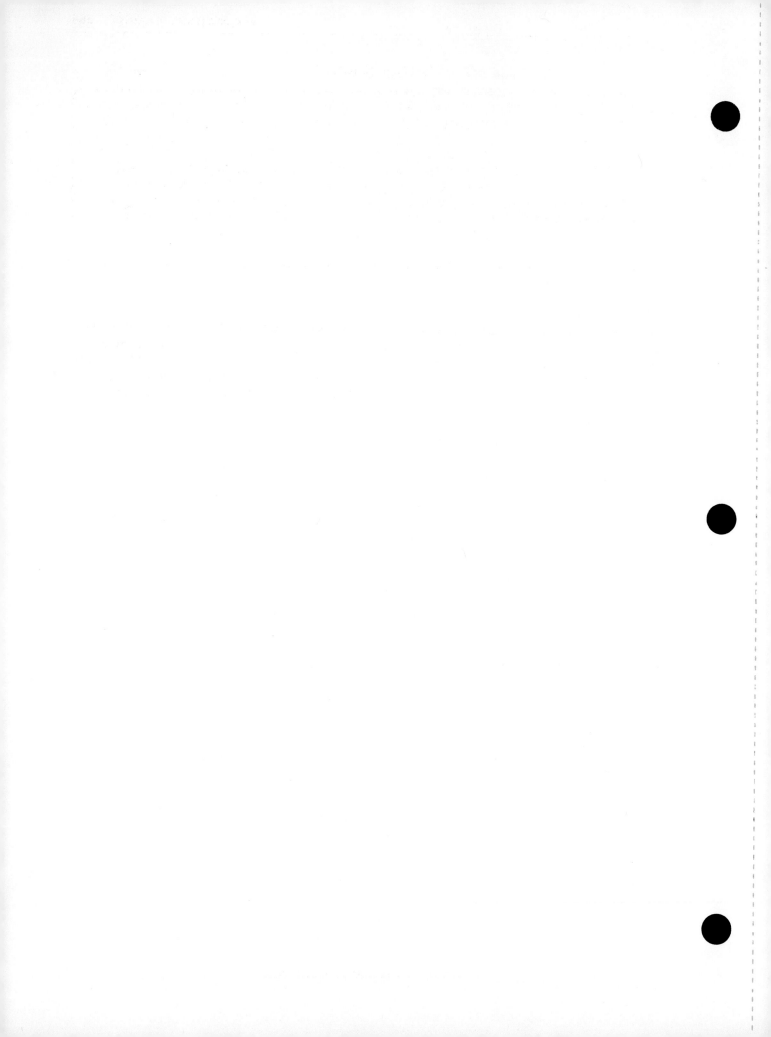

Case Study 8

Name ______________________ Class/Group __________ Date __________

Group Members ____

INSTRUCTIONS: All questions apply to this case study. Your responses should be brief and to the point. Adequate space has been provided for answers. When asked to provide several answers, they should be listed in order of priority or significance. Do not asume information that is not provided. Please print or write clearly. If your response is not legible, it will be marked as ? and you will need to rewrite it.

Scenario

J.F. is an 18-year-old single black gravida 1 para 0 at 38 weeks' gestation. This morning in clinic she presented with a blood pressure of 142/94, pulse 88, edema +2, headache, deep tendon reflexes (DTRs) +2, no clonus, proteinuria +2. Her physician is admitting her for induction of labor. She felt fine until 2 days ago, when she noticed swelling in her hands, feet, and face. She complains of a frontal headache, which started yesterday and hasn't abated with acetaminophen (Tylenol). She says she feels irritable and doesn't want the overhead lights on.

1. What other questions would you ask her at this time?

2. What information would you obtain from her obstetric record?

3. What laboratory values should be considered at this time?

4. What are the possible complications with preeclampsia?

5. Why is J.F. at risk for preeclampsia?

6. What measures are likely to be implemented?

J.F. progresses in labor and at 4 cm dilation her membranes spontaneously rupture. The small amount of amniotic fluid is green, indicating the fetus has had a meconium bowel movement.

7. What does this indicate? What are the risks?

8. J.F. delivers 5 hours later a 6-pound, 8-ounce boy, with Apgar of 7-8. What are your responsibilities at this time?

8. What neuroanatomic changes are seen in individuals with Alzheimer's disease?

9. A number of diagnostic tests have been ordered for K.B. From the tests listed below, which would be used to diagnose dementia?

Mental status examinations	Toxicology screen
Mini-Mental State Examination	ECG (electrocardiogram)
CMP (complete metabolic panel)	CBC (complete blood count) with differential
Thyroid function tests	Colonoscopy
RPR (rapid plasma reagin)	Serum B_{12}
Bleeding time	HIV (human immunodeficiency virus) screening
CT (computed tomography)	MRI (magnetic resonance imaging)

10. List at least three interventions would you plan for K.B. .

Available websites for additional information:
www.alzheimers.org
www.nlm.nih.gov/medlineplus/dementia.html

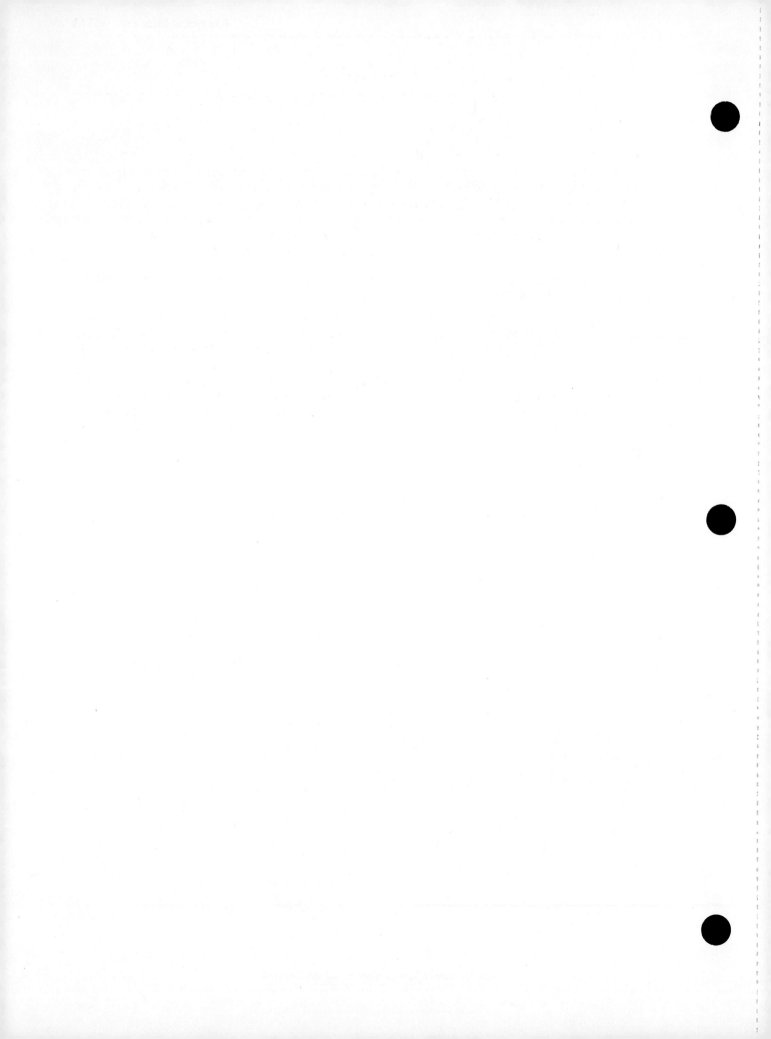

Case Study 2

Name ____________________ Class/Group __________ Date __________

Group Members ____

INSTRUCTIONS: All questions apply to this case study. Your responses should be brief and to the point. Adequate space has been provided for answers. When asked to provide several answers, they should be listed in order of priority or significance. Do not asume information that is not provided. Please print or write clearly. If your response is not legible, it will be marked as ? and you will need to rewrite it.

Scenario

You are working the day shift on a medicine inpatient unit. You are discussing discharge instructions with J.B., an 86-year-old male who was admitted for mitral valve repair. His serum blood sugar had been averaging 250 mg/dl or higher for the past several months. During this admission, his dosage of insulin was adjusted, and he was given additional education in managing his diet. In giving these instructions, J.B. tells you his wife died 9 months ago. He becomes tearful when telling you about that loss and the loneliness he has been feeling. He tells you he just doesn't feel good lately, feels sad much of the time, and hasn't been involved in his normal activities. He has very few friends left in the community, as most of them have passed away. He also tells you that he has been feeling so down the past few months that he has had thoughts about suicide.

1. What other information should you ask J.B. regarding his thoughts of suicide?

2. What characteristics of J.B. put him at high risk for suicide?

3. Which psychiatric disorders can result in suicidal ideations or gestures?

4. What questions would you ask J.B. to determine if he is clinically depressed?

5. List five of the most common signs of depression.

6. Identify two treatments that are available for depression.

7. If J.B. were started on an SSRI such as fluoxetine (Prozac) or sertraline (Zoloft), what special instructions would you give him regarding that class of medication?

8. What advantages does ECT hold over the other treatments of depression?

9. ECT is a highly stigmatized treatment; many people are reluctant to consent to initiate treatment. What are the most common untoward effects of ECT?

10. What immediate interventions would you carry out for J.B.?

Websites for additional information:
www.nimh.nih.gov/publicat/depressionmenu.cfm
www.depression-screening.org

Case Study 3

Name ____________________ Class/Group __________ Date __________

Group Members ______________________________

INSTRUCTIONS: All questions apply to this case study. Your responses should be brief and to the point. Adequate space has been provided for answers. When asked to provide several answers, they should be listed in order of priority or significance. Do not asume information that is not provided. Please print or write clearly. If your response is not legible, it will be marked as ? and you will need to rewrite it.

Scenario

You are the RN case manager in an outpatient mental health clinic. S.T. is here today for her outpatient mental health appointment. She has a diagnosis of bipolar disorder and has been stable for the past 3 years. Her last episode was an episode of mania that required hospitalization. She is 29 years old, married, with two children ages 2 and 4. She reports that her mood is better than it has been in a long time and she has lots of energy. When asked if she thinks this is a recurrence of mania she says no, she just thinks that things are finally getting better.

1. What other information would be important to ask S.T.?

2. What other information would help determine if S.T. presents with the onset of a manic or hypomanic episode?

3. Bipolar disorder is a disorder of mood, characterized by episodes of either depression, mania, or hypomania. What symptoms might you see if S.T. is experiencing mania or hypomania? (DSM-IV-TR: *Diagnostic and Statistical Manual of Mental Disorders*, IV edition, Text Revision)

4. How is hypomania different from mania?

Lithium is commonly used to treat bipolar disorder. S.T. has been taking lithium for several years.

5. When S.T. first started taking lithium she would have been cautioned to report side effects. Identify five symptoms she should report.

6. Lithium toxicity can occur in patients taking lithium. What are the symptoms of lithium toxicity?

7. What laboratory exams should S.T. have drawn routinely while taking lithium?

8. What instructions should have been given to S.T when she began lithium therapy?

9. Given her history of bipolar disorder, what should you teach S.T. to minimize mood swings?

Case Study 4

Name ______________________ Class/Group __________ Date __________

Group Members ____

INSTRUCTIONS: All questions apply to this case study. Your responses should be brief and to the point. Adequate space has been provided for answers. When asked to provide several answers, they should be listed in order of priority or significance. Do not asume information that is not provided. Please print or write clearly. If your response is not legible, it will be marked as ? and you will need to rewrite it.

Scenario

You are working on an inpatient psychiatric unit, and are to do an initial assessment on R.B., who has just been admitted. He has a diagnosis of schizophrenia, paranoid type. He is 22 years old and has been attending the local university and living at home with his parents. He has always been a good student, and has been active socially. Last semester his grades began declining and he became very withdrawn. He spends most of his time alone in his room. His grooming has deteriorated; he may go days without bathing. For several weeks prior to admission he insisted on keeping all of the blinds and curtains in the house closed. For the past 2 days he has refused to eat, saying, "They have contaminated the food." As you approach R.B., you note that he appears to be carrying on a conversation with someone but there is no one there. When you talk to him, he looks around and answers in a whisper but gives you very little information.

1. What are the "negative symptoms" of schizophrenia that R.B. is/may be experiencing? You should be able to identify at least three. (DSM-IV-TR)

2. Identify one "positive symptom" of schizophrenia that R.B. is experiencing?

3. Give an example of each of the following types of delusional thinking: thought broadcasting, thought insertion, grandiosity, ideas of reference.

4. What symptoms would indicate that R.B. has paranoid schizophrenia?

5. Why is it important to know R.B.'s history before he is diagnosed with schizophrenia?

6. What diagnostic screening would be important in evaluating R.B.?

7. What medications are commonly used to treat the symptoms of schizophrenia? Organize your answers according to typical and atypical antipsychotics.

8. R.B. is started on some typical antipsychotics. You inform R.B. and his family about the common side effects of the typical antipsychotics. Identify at least four symptoms.

9. What types of psychosocial treatments may be used to treat R.B.'s schizophrenia?

11. What would be the most important initial interventions in treating R.B.?

Case Study 6

Name ______________________ Class/Group __________ Date __________

Group Members ____

INSTRUCTIONS: All questions apply to this case study. Your responses should be brief and to the point. Adequate space has been provided for answers. When asked to provide several answers, they should be listed in order of priority or significance. Do not asume information that is not provided. Please print or write clearly. If your response is not legible, it will be marked as ? and you will need to rewrite it.

Scenario

You are working the evening shift in an inpatient psychiatric unit. The patients are in the day room watching a movie when suddenly someone starts yelling. You and other staff rush to the day room to find J.J., a 55-year-old male patient, crouched down in the corner behind a chair yelling at the other patients, "Get down. Get down quick.". You and the other staff are able to calm J.J. and the other patients and take J.J. to his room. He apologizes for his outburst and explains to you that the movie brought back memories of Vietnam. He had forgotten where he was and thought he was in combat again. He describes to you in detail the memory he had of being ambushed by the enemy and watching several of his comrades be killed. You remember hearing in report that J.J. is a Vietnam War veteran.

1. What is the most likely cause of J.J.'s behavior?

2. According to the DSM-IV, name three criteria that must be present to diagnose PTSD.

3. What is the difference between PTSD and acute stress disorder according to the DSM-IV?

4. Which symptom(s) of PTSD did J.J. most likely experience?

5. What therapeutic measures could be done to help J.J. during your shift this evening?

Note: When a clinician is faced with a patient who has experienced a significant trauma, major treatment approaches are support, encouragement to discuss the event, and education regarding a variety of treatments including relaxation techniques, psychotherapy, and medication.

6. Give examples of common antianxiety agents used to sedate a person experiencing severe anxiety.

Note: Some anxiolytics are controlled substances and should be used with caution, i.e., benzodiazepines such as lorazepam, alprazolam, diazepam, chlordiazepoxide, and clonazepam.

7. What are the adverse effects of long-term use of benzodiazepine anxiolytics?

8. What types of medications can be used safely for chronic anxiety disorders such as PTSD? Give examples of each.

9. List some relaxation techniques that could be implemented or taught to J.J. to help relieve J.J.'s anxiety.

10. What other treatment modalities could J.J. be referred to after his hospitalization to help treat his PTSD and related problems?

Case Study 7

Name ______________________ Class/Group __________ Date __________

Group Members ____

INSTRUCTIONS: All questions apply to this case study. Your responses should be brief and to the point. Adequate space has been provided for answers. When asked to provide several answers, they should be listed in order of priority or significance. Do not asume information that is not provided. Please print or write clearly. If your response is not legible, it will be marked as ? and you will need to rewrite it.

Scenario

J.G., a 49-year-old male, seen in the ED 2 days ago, was diagnosed (Dx) with alcohol intoxication and released after eight hours to his brother's care. He was brought back to the ED 12 hours ago with an active GI bleed and is being admitted to ICU; his Dx is upper GI bleed and alcohol intoxication.

You are assigned to admit and care for J.G. for the remainder of your shift. According to the ED notes, his admission vital signs (VS) were BP 84/56, P 110, R 26 and he was vomiting bright red blood. His labs were remarkable for Hct 23%, ALT 69 IU/ml, AST 111 IU/ml, and serum ETOH 271. He was given IV fluids and transfused 6 units of packed red cells (PRCs) in the ED. On initial assessment, you note that J.G.'s VS are BP 154/90, P 98, he has a slight tremor in his hands, and he appears anxious. He complains of a headache and appears flushed. You note that he has not had any emesis and has not had any frank red blood in his stool or "black tarry stools" over the past 5 hours. In response to your questions, J.G. denies that he has an alcohol problem but later admits to drinking approximately a fifth of vodka daily for the past 2 months. He reports having been drinking just prior to his admission to the ED. He admits to having had seizures while withdrawing from alcohol in the past.

1. Which data from your assessment of J.G. is of concern to you?

2. What are two most likely causes of J.G.'s symptoms?

3. When is it most likely for someone to have withdrawal symptoms after abrupt cessation of alcohol?

4. You note that J.G.'s physician has not diagnosed J.G. as having alcohol dependence and his orders do not include treatment for alcohol withdrawal. As an RN what action is necessary before you continue to care for J.G.?

5. According to the DSM-IV, what is the difference between alcohol dependence and alcohol abuse?

6. What would be helpful for J.G.'s physician to know regarding J.G.'s substance abuse history?

7. Which clinical assessment tool is commonly used to monitor for withdrawal symptoms? Explain how it is used.

8. What medications are commonly prescribed for patients withdrawing from alcohol?

9. What chronic health problems are associated with alcoholism?

10. What other medical problems will J.G.'s physician need to be aware of as he provides J.G.'s treatment for alcohol withdrawal? How could you help assess for these problems?

11. What lab tests might the physician order to assess for nutritional deficiencies or other medical problems J.G. is experiencing?

12. What types of education and referral should be done prior to J.G.'s discharge from the hospital?

13. What medications might be prescribed to J.G. to assist him with sobriety? What side effects and precautions should you educate the patient with each?

Case Study 8

Name ____________________ Class/Group __________ Date __________

Group Members ________________________________

INSTRUCTIONS: All questions apply to this case study. Your responses should be brief and to the point. Adequate space has been provided for answers. When asked to provide several answers, they should be listed in order of priority or significance. Do not asume information that is not provided. Please print or write clearly. If your response is not legible, it will be marked as ? and you will need to rewrite it.

Scenario

It is 1000 in the ED when the ambulance brings in G.G., a 35-year-old male who is having difficulty breathing. He complains about chest pain/tightness, dizziness, palpitations, nausea, paresthesias, feelings of impending doom, unreality, and is having trouble thinking clearly. He tells you, "I don't think I'm going to make it. I must be having a heart attack." He is diaphoretic and trembling. His vital signs are 184/92, 104, 28, 98.4° F. This episode began at work during a meeting at approximately 0920 and became progressively worse. A coworker called 911 and stayed with the patient until medical help arrived. The patient has no history of cardiac problems.

1. What would the highest medical priorities be for G.G.?

2. After a full medical work-up, it is determined that G.G. is stable. His shortness of breath (SOB) and anxiety are resolved after giving lorazepam 1 mg intravenous push (IVP). There is no evidence of any physical disorder and the Dx of panic attack has been made. G.G. admits to having had three similar episodes in the past 2 weeks; however, not nearly as severe or lasting as long. How do you think this diagnosis was determined?

3. G.G. shares with the ED staff that he has been under severe stress at work and home. He tells them he is going through a divorce, lost a child last summer in a motor vehicle accident (MVA), and his company is downsizing. He will probably be out of a job soon. He hasn't been sleeping well for the past couple of months and has lost about 20 pounds. Identify five additional triggers that could cause anxiety to build to the point of panic.

4. G.G. wants to know what causes panic attacks/disorder. Using etiologic theories regarding anxiety, what will you tell him?

5. G.G. has questions regarding the differences between panic attacks and panic disorder. According to the DSM-IV, what are the differences?

6. What medications are used to treat panic attacks? What will your patient teaching include?

7. G.G. expresses fear of panic attacks returning and wants to know what techniques would help him cope.

8. What is systematic desensitization?

9. What actions/interventions are most indicated in the treatment of panic disorder?

10. G.G. wants to know how he will be able to tell if he is successfully managing his anxiety disorder. What should you tell him?

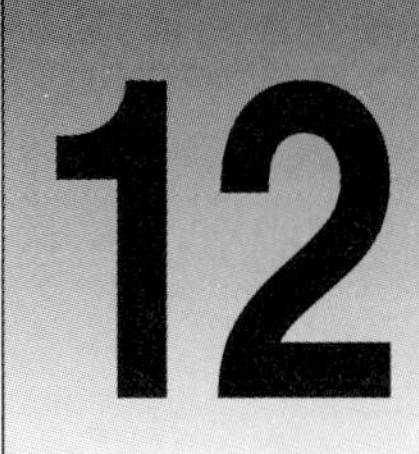

Alternative Therapies

Case Study 1

Name ______________________ Class/Group __________ Date __________

Group Members ____

INSTRUCTIONS: All questions apply to this case study. Your responses should be brief and to the point. Adequate space has been provided for answers. When asked to provide several answers, they should be listed in order of priority or significance. Do not asume information that is not provided. Please print or write clearly. If your response is not legible, it will be marked as ? and you will need to rewrite it.

Scenario

J.B., a 45-year-old female, is an office manager for a busy law firm and single mother of two children. While cleaning a shower stall she experienced a sharp pain in her lower back. Over the next few hours her lower back became increasingly more painful. By the time she picked up the children from their sporting event and drove to the nearest instacare, she had a sharp shooting pain into her right buttocks. Her spinal x-rays were not significant and she was diagnosed with acute musculoskeletal strain and given antiinflammatories, hydrocodone 5 mg/acetaminophen 500 mg (Lortab) by mouth (PO) every 6 hours as needed (PRN) for pain, and instructed to rest her back for the next 24 hours.

Monday morning she called in sick at work because she couldn't think clearly because of the pain medication. She developed stomach pain and her back pain was only slightly improved. She called a friend who had experienced a similar episode and related a very favorable outcome after being treated with acupuncture. J.B. comes to your alternative medicine clinic for her acupuncture appointment.

1. As you complete her intake interview, she asks, "What is acupuncture?" What would you tell her?

2. J.B. wants to know how acupuncture works. How should you explain acupuncture to her?

3. J.B. asks how acupuncture can help her back pain. Explain how acupuncture differs from traditional Western medicine in the treatment of back pain.

4. J.B. asks, "What does it feel like? Does it hurt?" How should you respond?

5. J.B. asks if she will have more than one treatment. Explain

6. J.B. asks, “Does insurance cover the cost?” Provide a response.

7. List possible risks and complications of acupuncture.

8. What types of condition can be treated with acupuncture?

9. J.B. asks where he could find an acupuncture practitioner.

For more information about acupuncture and acupuncture research contact the National Institutes of Health (NIH) National Library of Medicine (NLM). The bibliography is available on the Internet at www.nim.nih.gov/pubs/cbm/acupuncture.html or call the toll-free telephone number: 888-346-3056.

For a database of research on complementary and alternative medicine, including acupuncture, access the CAM Citation Index on the National Center for Complementary and Alternative Medicine (NCCAM) website at http://altmed.od.hih.gov/nccam.

Case Study 2

Name ______________________ Class/Group __________ Date __________

Group Members ____

INSTRUCTIONS: All questions apply to this case study. Your responses should be brief and to the point. Adequate space has been provided for answers. When asked to provide several answers, they should be listed in order of priority or significance. Do not asume information that is not provided. Please print or write clearly. If your response is not legible, it will be marked as ? and you will need to rewrite it.

Scenario

One month ago J.P., a 50-year-old male, came to the outpatient clinic with complaints of (C/O) mild shortness of breath (SOB) and some mild intermittent chest pain (CP). He described himself as a high-stress, type A personality who owns his own business and works long hours. He has smoked 1 pack per day (PPD) for the past 30 years. He has tried to quit several times and has been successful for as long as 6 months at a time but when business becomes stressful, he starts smoking again. Also, J.P. said he has been trying to lose the extra 30 pounds he is carrying but stated it is difficult to exercise due to the long hours of work.

The cardiac workup is negative for coronary artery disease (CAD) and he has returned for a follow-up (F/U) visit. During the discussion about lifestyle changes, J.P. expresses interest in medical hypnosis for stress management, smoking cessation, and weight loss. He would like more information. You are the case manager for the clinic and meet with J.P. to discuss medical hypnosis.

1. J.P. asks, “What is hypnosis?” What should you tell him?

2. J.P. asks what you mean by “trance state.” Explain the term.

3. J.P. wants to know what you mean by subconscious mind. Explain.

4. J.P. asks, "How does hypnosis work to help someone change a subconscious belief?"

5. J.P. states he has seen TV shows where people did silly things on stage. He wants to know how medical hypnosis is different than TV hypnosis. Explain.

6. J.P. asks how you can tell if hypnosis will work for a patient. Please respond.

7. J.P. wants to know how hypnosis is done, what happens during a session? You inform him that medical hypnosis has several components: patient preparation and education, establishing a rapport and trusting relationship, induction and deepening, hypnosis suggestions, and reawakening from the trance state. Briefly explain each step.

8. J.P asks what types of medical conditions can be helped by hypnosis. How should you respond?

9. J.P. asks if hypnosis is contraindicated for anyone. Please respond.

10. J.P. apologizes for being full of questions but wants to know if hypnosis can be done in a group or if it is one on one? Please respond.

11. J.P asks how he would go about finding a hypnotist. Formulate an answer.

For more information contact:
American Board of Hypnotherapy
16842 Von Karman Avenue, Suite 475
Irvine, CA 92714
(714) 261-4632
aih@hypnosis.com

American Psychological Association
Division 30, Psychological Hypnosis
750 First Street NE
Washington, DC 20002-4242
(202) 336-6013
www.apa.org/divisions/div30

American Society of Clinical Hypnosis
30 West Grand Avenue, Suite 402
Chicago, IL 60610
(312) 645-9810
info@asch.net

National Board for Certified Clinical Hynotherapist
8750 Georgia Avenue, Suite 14E
Silver Springs, MD 20901
nbcc@natboard.com

Recommended Journals:
American Journal of Clinical Hypnosis
C/O American Society of Clinical Hypnosis
33 West Grant Avenue, Suite 402
Chicago, IL 60610
www.asch.net/ajchform.htm
International Journal of Clinical and Experimental Hypnosis
Sage Publications
2455 Teller Road
Thousand Oaks, CA 91320
(805) 499-9774

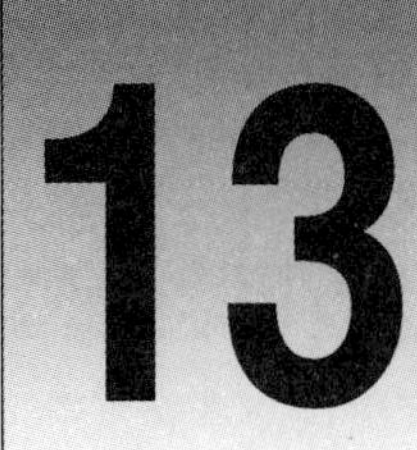

Multiple System Disorders

Case Study 1

Name ______________________ Class/Group __________ Date __________

Group Members ____

INSTRUCTIONS: All questions apply to this case study. Your responses should be brief and to the point. Adequate space has been provided for answers. When asked to provide several answers, they should be listed in order of priority or significance. Do not asume information that is not provided. Please print or write clearly. If your response is not legible, it will be marked as ? and you will need to rewrite it.

Scenario

You are working the day shift on the medical-surgical unit in a small rural community hospital. Your assignment includes an 18-year-old woman, A.N., admitted at night. A.N. was burned in a house fire and sustained burns over 30% of body surface area, with partial-thickness burns on her legs and back.

1. A.N. is undergoing burn fluid resuscitation using the standard Baxter (Parkland) formula. She was burned at 0200 and admitted at 0400. She weighs 110 pounds. Calculate her fluid requirements, and specify how much will be given and what time intervals will be used.

2. A.N. was sleeping when the fire started and managed to make her way out of the house through thick smoke. You are concerned about possible smoke inhalation. What assessment findings would corroborate this concern?

3. A.N. is very concerned about visible scars. What will you tell her to allay her fears?

4. A.N. is in severe pain. What is the drug of choice for pain relief following burn injury, and how should it be given?

5. A.N.'s burns are to be treated by the open method with topical application of silver sufadiazine (Silvadene). What is the major drawback to this method of treatment?

6. A special burn diet is ordered for A.N. She has always gained weight easily and is concerned about the size of the portions. What diet-related teaching will you provide?

7. Tissues under and around A.N.'s burns are severely swollen. She looks at you with tears in her eyes and asks, "Will they stay this way?" What is your answer?

8. Following significant burn injury, the patient is at high risk for infection. What measures will you institute to prevent this?

9. A.N. has one area of circumferential burns on her right lower leg. What complication is she in danger of developing, and how will you monitor for it?

Case Study 2

Name ______________________ Class/Group __________ Date __________

Group Members ____

INSTRUCTIONS: All questions apply to this case study. Your responses should be brief and to the point. Adequate space has been provided for answers. When asked to provide several answers, they should be listed in order of priority or significance. Do not asume information that is not provided. Please print or write clearly. If your response is not legible, it will be marked as ? and you will need to rewrite it.

Scenario

You are admitting a 30-year-old woman, J.L., to your telemetry unit with the diagnosis of status postcardiac transplantation and fever of unknown origin (FUO). She was healthy until the birth of her only child at 27 years of age. She developed idiopathic cardiomyopathy following childbirth and underwent cardiac transplantation at 29 years of age. There is a family history of early death from "heart problems."

1. Admitting has assigned J.L. to a semiprivate room. Her roommate is on day 4 of intravenous antibiotic treatment for pneumonia and now has a near normal white blood cell count (WBC) level. Is this assignment appropriate? What is your response?

2. Fever is a sign of two major complications of organ transplantation. What are they?

3. What other signs and symptoms (S/S) of organ rejection should the nurse assess for in this patient?

4. What other S/S of sepsis should the nurse assess for in J.L.?

5. While you are assessing J.L., she tells you that she always urinates frequently because of her diuretics. However, she has experienced burning with urination for the past 2 days. You wish to collect a urine specimen for laboratory analysis. What do you suspect may be causing the burning, and what type of urine specimen should you obtain?

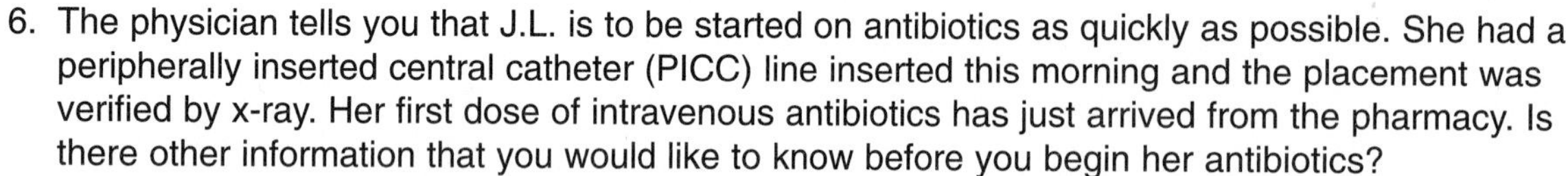

6. The physician tells you that J.L. is to be started on antibiotics as quickly as possible. She had a peripherally inserted central catheter (PICC) line inserted this morning and the placement was verified by x-ray. Her first dose of intravenous antibiotics has just arrived from the pharmacy. Is there other information that you would like to know before you begin her antibiotics?

7. Because J.L.'s heart was transplanted, there is no nerve connection. What happens to her heart rate with increased activity?

8. J.L. tells you that her husband's parents have given her son a pet cat. She jokingly says, "They gave him the play and me the work! My husband is going to have to help. I'm not up to looking after a cat, too." What job does her husband need to do?

9. You would like to teach J.L. some practical things she can do to protect herself from infection. List five. (Hint: This list should include many of the same things cancer patients on chemotherapy are taught.)

Case Study 3

Name ______________________ Class/Group __________ Date __________

Group Members ____

INSTRUCTIONS: All questions apply to this case study. Your responses should be brief and to the point. Adequate space has been provided for answers. When asked to provide several answers, they should be listed in order of priority or significance. Do not asume information that is not provided. Please print or write clearly. If your response is not legible, it will be marked as ? and you will need to rewrite it.

Scenario

You are working evenings on an orthopedic floor. One of your patients, J.O., is a 25-year-old man who was a new admission on day shift. He was involved in a motor vehicle accident (MVA) during a high-speed police chase. His admitting diagnosis is status post (S/P) open reduction and internal fixation (ORIF) of the right femur (which was performed under general anesthesia), multiple rib fractures, sternal bruises, and multiple abrasions. He speaks some English but is more comfortable with his "home" language. He is under arrest for narcotics trafficking, so one wrist is shackled to the bed and he has a guard with him continuously. Another drug dealer has told him "he's coming to get him." Hospital security is aware of the situation.

Your initial assessment reveals stable VS of 116/78, 84, 16, 98.6° F. His only complaint is pain, for which he has a PCA pump. He has crackles in lung bases bilaterally. His abdomen is soft and nontender. He has a NGT (nasogastric tube) connected to LWS (low wall suction). His IV of D_5LR is infusing in the proximal port of a left subclavian triple-lumen catheter; the remaining two ports are heparin-locked. His right femur is connected to skeletal traction. The dressing is dry and intact over the incision site.

1. J.O. wants to smoke a cigarette. He usually smokes a pack a day and has had none since the accident. He is irate because the day nurse would not let him smoke. What is your major concern about J.O.'s smoking?

2. Do you think J.O. would be a good candidate for a nicotine patch? Why or why not? State your rationale.

3. J.O.'s right leg is connected to 10 pounds of skeletal traction. As you troubleshoot the system, you note that the ropes are knotted at connection sites, the pulleys have rope running along the center tracts, the leg is slightly flexed at the knee, the leg is 6 inches above the mattress, and the 10-pound weight is resting on the floor. Are any of these findings of concern to you? If so, how would you fix it?

The nurse in the emergency department (ED) phones to tell you that J.O.'s immunization status could not be determined when he arrived so no tetanus immunization was given. When you ask J.O. the date of his last tetanus shot, he looks puzzled and asks you what a tetanus shot is. When asking about his childhood, you find that he was born and raised in Colombia. He immigrated to the United States 5 years ago. He does not know if he has ever had a tetanus shot. You inform the physician and he orders diphtheria/tetanus toxoid 0.5 ml IM and tetanus immune globulin (Hypertet) 250 units deep IM.

4. Why is J.O. getting two injections?

5. J.O. has a Foley catheter inserted to drain his urine. What should the nurse assess for in relation to the Foley catheter?

6. While assessing distal to the fractured femur, the nurse notes that his toes are cold to the touch. What other assessment findings should be gathered?

7. J.O. has an antiembolism stocking ordered for his left leg. What is the rationale for putting stockings on only one leg?

8. At 1800 J.O.'s guard summons you to his room. J.O. is cold and clammy, groaning, pale, agitated, and slightly confused. VS are 70/palp, 140, 28, 98.0° F. His pulse is weak and thready. His abdomen is painful and appears to be increased in size. You summon the physician. What else can you do?

9. The physician arrives and wishes to perform a peritoneal lavage. Explain why peritoneal lavage is being done, and describe the procedure.

10. What are the nurse's responsibilities in preparation for this procedure (in order)?

11. The physician begins the diagnostic peritoneal lavage procedure. Upon insertion of the trochar into the abdomen, bright red blood under pressure returns. What happens next?

12. In view of the threat made on J.O.'s life and his vulnerable situation, what precautions should the nursing unit take to protect him?

J.O. recovered for several weeks in the hospital before being sent to jail to await trial. Shortly before his trial date, he was found stabbed to death in his cell. Although there was an investigation, the murder weapon was never found, and no one was ever charged in his death.

Case Study 4

Name ______________________ Class/Group __________ Date __________

Group Members ____

INSTRUCTIONS: All questions apply to this case study. Your responses should be brief and to the point. Adequate space has been provided for answers. When asked to provide several answers, they should be listed in order of priority or significance. Do not asume information that is not provided. Please print or write clearly. If your response is not legible, it will be marked as ? and you will need to rewrite it.

Scenario

You are working on a telemetry unit and have just received a transfer from the ICU. The 50-year-old male patient, T.A., had a repair of an AAA measuring 8 cm in diameter. This is his second postoperative day. He is an attorney with a very active practice. He considered himself to be healthy before diagnosis of the aneurysm, although he took medication for gastritis. He has had progressive weakness of his lower extremities and decreasing urine output since surgery. T.A. also has a 10-year history of type 2 DM; he has been requiring insulin the past 6 months to keep his glucose levels under control.

1. T.A. has questions about his surgery. He asks you, "I was fine before surgery. I'd still be fine now if I hadn't been operated on, wouldn't I?" Based on your knowledge of AAA, what should your response be?

Because the AAA is clamped during the most crucial part of the surgery, nerve damage to the legs and blood clots are a risk with this surgery and require frequent assessment.

2. You are performing your initial assessment of T.A.'s legs. What findings should you record?

3. Four hours after admission to your floor, you note that T.A. has had a urine output of 75 ml of dark amber urine. You examine the catheter and tubing for obstructions, and there are none. What other assessment data should you gather to determine whether or not a problem exists?

4. Laboratory tests reveal renal damage. T.A. is placed on fluid restriction and a renal diet. T.A. asks what he is going to be able to eat on his diet. What is your reply?

Note: An RD can work with T.A. to incorporate many of his favorite foods in a reasonable diet that he can live with.

5. T.A. has a dialysis catheter inserted into his left subclavian vein. You are preparing to administer an IV antibiotic and find that his only other IV access, a peripheral line, is obstructed. What should you do?

6. Upon return from his first dialysis, T.A. complains of (C/O) headache and nausea. He is restless and slightly confused, and he has an elevated blood pressure (BP). You suspect disequilibrium phenomenon. You notify the physician. What measures can you institute at this point?

7. T.A. has an episode of severe vomiting. His abdominal wound dehisces, and a loop of his intestines eviscerates. Another staff member has summoned the physician. What care should you render before the physician's arrival?

T.A. returns from the OR. You note that his blood sugars have ranged from 62-387 mg/dL over the last 7 days.

8. A sliding scale with regular insulin has been ordered. He comments, "That's funny, you're giving me about the same amount of insulin that I give myself at home. I don't understand why it's not working." How should you respond?

9. T.A.'s wound is not healing. You call the enterostomal therapy (ET) registered nurse (RN) to evaluate what can be done. After looking at T.A.'s wound, he looks at the chart, sighs, and points to the glucose levels. "Here's your problem," he says. "The way this is going, he'll never heal." Based on recent findings in diabetes management, explain what he means. What other health care professionals may help you with T.A.'s glucose regulation?

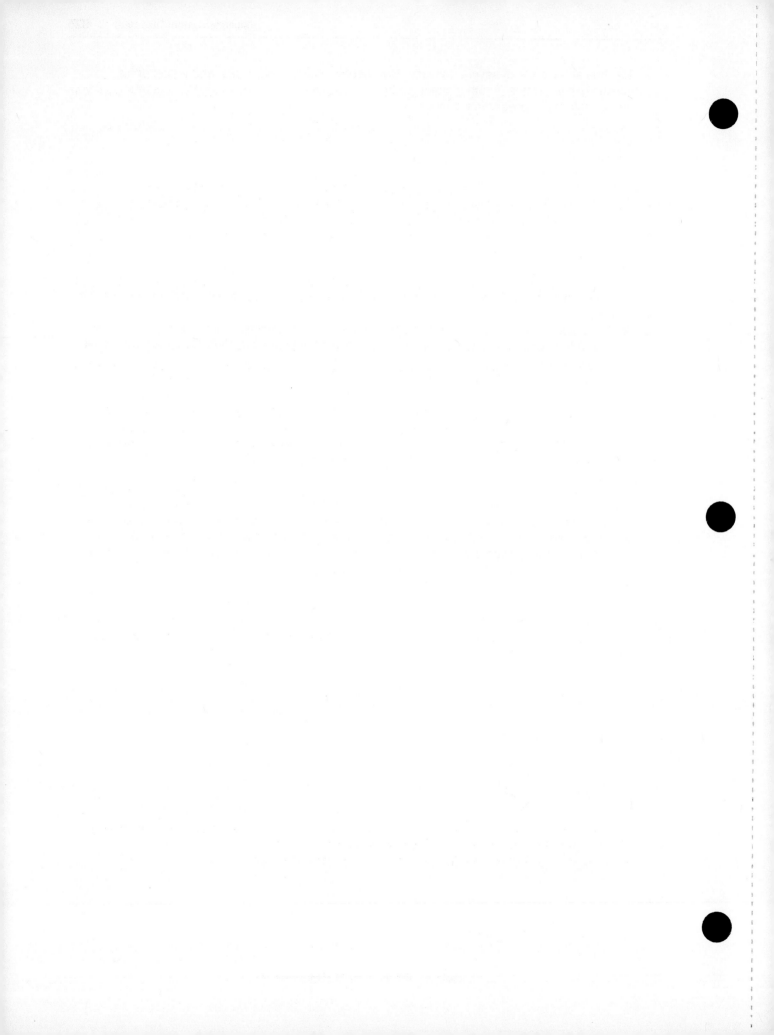

Case Study 5

Name ______________________ Class/Group __________ Date __________

Group Members ____

INSTRUCTIONS: All questions apply to this case study. Your responses should be brief and to the point. Adequate space has been provided for answers. When asked to provide several answers, they should be listed in order of priority or significance. Do not asume information that is not provided. Please print or write clearly. If your response is not legible, it will be marked as ? and you will need to rewrite it.

Scenario

You are a nurse working in the medical intensive care unit (MICU) and take the following report from the ED RN. We have a patient for you; R.L. is an 82-year-old frail woman who has been in a nursing home. Her admitting diagnosis (Dx) is sepsis, pneumonia, dehydration, and she has a stage III pressure ulcer. Past medical history (PMH) includes remote Hx CVA with residual right-sided weakness and paresthesia, remote MI, and PVD. Her VS are 98/62, 88, R 38 and labored T 100.4. Labs have been drawn and are pending; she has O_2 at 10 L via face mask, an IV of D_5.45NS at 100 ml/hr, and an indwelling Foley. The infectious disease doctors have been notified, and respiratory therapy is with the patient—they are just leaving the ED and should arrive shortly.

1. Knowing that L.R. is frail, has right-sided weakness and pressure ulcer, what consults would you initiate?

2. As you conduct your skin assessment, what areas of the patient's body will you pay particular attention to?

During your admission skin assessment you note that she has very dry, thin, almost transparent skin. There are several areas of ecchymosis on her upper extremities.

3. What interventions would you initiate to prevent further skin breakdown?

4. What does it mean to "stage a pressure ulcer"?

5. What factors increase risk for the development of tissue breakdown and the formation of pressure-induced ulcers?

Many facilities have a policy for using a validated risk assessment tool, i.e., Braden, Norton, or Gosnell scale, when a patient is admitted to their facility. All facilities have protocols dictating frequency of skin assessment.

6. What are the advantages of using a validated risk assessment tool to document the patient's skin condition on admission?

7. What does a stage I pressure ulcer look like?

8. What tissues are involved with stage II through IV ulcers?

9. What are the limitation/restrictions of staging pressure ulcers?

As you proceed with the assessment, an ET and wound nurse specialist comes in. She knows R.L. from a prior admission and had ordered a specialty mattress as soon as she received the wound/bed consult. She states she has ordered an air overlay and it should be delivered to your unit before your shift ends.

10. Why is a specialty bed or mattress used for immobile or compromised patients?

There are classifications of specialty beds/mattresses, with general guidelines for placement based on a patient's condition/risk. At one end of the spectrum are foam mattress/mattress replacements and gel overlays. Then there are several types of air overlay mattresses and beds: static air, dynamic air, low air loss, and fluidized air. Often they are referred to in terms of pressure relief or reduction.

11. What are the essential points all nurses should know about the patient's bed?

12. Why do patients placed on a specialty mattress/bed remain at risk for breakdown?

13. Why do the heels have the greatest incidence of breakdown, even when the patient is on the most advanced specialty bed?

14. What intervention can you initiate to protect R.L.'s heels?

15. R.L. has limited mobility secondary to her stroke. Her current illness may have further compromised her mobility and activity. What measures should you include in her plan of care?

16. What risk factor does the drawsheet prevent/minimize?

Pressure, friction, and shear are all mechanical injuries. Shear is a force applied parallel to the plane of an object but in the opposite direction to the force being applied. Shear is the result of gravity and resistance. For example: The head of the bed is elevated and the patient slowly slides toward the foot of the bed. The skin of the sacrum meets the resistance of the bed surface while gravity pulls the patient's body toward the foot of the bed. This means the skin and the bones are going in opposite directions, thereby pulling and stretching tissue and distorting vessels within the area, causing destruction of both. Undermining is thought to be the direct result of shear insult to pressure-induced injury. Friction can happen without shear, but shear always begins with friction.

17. What intervention is needed to reduce the possibility of shear?

The wound nurse gently removes the old dressing, using the push-pull method and adhesive remover wipes. After she takes off the outside dressing, often called a secondary dressing, she pulls out the primary dressing and tells you it was "packed" too hard.

18. What problems can packing a wound too full create?

19. What is considered the best-practice protocol for swab culture?

After culturing of the wound, you watch the nurse do a systematic assessment of the wound as per the recommended guidelines provided by the AHCPR/AHCRQ and NPUAC. The wound nurse will chart the findings and make recommendations for management.

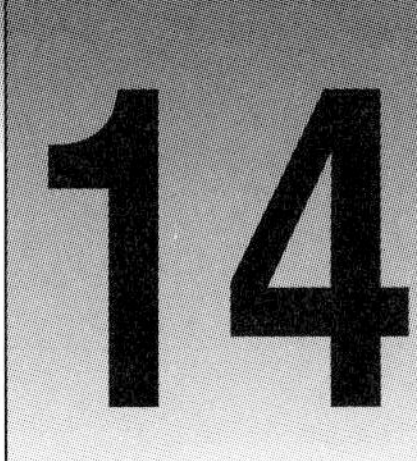

Emergency Situations

Case Study 1

Name ________________________________ Class/Group ___________ Date ___________

Group Members ____

INSTRUCTIONS: All questions apply to this case study. Your responses should be brief and to the point. Adequate space has been provided for answers. When asked to provide several answers, they should be listed in order of priority or significance. Do not asume information that is not provided. Please print or write clearly. If your response is not legible, it will be marked as ? and you will need to rewrite it.

Scenario

You are on duty in the emergency department (ED) when a "code blue" is called overhead. As the code nurse, you grab the crash cart and run to the code, which is in the employee lounge of the operating room (OR). On the couch you find a nurse, Z.H., unconscious, cyanotic, and barely breathing. Her scrub shirt has been cut off, and you attach electrocardiogram (ECG) leads to her chest. Her pulse is 45; respirations are 8 and shallow. She is intubated, an intravenous (IV) line is started with 0.9% NS (normal saline), and she is given an ampule of 50 ml D_5W, 0.4 mg naloxone (Narcan), and 0.5 mg atropine intravenous push (IVP). Her respirations improve slightly, and pulse increases to 56. She is transported to the ED.

1. What is the purpose of giving the three drugs mentioned in this case?

After additional naloxone, the patient wakes up and is extubated.

2. What additional information do you want to know?

In response to your questions, Z.H. tells you that she took fentanyl (Duragesic) IM (intramuscular). She then asks you to call a friend to come stay with her.

3. What information would you give her friend over the phone?

4. The friend asks you what is wrong. How do you respond?

5. Identify four problems relating to Z.H.'s care that apply to this situation.

Z.H. is admitted to the intensive care unit (ICU) for 24-hour observation and then transferred to the chemical dependency unit.

6. What is chemical dependency?

One of Z.H.'s colleagues calls on the phone to ask how she is. She tells you that she thought something was wrong with Z.H. because her behavior was so erratic, but "I had no idea it was drugs. I didn't think Z.H. would ever do anything like that!" Keep in mind that patient confidentiality extends to health care professionals not directly involved in Z.H.'s care. You cannot give information on how Z.H. is doing. (For more information see HIPAA [Health Insurance Portability and Accountability Act] guidelines.)

7. What is the profile of an impaired nurse? (List five characteristics.)

8. What four problems are associated with impaired nurses who are practicing?

Z.H. asks her nurse what is going to happen to her career.

9. What are the regulatory issues related to (R/T) impaired nurses that will guide your response? (List at least five.)

Note: These stipulations vary according to individual state regulatory laws and nurse practice acts. Encourage students to become familiar with the policies of your state.

Z.H. successfully completes treatment and continues to practice as a nurse. She is now serving as a sponsor for another nurse undergoing treatment for chemical dependency.

Case Study 2

Name ____________________ Class/Group __________ Date __________

Group Members ____________________________________

INSTRUCTIONS: All questions apply to this case study. Your responses should be brief and to the point. Adequate space has been provided for answers. When asked to provide several answers, they should be listed in order of priority or significance. Do not asume information that is not provided. Please print or write clearly. If your response is not legible, it will be marked as ? and you will need to rewrite it.

Scenario

It is 0800, and the outpatient clinic where you work as an RN has just opened. R.W., a 40-year-old man, hops into the clinic and complains of (C/O) severe pain and swelling in his right lower leg. He tells you he was walking between two cars the night before, when one of the cars backed up, catching his lower leg between the bumpers. He states he didn't think it was "hurt that bad" and went home to wash the abrasions. He woke up at approximately 0400, and states, "My leg was killing me."

1. How would you transport R.W. to the examining room?

R.W. is placed in the examining room and asked to remove his trousers and put on a gown. R.W. is unable to lay his leg on the exam table without pain. You observe that his right lower leg is grossly edematous and pale.

2. What should your next priority be?

There are no pulses in the distal extremity, sensation is diminished, the extremity is cold to touch, and any movement is extremely painful.

3. What should your next action be?

4. The physician is with another patient, and asks you to wait a minute. How should you respond?

After assessing the patient, the physician determines that R.W. should be transported to the nearest ED. The clinic physician notifies the ED physician that R.W. is coming in by ambulance with possible compartment syndrome of the right lower leg.

5. Explain the pathophysiology of compartment syndrome and clarify its significance.

6. How is compartment syndrome treated?

7. While waiting for the ambulance, R.W. starts to tell you "one-leg" jokes. How will you respond?

8. How would a nurse manage the fasciotomy once it has been performed?

9. Given that this is a crush injury, the physician orders a urine for myoglobin on R.W. What is the rationale behind this order?

10. How is rhabdomyolysis treated?

After an uneventful 5-day stay on the surgical unit, R.W. is being discharged to home care services and has been referred for PT.

11. As the nurse questions him about his living conditions, she discovers that R.W. lives alone in a third-story apartment; there are no elevators. What other information would she need from R.W. in preparation for discharge?

Case Study 3

Name ______________________ Class/Group __________ Date __________

Group Members ____

INSTRUCTIONS: All questions apply to this case study. Your responses should be brief and to the point. Adequate space has been provided for answers. When asked to provide several answers, they should be listed in order of priority or significance. Do not asume information that is not provided. Please print or write clearly. If your response is not legible, it will be marked as ? and you will need to rewrite it.

Scenario

You are the nurse on a medical unit taking care of a 40-year-old man, T.Z., who has been admitted with peptic ulcer disease (PUD) secondary to chronic alcoholism. You enter T.Z.'s room and find him having a generalized convulsive (tonic-clonic) seizure.

1. List five things you would do.

Note: Placing any objects, including an airway, into the patient's mouth at this point is contraindicated because of the possibility of patient or caregiver harm.

T.Z.'s seizure activity does not appear to be subsiding, and he is becoming cyanotic. The physician is notified and orders lorazepam (Ativan) 4 mg IV over 2 to 5 minutes, repeat once in 1- to 15 minutes prn (as needed).

2. What is the rationale for giving T.Z. lorazepam?

3. What is status epilepticus?

4. List one thing you would be particularly alert for when giving lorazepam intravenously.

By the time the physician arrives, T.Z.'s seizure activity has not subsided. The physician administers an additional 4 mg of lorazepam, without effect. Fifteen minutes have elapsed since you found T.Z. having seizure activity.

5. What is the significance of this?

The physician decides to administer succinylcholine (Anectine) and intubate T.Z. to protect his airway.

6. What is succinylcholine, and why is it being administered to T.Z.?

T.Z. has been intubated; the physician orders a phenytoin (Dilantin) 20 mg/kg IV loading dose and transport to ICU.

7. What is the rationale behind giving phenytoin?

8. List two problems related to T.Z.'s care.

9. Given T.Z.'s history, state at least two possible causes for his grand mal seizure.

T.Z's seizure is successfully treated with lorazepam and phenytoin, and he has no further seizure activity. As you are writing up his discharge papers, you overhear T.Z. telling his girlfriend to have his car brought to the hospital so he can drive home.

10. How should you respond to this situation?

Case Study 4

Name ______________________ Class/Group __________ Date __________

Group Members ____

INSTRUCTIONS: All questions apply to this case study. Your responses should be brief and to the point. Adequate space has been provided for answers. When asked to provide several answers, they should be listed in order of priority or significance. Do not asume information that is not provided. Please print or write clearly. If your response is not legible, it will be marked as ? and you will need to rewrite it.

Scenario

You are working in the ED when a patient comes in with an allergic reaction to bee pollen she has eaten. She brought the jar of bee pollen with her. M.W., your nurse colleague, is curious about how bee pollen tastes and ingests a small amount. A few minutes later M.W. begins to experience itching in her throat and ears, hives, and mild respiratory distress. The respiratory distress rapidly progresses to audible wheezing. You notice that she appears to be in distress.

1. What do you think is wrong with M.W.?

2. Given that your colleague is having a possible allergic reaction, what actions should you take? (List five.)

3. What is the rationale behind giving the medications you identified in your answer to question 2? List their usual dosages.

M.W. begins to improve. She states that the itching has subsided and the hives are fading. She reports that she no longer has acute SOB (shortness of breath). On auscultation of her lungs, you note that the wheezing has resolved. She wants to return to work.

4. Is it appropriate to allow her to return to duty? Why?

A decision is made to discharge M.W. to her home.

5. What issues should you address in discharge teaching of this nurse? (List three.)

6. Should you allow M.W. to drive herself home? Why?

A friend is called to come and drive M.W. home, and she is discharged. She lives to nurse another day!

Case Study 5

Name ________________________________ Class/Group ___________ Date ___________

Group Members ____

INSTRUCTIONS: All questions apply to this case study. Your responses should be brief and to the point. Adequate space has been provided for answers. When asked to provide several answers, they should be listed in order of priority or significance. Do not asume information that is not provided. Please print or write clearly. If your response is not legible, it will be marked as ? and you will need to rewrite it.

Scenario

You are working on the intermediate cardiac care unit in a large hospital. You are taking care of R.J., who was admitted for a chest contusion he sustained in an auto accident; he fractured the fourth and fifth ribs on his left side. About 2000, his wife runs up to you at the nurse's station and says, "I think my husband just had a heart attack. Come quick!" She follows you into his room, where you find him face down on the floor. He is breathing and is cyanotic from the neck up. His pulse is very weak.

1. What should your first action be?

2. Suddenly, you remember R.J.'s wife, who is anxiously hovering over you in the room. What are you going to do?

The code team arrives. R.J.'s trauma surgeon is making rounds on your unit when the code is called, and he runs to the room. R.J. is intubated, and the normal saline (NS) lock is changed to an IV of lactated Ringer's (LR). The trauma surgeon recognizes Beck's triad and calls for a cardiac needle and syringe. He inserts the needle below the xiphoid process and aspirates 50 ml of unclotted blood.

3. What is Beck's triad, and what causes it?

4. Explain the rationale for the surgeon performing a pericardiocentesis.

R.J. is transferred to the thoracic ICU (TICU) for observation.

5. As the team prepares R.J.'s transfer, you go to find R.J.'s wife to thank her for alerting you to the emergency so promptly and to tell her what has happened. Briefly, and in everyday terms, how would you explain what happened to her husband?

6. As you both get up to leave, Mrs. J. suddenly turns pale and says she feels very dizzy. What are you going to do?

Case Study 6

Name ________________ Class/Group ________ Date ________

Group Members ________________________________

INSTRUCTIONS: All questions apply to this case study. Your responses should be brief and to the point. Adequate space has been provided for answers. When asked to provide several answers, they should be listed in order of priority or significance. Do not asume information that is not provided. Please print or write clearly. If your response is not legible, it will be marked as ? and you will need to rewrite it.

Scenario

You are the nurse on duty on the intermediate care unit, and you are scheduled to take the next admission. The ED nurse calls to give you the following report, "This is Barb in the ED, and we have a 42-year-old man with lower GI bleeding. He is a sandblaster with a 12-year history of silicosis. He is taking 40 mg of prednisone per day. During the night he developed severe diarrhea. He was unable to get out of bed fast enough and had a large maroon-colored stool (hematochezia) in the bed. His wife 'freaked' and called the paramedics. He is coming to you. His VS are stable: 110/64, 110, 28, and he's a little agitated. His temperature is 36.8° C. He hasn't had any stools since admission, but his rectal exam was guaiac-positive and he is pale but not diaphoretic. We have him on 5 L O_2/NC. We started a 16-gauge IV with LR at 125/hr. He has an 18-gauge Salem sump to continuous low suction; the drainage is guaiac-positive. We have done a hemogram with differential, advanced metabolic panel, PT/INR and PTT, and a T&C for four units RBCs and a UA. He's all ready for you."

1. How should you prepare for this patient's arrival?

K.L. arrives on your unit. As you help him transfer from the ED stretcher to the bed, K.L. becomes very dyspneic and expels 800 ml of maroon stool.

2. What are the first three actions you should take?

K.L. reports that he is getting nauseated but not thirsty. VS are 106/68, 116, 32.

3. What additional interventions would you need to institute?

ABG results are as follows (these results reflect values at sea level): pH 7.45; $Paco_2$ 33 mm Hg; Pao_2 65 mm Hg; HCO_3 23 mmol/L; BE +1.0; Sao_2 91%.

4. Interpret the preceding ABGs. What do they tell you?

The gastroenterologist is notified by K.L.'s physician and arrives on the unit to perform a colonoscopy and endoscopy. You are going to give K.L. midazolam (Versed) and meperidine (Demerol) IV during the procedures.

5. Given the above history, what do you think significantly contributed to the GI bleed?

6. What are midazolam and meperidine, and why are they being given to K.L.?

During the colonoscopy, K.L. begins passing large amounts of bright red blood. He becomes more pale and diaphoretic and begins to have an altered level of consciousness (LOC).

7. Identify five immediate interventions you should initiate.

K.L. has been stabilized with fluids, blood, and FFP. There has been no further evidence of active bleeding. He received ranitidine (Zantac) 150 mg IV push, and is receiving an infusion of 8 mg/hr via infusion pump.

8. Later, when he seems to be feeling better, K.L. tells you he's really embarrassed about the mess he made for you. How are you going to respond to him?

It is concluded that the GI hemorrhage was prednisone induced. The prednisone is being used to suppress the progression of silicosis. The physician will discharge K.L. and attempt to decrease his maintenance dose of prednisone while monitoring his respiratory status.

Case Study 7

Name ______________________ Class/Group __________ Date __________

Group Members ____

INSTRUCTIONS: All questions apply to this case study. Your responses should be brief and to the point. Adequate space has been provided for answers. When asked to provide several answers, they should be listed in order of priority or significance. Do not asume information that is not provided. Please print or write clearly. If your response is not legible, it will be marked as ? and you will need to rewrite it.

Scenario

J.R. is a 28-year-old man who is doing home repairs. He falls from the top of a 6-foot stepladder, striking his head on a large rock. He experiences momentary loss of consciousness. By the time his neighbor gets to him, he is conscious but bleeding profusely from a laceration over the right temporal area. The neighbor drives him to the ED of your hospital. As the nurse, you immediately apply a cervical collar, lay him on a stretcher, and take J.R. to a treatment room.

1. What steps should you take to assess J.R.?

2. List at least five components of a neurologic examination.

You complete your neurologic examination and find the following: GCS 15, pupils equal, round, react to light (PERRL), and full sensation. J.R. C/O a headache and is becoming increasingly drowsy.

3. As the radiology technician performs a portable cross-table lateral C-spine x-ray, J.R. begins to speak incoherently and appears to drift off to sleep. What is the next action you would take?

You find J.R. has become unresponsive to verbal stimuli and responds to painful stimuli by abnormally flexing his extremities (decorticate movement). He has no verbal response. The right pupil is larger than the left, and does not respond to light.

4. What is J.R.'s GCS score at this time? Indicate what this means.

5. Based on his GCS score, what are the next steps you should take?

6. What is the significance of the dilated and fixed pupil on the right?

The physician orders 500 ml of 25% mannitol solution IV.

7. What is mannitol, and why is it being used on J.R.?

J.R. is transported to x-ray for helical or spinal CT scan, where he is found to have a large epidural hematoma on the right with a hemispheric shift to the left. He will be taken straight to the OR for evacuation of a right epidural hematoma.

While en route from the CT scan to the OR, the physician instructs the respiratory therapist to initiate hyperventilation of the patient to "blow off more CO_2."

8. What is the rationale for this action?

9. Explain at least six interventions you would use to prevent increased ICP in the first 48 postoperative hours.

While he is in surgery, J.R.'s family arrives at the ED. They ask that their faith healer anoint J.R. and pray over him.

10. What should the nurse say?

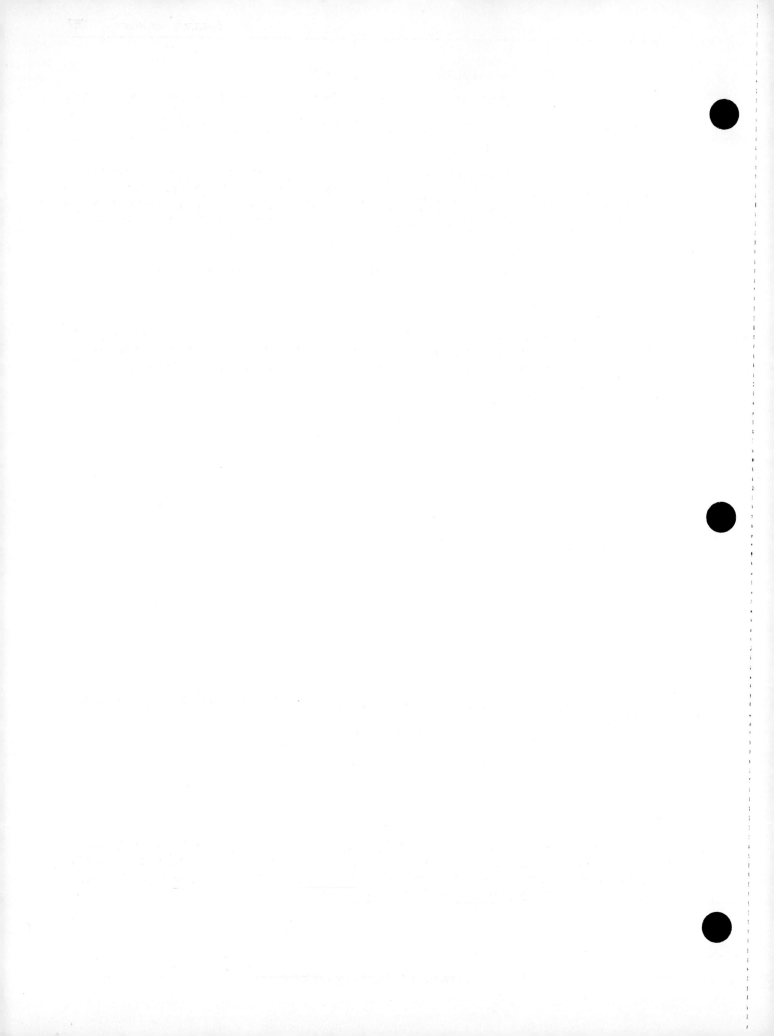

Case Study 8

Name ______________________ Class/Group __________ Date __________

Group Members ______________________

INSTRUCTIONS: All questions apply to this case study. Your responses should be brief and to the point. Adequate space has been provided for answers. When asked to provide several answers, they should be listed in order of priority or significance. Do not asume information that is not provided. Please print or write clearly. If your response is not legible, it will be marked as ? and you will need to rewrite it.

Scenario

B.J. is a 34-year-old woman who has been thrown from a galloping horse in a remote area. She was flown to the trauma center by helicopter from a rural hospital with spinal cord compression due to spinal fracture and disk fragments in her lumbar spine. Her cervical spine is free from injury. She arrives strapped to a rigid backboard and begins to vomit.

1. What would you do to keep B.J. from aspirating?

2. What would you do to assess B.J.?

You find that B.J. is hypotensive and bradycardic. She has an IV of 1000 ml LR with a large-bore catheter at 75 ml/hr.

3. What is causing the hypotension and bradycardia?

The neurosurgeon arrives in the ED and examines B.J. He finds her areflexic below the lumbar region of the spinal cord. There is absence of sweating in the region and no sensation below the level of the lesion. He writes the following orders: CT scan of the spine; myelogram; prepare for surgery; admit to ICU; 10 mg dexamethasone (Decadron) IV now.

4. Why did the physician order both a CT scan and a myelogram? Differentiate between the diagnostic value of each.

5. What is dexamethasone, and why is it being used on B.J.?

6. List four problems relevant to B.J.'s care.

7. What are complications and problems associated with spinal cord shock? (List at least six.)

8. List six ways you would detect complications from spinal cord shock.

9. What are seven interventions that could be initiated to prevent or treat complications from spinal cord shock?

B.J. went to surgery directly from x-ray for decompression of her spinal cord, and was admitted to ICU on absolute bed rest. From ICU she was transferred to the surgical unit and fitted for a back brace; she began physiotherapy. After undergoing surgery for a bone graft and spinal fusion, she was transferred to a rehabilitation facility. After months of intense physiotherapy, B.J. regained the use of her legs and basic functioning and was discharged to home.

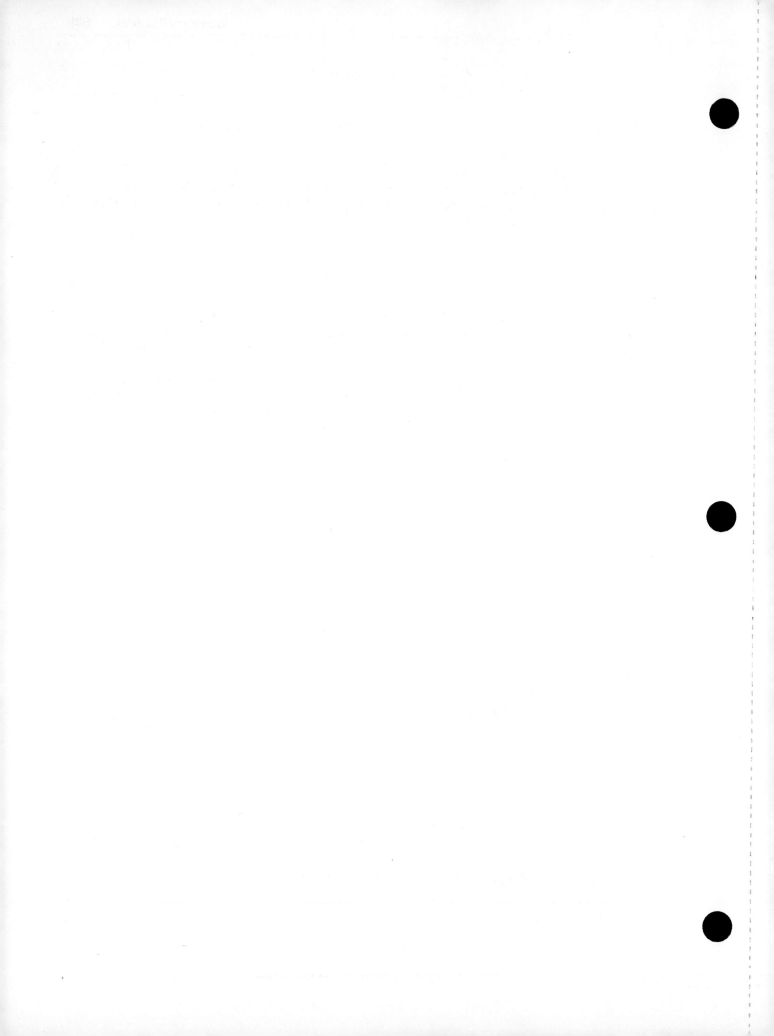

Case Study 9

Name ______________________ Class/Group __________ Date __________

Group Members ____

INSTRUCTIONS: All questions apply to this case study. Your responses should be brief and to the point. Adequate space has been provided for answers. When asked to provide several answers, they should be listed in order of priority or significance. Do not asume information that is not provided. Please print or write clearly. If your response is not legible, it will be marked as ? and you will need to rewrite it.

Scenario

You are working in an outpatient clinic when a mother brings in her 20-year-old-daughter, C.J., who has type 1 DM and has just returned from a trip to Mexico. She's had a 3-day fever and diarrhea with nausea and vomiting (N/V). She has been unable to eat and has tolerated only sips of fluid. Because she has been unable to eat, she has not taken her insulin.

Because C.J. is unsteady, you bring her to the examining room in a wheelchair. While assisting her onto the examining table, you note that her skin is very warm and flushed. Her respirations are deep and rapid, and her breath is fruity smelling. C.J. is drowsy and unable to answer your questions. Her mother states, "She keeps telling me she's so thirsty, but she can't keep anything down."

1. List four pieces of additional information you need to elicit from C.J.'s mother.

2. Describe the pathophysiology of DKA (diabetic ketoacidosis).

3. Explain the patient's presenting S/S. (List six.)

4. Her current VS are 90/50, 124, 36 and deep; temperature is 101.3° F (tympanic). Are these VS appropriate for a woman of C.J.'s age? Why or why not? Discuss your rationale.

A decision has been made to transport C.J. by ambulance to the local ED. After evaluating C.J., the ED physician writes the following orders.

5. Carefully review each order. Mark with an "A" if the order is appropriate; mark with an "I" if inappropriate. For each order you mark as "I," explain why it is inappropriate and correct the order.
   ___ 1000 ml LR IV STAT.
   ___ Give 36 units lente insulin and 20 units regular insulin SC (subcutaneously) now.

___ CBC with differential; CMP, blood cultures × two sites; clean-catch urine for UA and culture and sensitivity (C&S); stool for ova and parasites, *Clostridium difficile* toxin, and C&S; serum lactate, ketone, and osmolality; ABGs on room air
___ 1800-calorie American Diabetes Association (ADA) diet
___ Ambulate qid
___ Acetaminophen (Tylenol) 650 mg (10 gr) PO
___ Furosemide (Lasix) 60 mg IVP now
___ Urine output every hour
___ VS every shift

All orders have been corrected and initiated. C.J. has received fluid resuscitation and is on a sliding scale insulin drip via infusion pump. Her latest glucose was 347 mg/dl.

6. What is the rationale behind using an infusion pump for the insulin drip?

C.J. is ready for transport to the medical ICU. C.J.'s mother is beginning to realize that C.J. is more acutely ill than she thought. She leaves the room and begins to cry. Reassure her that C.S. will be okay.

7. How would you handle this situation?

8. C.J.'s mother asks where she can get more information on how C.J. can control her diabetes. What are some resources she may find useful?

C.J. is transported to the MICU in slightly improved condition. She continues to improve and is discharged from the hospital 3 days later.

Case Study 10

Name ______________________________ Class/Group __________ Date __________

Group Members ____

INSTRUCTIONS: All questions apply to this case study. Your responses should be brief and to the point. Adequate space has been provided for answers. When asked to provide several answers, they should be listed in order of priority or significance. Do not asume information that is not provided. Please print or write clearly. If your response is not legible, it will be marked as ? and you will need to rewrite it.

Scenario

T.R. is a 22-year-old college senior who lives in the dormitory. His friend finds him wandering aimlessly about the campus appearing pale and sweaty. He engages T.R. in conversation and walks him to the campus medical clinic, where you are on duty. It is 10:50 AM. The friend explains to you how he found T.R. and states that T.R. has diabetes and takes insulin. T.R. is not wearing a medical warning tag.

1. What do you think is going on with T.R.?

2. What is the first action you would take?

3. Because the glucometer reading is 50 mg/dl, what would your next action be?

4. When you enter the room to administer the orange juice, T.R. is unresponsive. What should your next action be?

5. T.R. is breathing at 16 breaths per minute, has a pulse of 85 and regular, but remains unresponsive. What should your next action be if (1) your clinic is well equipped for emergencies or (2) your clinic has no emergency supplies?

A few minutes after dextrose is administered, T.R. begins to awaken. He becomes alert and asks where he is and what happened to him. You orient him, then explain what has transpired.

6. What questions would you ask to find out what precipitated these events?

T.R. tells you he took 35 units NPH insulin and 12 units of regular insulin at 0745. He says he was late to class so he just grabbed an apple on the way. He adds this has happened twice in the past, but he recognized it, treated it with candy, and then ate a meal. He says he is on a 2000-calorie ADA diet.

7. Based on your knowledge of different types of insulin, when would you expect T.R. to experience an insulin reaction?

8. List at least four important points that you would stress in discussing your teaching plan with T.R.

Case Study 11

Name ________________________ Class/Group __________ Date __________

Group Members ____

INSTRUCTIONS: All questions apply to this case study. Your responses should be brief and to the point. Adequate space has been provided for answers. When asked to provide several answers, they should be listed in order of priority or significance. Do not asume information that is not provided. Please print or write clearly. If your response is not legible, it will be marked as ? and you will need to rewrite it.

Scenario

S.K., a 51-year-old roofer, was admitted to the hospital 3 days ago after falling 15 feet from a roof. He sustained bilateral fractured wrists and an open fracture of the left tibia and fibula. He was taken to surgery for open reduction and internal fixation (ORIF) of all his fractures. He is recovering on your orthopedic unit. You have instructions to begin getting him out of bed and into the chair today. When you enter the room to get S.K. into the chair, you notice that he is very agitated and dyspneic and says to you, "My chest hurts real bad. I can't breathe."

1. Identify five possible reasons for S.K.'s symptoms.

You auscultate S.K.'s breath sounds. You find that they are diminished in the left lower lobe (LLL). S.K. is diaphoretic and tachypneic and has circumoral cyanosis. His apical pulse is irregular and 110 bpm.

2. List in order of priority three actions you should take next.

The physician orders the following: ABGs, chest x-ray (CXR), ECG, and $\dot{V}/\dot{Q}$ (ventilation/perfusion) lung scan. The blood gas results come back as follows (these results reflect values at sea level): pH 7.47, $Paco_2$ 33.6 mm Hg, Pao_2 52 mm Hg, HCO_3 24.2 mmol/L, BE –3, Sao_2 83%, and A-a (alveolar-arterial oxygen gradient) gradient 32 mm Hg.

3. What is your interpretation of the blood gases? Give your rationale.

4. Based on the ABGs and your assessment findings, what do you think is wrong with S.K.?

5. The physician writes the following orders for S.K. Carefully review each order. Mark with an "A" if the order is appropriate; mark with an "I" if the order is inappropriate. Correct all inappropriate orders, and provide rationales for your decisions.
   ___ Transfer to MICU
   ___ Heparin 20,000 units IVP now, and 20,000 units in 1000 ml/D_5W to run at 1000 units per hour
   ___ PT/INR and PTT q4h. Call house officer with results.
   ___ 3 L O_2/NC
   ___ Patient-controlled analgesia (PCA) pump with morphine sulfate: loading dose 10 mg; dose 2 mg; lock-out time 15 minutes; maximum 4-hour dose 30 mg
   ___ Streptokinase 250,000 IU IV over 30 minutes, then 100,000 IU per hour × 24 hours
   ___ Prednisolone (Solu-Cortef) 1 g IV now
   ___ Albuterol (Proventil) metered-dose inhaler (MDI), two puffs q6h

All orders have been corrected. S.K.'s $\dot{V}/\dot{Q}$ scan indicates a PE in the LLL, and heparin therapy is initiated. Repeat ABGs show the following values (these results reflect values at sea level): pH 7.45, $Paco_2$ 35 mm Hg, Pao_2 82 mm Hg, HCO_3 24 mmol/L, BE −2.4, Sao_2 90%, A-a gradient 28 mm Hg.

6. What do these gases generally indicate?

The physician orders furosemide (Lasix) 20 mg IV now.

7. Why do you think the physician ordered furosemide for S.K.?

S.K. is watched very closely for the next several days for the onset of pulmonary edema. Thrombotic therapy (heparin), oxygen, pulse oximetry, daily CXRs and ABG analysis, and pain management are continued. When he is stable, S.K. is transferred back to your orthopedic unit.

8. The next day S.K. suddenly explodes and throws the physical therapist (PT) out of his room. He yells, “I'm sick and tired of having everyone tell me what to do.” How are you going to deal with this situation?

Case Study 12

Name ______________________ Class/Group __________ Date __________

Group Members ____

INSTRUCTIONS: All questions apply to this case study. Your responses should be brief and to the point. Adequate space has been provided for answers. When asked to provide several answers, they should be listed in order of priority or significance. Do not asume information that is not provided. Please print or write clearly. If your response is not legible, it will be marked as ? and you will need to rewrite it.

Scenario

D.V., a 38-year-old woman diagnosed with ruptured appendix, was hospitalized for an appendectomy. She developed peritonitis and was discharged 9 days later with a left peripherally inserted central catheter (PICC) line to home care for IV antibiotic therapy. You work for the home care department of the hospital. You have been assigned to D.V.'s case, and this is your first home visit. You are to do a full assessment on D.V. During the assessment, you notice a large ecchymotic area over the right upper arm. You question her about the bruise and she tells you, "The nurses took my BP so many times it bruised."

1. Do you accept D.V.'s explanation? Why or why not?

In examining D.V. further, you find a fine, nonraised, dark red rash over her trunk (petechiae).

2. What questions would you ask D.V. to elicit additional information?

D.V. hadn't noticed the petechiae before you pointed it out. The rash does not itch or cause pain. She has never had one like it before.

3. What other information would you want to gather?

The wound is not discolored or draining; the abdomen is tender to palpation. There is oozing of serosanguineous fluid around the PICC insertion site. The rash is confined to the trunk. You make a decision to call the physician regarding your findings.

4. What vital information will you relay to the physician? (Always start by identifying yourself.)

The physician orders blood to be drawn for coagulation studies and a complete blood count (CBC) with differential. He says he would like to evaluate D.V. for DIC.

5. What laboratory tests would you expect to see performed in coagulation studies?

You give D.V. her antibiotic, draw her blood, and take it to the lab. You return 6 hours later to administer another dose of antibiotics. D.V. greets you at the door. She is very upset and ushers you to the bathroom, where you find blood in the toilet. She tells you that she has been urinating blood for the past 2 or 3 hours. She also shows you a tissue in which she has bloody-appearing sputum. She tells you she has been coughing up blood. You notify the physician, who instructs you to call 911 and get the patient to the ED immediately. You call the ED and give report to the triage nurse on duty.

6. What are you going to tell the triage nurse?

7. Are the patient's presenting S/S consistent with DIC? Explain.

The following labs were prolonged: PT/INR, PTT, split fibrin products, and D-dimer. The following labs were decreased: platelets, platelet aggregation time, clot retraction time, and fibrinogen level. The WBC was 12.5/cmm and platelet count 46/cmm. D.V. is diagnosed with DIC.

8. List at least three priority needs for D.V.

D.V. is stabilized with oxygen, fluids, and blood products; and medication therapy is initiated. She is transferred to the ICU in guarded condition.

Note: The prognosis for someone with DIC depends on the underlying cause.

Case Study 13

Name ______________________ Class/Group __________ Date __________

Group Members ____

INSTRUCTIONS: All questions apply to this case study. Your responses should be brief and to the point. Adequate space has been provided for answers. When asked to provide several answers, they should be listed in order of priority or significance. Do not asume information that is not provided. Please print or write clearly. If your response is not legible, it will be marked as ? and you will need to rewrite it.

Scenario

You are the trauma nurse working in a busy tertiary care facility. You receive a call from the paramedics that they are en route to your facility with the victim of multiple gunshot wounds to the chest and abdomen. The paramedics have started two large-bore IV lines with LR, O_2 by mask at 15 L/min. The patient has a sucking chest wound on the left and a wound in the upper right quadrant of the abdomen. VS are 80/36, 140, 42. The patient is diaphoretic, very pale, and confused. Estimated time of arrival (ETA) is 4 minutes.

1. List at least six things you will do to prepare for this patient's arrival.

On arrival to the ED, your patient, B.W., is cyanotic and in severe respiratory distress. When he is transferred to the trauma stretcher, you notice that there is an occlusive dressing over the sucking chest wound. It is taped down on all sides.

2. Is taping the occlusive dressing on all sides appropriate? Explain.

3. Who usually responds to a trauma code, and what are the functions of the people from the various departments?

4. Prioritize the actions of the physicians and nurses in the trauma situation.

B.W. is to have a CT scan of the abdomen. His abdomen has become distended and rigid.

5. What are the possible reasons for the abdominal distention and rigidity?

The abdominal CT scan shows a large liver laceration. B.W. will be taken directly to the OR for an exploratory laparotomy with repair of liver laceration, then to the ICU. When you return from transporting the patient to the OR, B.W.'s wife is in the ED very upset and frightened. The social worker has been called to another emergency.

6. How would you interact with B.W.'s wife?

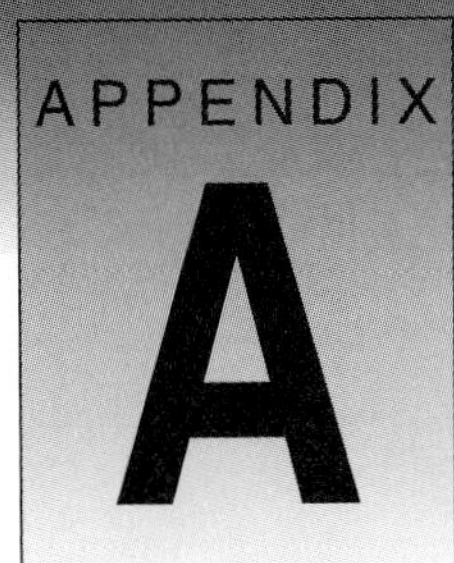

Appendix A
Pointers for Students—How to Look Like You Know What You're Doing

Pointers for Students: How to Look Like You Know What You're Doing

Clinical experiences can be overwhelming and confusing; the environment is filled with distractions. What you experience often doesn't resemble what you have read in the book! We want to help you become a good clinician. The following are "tips and tricks" contributed by the writers of these cases. They are presented in no particular order of importance. Don't read all of them at once; read a few here and there, think about them, and apply them as you get the opportunity.

General Suggestions

- There are five instruments every nursing student should carry at all times. Never lend these items to anyone unless you can afford to replace one or more without complaint. These five essential items are a good black-ink ballpoint pen; a high-quality stethoscope; a pocket penlight (preferably with pupil sizes or centimeter ruler on the side); a medium-sized hemostat (straight Kelly); and a pair of bandage scissors.
- Purchase a high-quality stethoscope. Try listening with several different types, and choose the one that is best for you. Engrave your name on it. Your stethoscope is a very important tool.
- Staying hydrated will help you stay more alert. Drink plenty of fluids. (Besides the health benefits, this gives you an excuse to go to the bathroom for 30-second breaks!)
- Keep a quick snack handy. Sometimes you need a pick-me-up and don't have time for meals or to leave the unit to get something.
- Plan something special you can do to help alleviate stress—and use it on a regular basis.
- Avoid use of slang or words that could offend patients and families. Be aware of your patient's comfort level. Do not call patients by their first name unless they have given you permission.
- Assume nothing and take nothing for granted.
- Listen and observe carefully. Be aware of changes and try to anticipate their significance.
- Watch how nurses you work with do things, and pick out things that work best for you.
- You can also learn from a negative example. If nothing else, you learn how *not* to do something!
- Projecting confidence and a "matter of fact" manner will usually put the patient, and yourself, at ease.
- Take care to respect each patient's confidentiality. Conduct interviews and examinations in a private and professional manner.
- Be sensitive to hesitation and nonverbal cues when gathering information. What is left unsaid may be extremely important. Use phrases such as "Could you tell me more?" or "Could you help me understand?" to elicit more information.
- Watch for physical or emotional scars. Health care touches on the most intimate experiences of our lives. Individuals—both men and women—who have been subjected to the degradation of sexual abuse and molestation may be especially prone to shame, aversion, or aggressive reactions.
- Don't be surprised when you discover that many adults are not knowledgeable about the basics of elimination and sexual functioning. Their ignorance or discomfort often is covered up with humor or aggressive behavior.
- Documentation is critical: patient education handouts should be simple to use and developed for use at a sixth-grade reading level.
- If you have a limited budget and a clinical setting of patients who speak more than one language, ask for volunteers to help translate educational material—and then have that work double-checked. Local ethnic clubs or support groups can be a good source of translators.
- As the patient's resting respiratory rate doubles from baseline, he or she will need to be intubated and placed on mechanical ventilation.
- Never trust equipment. Don't assume anything. Things tend to break down at the worst times.
- Double-check to be sure all equipment is functional.
- Treat the patient, not the monitoring devices or numbers.
- Not every patient with hepatitis or cirrhosis is an alcoholic.
- Not every alcoholic will go into DTs.
- Do not assume patients are anorexic just because they look malnourished.
- Do not assume patients are well nourished just because they are obese.

Assessment and Data Collection

- Learn to assess pain without leaving out important data. Suggestion: use the COLDERRA method where **C** = characteristics, **O** = onset, **L** = location, **D** = duration, **E** = exacerbation, **R** = relief, **R** = radiation, and **A** = associated signs and symptoms.
- Begin with the basics and keep reviewing them: airway, breathing, circulation (ABCs).
- When you see acute changes in level of consciousness, first check oxygenation status.
- Become a keen observer; use all your senses.
- Don't be distracted by the obvious. Keep looking!
- Formulate a systematic way of assessing patients and make it a habit. Go through the same sequence every time. You will be less likely to overlook or omit something.
- You can't find something if you don't look for it.
- Don't trust (1) machines, (2) numbers, or (3) what you can't see.
- Occasionally ask an experienced nurse or instructor to watch you do your assessments. Everyone, no matter how experienced, can benefit from objective suggestions for improvement. Over time, it is easy to become sloppy or start forgetting important things.
- With the first assessment of your shift, check the patient's ID bracelet and the rate and type of every fluid infusing—you are responsible for fluids under your control from the moment your shift begins until your shift is over.
- Remember to auscultate before palpating: Watch! Listen! *Then* Touch!
- Testing pH of nasogastric tube (NGT) drainage is easier if you slip the litmus paper into the end of the NGT and reconnect the tube to suction. Drainage will be pulled over the paper, which can then be removed. (Of course, antacids in the tube will negate this.)
- Any abrupt change in color or amount of drainage from wounds or drains needs to be explored and reported.
- Do not suggest words to describe feelings or events to your patients. You may miss subtle nuances if you jump to conclusions; listen to what your patients have to say and the words they use to say it.
- Perform a thorough psychosocial assessment that includes taking the values of patients and their significant others seriously.
- Include the significant others when you assess sleep patterns. They may be able to tell you more about snoring and other sleep disturbances than the patient can.
- Accurate recording of data, such as intake and output (I&O), is a must. Lawsuits have been won—and lost—over one single I&O sheet. Involve the patient and family in helping to keep accurate records. Ask them to let you know about foods or liquids brought in to the patient.
- Always double-check calculations: use a calculator, if necessary.
- Acute cardiovascular and musculoskeletal injuries require frequent evaluation and documentation of the five Ps: pulse, pallor, pain, paresthesia, and paralysis. Deterioration of status in any of these variables may indicate a medical emergency and requires a rapid response.
- Be alert for substance abuse as an underlying diagnosis in individuals whose hospitalization is sudden and unanticipated. Many nurses have been injured by patients in undiagnosed withdrawal. This may be a particular risk in motor vehicle accidents (MVAs) or medical crises in which alcohol or drug use may be contributing factors.
- Often patients and families will deny the existence of mental illness or abuse because of stigma or ignorance. Ask about family violence (verbal or physical) or suicide very carefully.

Understanding the Problem/Diagnoses

- You have gathered your information, now look at it. Do you see any patterns? Do the data fit the history? Do all medications fit the diagnoses? Are all diagnoses accounted for in the medications?
- Ask the following questions:
  - Do the data make sense in the context of this patient?
  - Do the data create a complete picture?
  - Do you need additional data?

- Use the data to formulate your list of patient problems.
- Prioritize specific problem statements, and guard yourself against distractions.
- Never think you are too smart to look something up.

Developing Strategies of Care

- Plan and coordinate care with your patient. By discussing interventions and priorities, you will learn to understand more about your patient's value system.
- Educate the patient as you carry out this process; process and outcome can and should be integrated. A better-educated patient is more prepared to cooperate with the medical and nursing care regimen.
- Always include relationships, cultural orientation, self-esteem, and emotional issues in planning care.
- Prevent infection. Teach your patients and their families to wash their hands properly. Take them to the sink in the room and demonstrate handwashing techniques that you were taught in Nursing 101. Show them how to use a paper towel to turn off the faucet. Have them practice.
- Watch other health care providers to make sure they wash their hands. If you are training others who are with you, leave the water running in the sink as you leave the room—it is a strong hint for them to wash their hands as they follow you out!
- Check equipment; double-check if you have any doubt. You are responsible for reporting equipment that is not in working order. Equipment not in working order can result in shock or other forms of injury to personnel as well as patients or families. Remove it from the room promptly, label it clearly with a brief description of what is wrong, and report it according to policy.
- Substance abuse is not an uncommon complication in the recovery of trauma patients. Consider a psychiatric nurse practitioner or social services consultation if you suspect this is a problem.
- Accidents or injuries can aggravate feelings and memories associated with earlier experiences of trauma and abuse. If responses to current health problems seem to be unusual or in excess of what is expected, consider consulting a psychiatric nurse practitioner or someone from social services.

Carrying Out the Plan of Care

- Frequently check your patient's charts for STAT orders.
- Document everything you do; if it isn't charted, you didn't do it.
- Document the patient's response to treatments, medications, and activities.
- Let the patient's values and preferences guide you.
- Get the family and significant others to help, if appropriate.

Evaluation and Reevaluation

- Monitor carefully for changes, whether dramatic and sudden, or subtle and gradual.
- Include the patient and families in helping to evaluate care. Ask, "Do you feel that what we are doing is helping you? What do you think?"
- Is the patient getting better? If so, continue with the plan. If not, reassess and revise the plan as needed.
- Evaluate patient and spousal cooperation. Never label patients as "noncompliant." Determine why patients do not take their medication, complete treatments, etc. Perhaps the side effects of treatment make patients feel worse than the disease, and they are exercising their right of choice. Remember, "noncompliance" on the part of patients is more often "knowledge deficit" or ignorance on our part! Noncompliance is rare when there is true teamwork, and it is a misleading term. Adherence is a better, more nonjudgmental word.
- Long-term problems, particularly fatigue and pain, often contribute to depression.
- Involve other health care professionals and pain specialists in addressing complex issues.

Teamwork is the Key to Survival

- When you graduate and start working as a nurse, you will be expected to be a team leader, coordinating the patient care given by certified nursing assistants, other nurses, and students, with the care given by many other professionals. Use this opportunity to observe the nurses you think are the most effective in promoting teamwork. Analyze why they are effective and try integrating those techniques into your own practice.
- Work at developing good relationships with other professionals. The health care system is complex and constantly changing. We all need and deserve respect. We also depend on one another.
- Getting to know the medical nutritionists (dietitians), pharmacists, physical and occupational therapists, psychologists, social workers, case managers, laboratory personnel, nurse practitioners, medical staff, pastoral counselors, and other professionals in your setting can make things a lot easier for you later on. While you are a student, learn as much as you can about the role of each professional and the most effective ways to interact with them. It all adds up to good patient care.
- Patient care settings can be very stressful, high-pressure environments, especially in emergency situations. Some of the most important things you can remember are:
  - Try to sort out the difference between fact and feelings.
  - Be forgiving.
  - Never take anything personally.

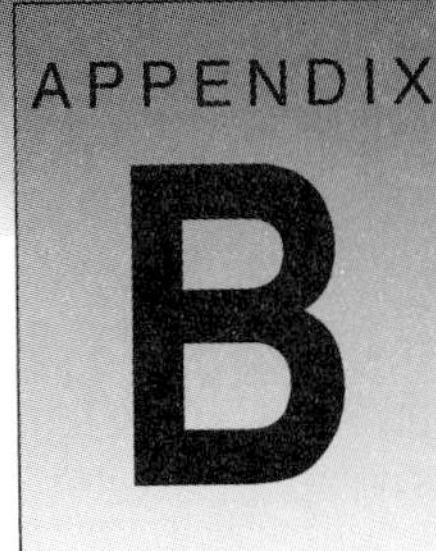

Case Study Worksheet

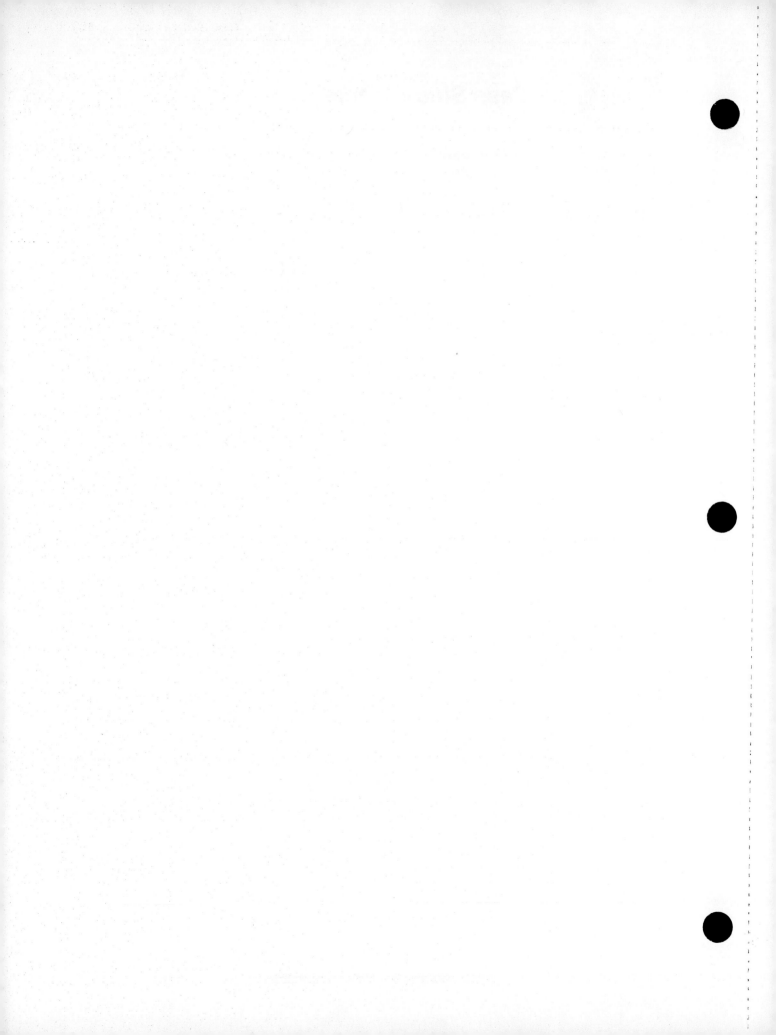

Name: ____________________ Chapter __________ Case __________ Date __________

Patient initials ____

Symbols/terms/abbreviations

Meaning/definition (diagnoses and medications go in following sections)

Diagnoses/medical conditions (+current and −past)

Description/meaning of diagnosis or medical problem (include possible significance)

Medications (brand and generic name if applicable)

Class, indications, contraindications, significant side effects, food and drug interactions

Treatments, interventions, and therapeutic procedures	Method of delivery, purpose/desired outcome, indications, contraindications, and precautions (include supplemental oxygen, tube feedings, therapeutic beds, etc.)

Laboratory tests and diagnostic procedures	What is it, when was it done, and why?

Cultural issues and their significance:

Notes:

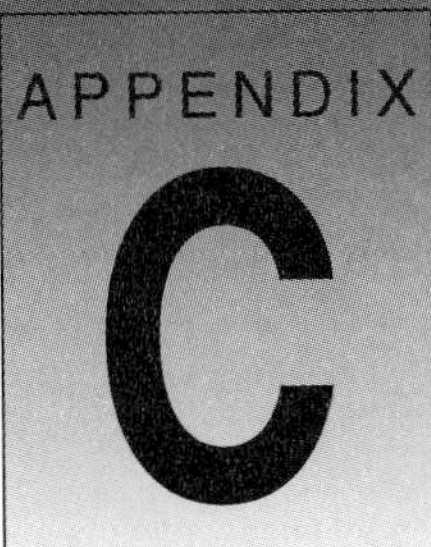

Abbreviations

AA	Alcoholics Anonymous
AAA	abdominal aortic aneurysm
A-a gradient	alveolar-arterial oxygen gradient
AAO	awake, alert, and oriented
ABCs	airway, breathing, circulation check(s)
ABGs	arterial blood gases
ABI	ankle-brachial index
ac	before meals
ACD	sickle cell disease
ACE I	angiotensin-converting enzyme inhibitor
Ach	acetylcholine
Ach R	acetylcholine receptor
ACTH	adrenocorticotropic hormone
AD	autonomic dysreflexia
ADA	American Dietetic Association
ADH	antidiuretic hormone
ADL	activities of daily living
ad lib	as directed
A-fib	atrial fibrillation
AGC (ANC)	absolute granulocyte count
AGE	advanced glycosylated end products
AIDS	acquired immunodeficiency syndrome
Alk Phos	alkaline phosphatase
ALL	acute lymphoblastic leukemia
ALP	alkaline phosphatase (serum)
ALS	amyotrophic lateral sclerosis
ALT (SGPT)	serum glutamic-pyruvic transaminase
AM	morning
AML	acute myelogenous leukemia
ANA	antinuclear antibody
ANC (AGC)	absolute neutrophil count
Anti-Sm	anti-smooth muscle antibody
aPTT	activated partial thromboplastin time
ARDS	adult respiratory distress syndrome
ASA	aspirin
ASAP	as soon as possible
AST (SGOT)	serum aspartate transaminase; aspartate serum transaminase
ATB	antibiotic
AV	atrioventricular/arteriovenous
AVS	aortic valve stenosis
BAL	blood alcohol level
BE	base excess
BiPAP	CPAP with mask over both mouth and nose
BM	bowel movement
BMI	body mass index
BMP	basic metabolic panel
BP	blood pressure
BPH	benign prostatic hyperplasia
bpm	beats per minute
brady	bradycardia
BR	bed rest
BRB	bright red blood
BRP	bathroom privileges
BS	bowel sounds; breath sounds
BSE	breast self-examination
BUN	blood urea nitrogen
Bx	biopsy
CABG	coronary artery bypass graft
CAD	coronary artery disease
C&DB	cough and deep breathe
cap	capsule
CAP	community acquired pneumonia
CAT scan	computerized axial tomography scan
CBC	complete blood count
CBC with diff	complete blood count with differential
CBD	common bile duct
CBR	complete bed rest
C/C	chief complaint
CCU	coronary care unit
CDE	certified diabetes educator
CHB	cystoscopy hydrodistention of bladder
CHF	congestive heart failure
CHO	carbohydrate(s)
Chol	cholesterol
CI	cardiac index
CK (CPK)	creatinine phosphokinase
CK-MM	CK isoenzymes
CLL	chronic lymphocytic leukemia
CM	case manager
CML	chronic myelogenous leukemia
CMP	complete metabolic panel; complete metabolic profile
CMV	cytomegalovirus
CNA	certified nursing assistant
CNS	central nervous system
CO	cardiac output
C/O	complaint(s) of
CO2	carbon dioxide
COPD	chronic obstructive pulmonary disease
CPAP	continuous positive airway pressure
CPR	cardiopulmonary resuscitation
CRF	chronic renal failure
C&S	culture and sensitivity
CSF	cerebrospinal fluid
CT	chest tube
CTA	clear to auscultation
CT scan	computed tomography scan
CV	cardiovascular
CVA	costovertebral angle; cerebrovascular accident
CVC	central venous catheter
CVP	central venous pressure
CWOCN	certified wound, ostomy, continence nurse
CXR	chest x-ray
DA	dopamine
DBP	diastolic blood pressure
DC; D/C	discontinue
DD	down drain
DEXA scan	duel-energy x-ray absorptiometry
DI	diabetes insipidus
DIC	disseminated intravascular coagulation

DKA	diabetic ketoacidosis
DM	diabetes mellitus
DNA	deoxyribonucleic acid
DO	doctor of osteopathy
DOE	dyspnea on exertion
DPT	diphtheria, pertussis, tetanus
DSA	digital subtraction angiography
DSM-IV-TR	Diagnostic & Statistical Manual of Mental Disorders, IV edition, Text Revision
D/T; d/t	due to
DTs	delirium tremens
DTRs	deep tendon reflexes
DVT	deep vein thrombosis
Dx	diagnosis
EBL	estimated blood loss
EC	emergency contraception
ECF	extended care facility
ECG	electrocardiogram
ECHO	cardiogram; cardiac ultrasound (sonogram)
ED	erectile dysfunction
Ecoli	*Escherichia coli*
ECT	electroconvulsive therapy
ECU	emergency care unit
ED/ER	emergency department; emergency room
EDC	estimated date of conception
EEG	electroencephalogram
EF	ejection fraction
EGD	esophagogastroduodenoscopy
EIA	enzyme immunoassay; exercise-induced asthma
ELISA	enzyme-linked immunosorbent assay
EMG	electromyogram
EMS	emergency medical system
EOMs	extraoccular eye movements
EPS	evoked potential studies
ER	estrogen receptor
ERS	erythrocyte sedimentation rate
ESRD	end stage renal disease
ET	enterostomal therapist
ETOH	alcohol
FBG	fasting blood glucose
FDA	U.S. Food & Drug Administration
FFP	fresh frozen plasma
Fio_2	fraction of inspired oxygen
FSH	follicle stimulating hormone
F/U	follow-up
FUO	fever of unknown origin
Fx	fracture
GBS	Guillain-Barré syndrome
GCS	Glasgow Coma Scale
GDM	gestational diabetes mellitus
GERD	gastroesophageal reflux disease
GGT	glucose glutamyl transferase (transpeptidase)
GH	growth hormone
GI	gastrointestinal
GTT	glucose tolerance test
GU	genitourinary
GXT	graded exercise (stress) test
HA	headache
HAV	hepatitis A virus
Hct	hematocrit
HbA1c	hemoglobin A1c; glycosylated hemoglobin test
HBAg	hepatitis B antigen
HBV	hepatitis B virus
HCl	hydrochloric acid
hCG	human chorionic gonadotropin
HCV	hepatitis C virus
HCO_3	bicarbonate ion
HCTZ	hydrochlorothiazide
HDL	high-density lipoprotein
HEENT	head, eyes, ears, nose, throat
HELLP	hepatic elevated liver enzymes
Hem/Onc	hematology/oncology
Hgb	hemoglobin
HgS	hemoglobin S
H/H	hemoglobin/hematocrit
HHH	hypervolemia, hypertension hemodilution
HIPAA	Health Insurance Portability & Accountability Act
HIV	human immunodeficiency virus
HLA	human leukocyte antigen
HMO	health maintenance organization
HO	house officer (physician)
HOB	head of bed
HPV	human papilloma virus
HRT	hormone replacement therapy (estrogen and progesterone)
HTN	hypertension
Hx	history
IBD	inflammatory bowel disease
IBS	irritable bowel syndrome
ICD/AICD	implantable cardioverter defibrillator/automatic ICD
IDCA	idiopathic dilated cardiomyopathy
ICP	intracranial pressure
ICU	intensive care unit
IFG	impaired fasting glucose
IGT	impaired glucose tolerance
IICP	increased intracranial pressure
IM	intramuscular
INR	International Normalized Ratio
I&O	intake and output
IS	incentive spirometer
IT	intrathecal
IUD	intrauterine device
IV	intravenous
IVP	intravenous pyelogram
IVDA	intravenous drug abuse
IVF	intravenous fluid
IVIG	intravenous immunoglobulin
IVP	intravenous push; intravenous pyelogram
IVPB	intravenous piggyback

JNC	Joint National Committee on Detection, Evaluation, and Treatment of High Blood Pressure
JP	Jackson-Pratt
JVD	jugular vein distention
kg	kilogram
KS	Kaposi's sarcoma
KVO	keep vein open
KUB	kidney, ureters, and bladder x-ray
lab(s)	laboratory; laboratory tests
LAD	left anterior descending coronary artery
lb(s)	pound(s)
LBBB	left bundle branch block
LDH	lactic dehydrogenase
LDL	low-density lipoprotein
LE	lower extremities
LFT(s)	liver function test (s)
LH	lutenizing hormone
LLL	left lower lobe (of lungs)
LLQ	left lower quadrant (of abdomen)
LMP	last menstrual period
LOC	level of consciousness
LPN	licensed practical nurse
LR	lactated Ringer's or Ringer's lactate
LUQ	left upper quadrant (of abdomen)
LV	left ventricle
LWS	low wall suction
MAE(W)	moves all extremities (well)
MAOI	monoamine oxidase inhibitor
MDI	multiple-dose injection; metered-dose inhaler
meds	medications
MD	doctor of medicine
MG	myasthenia gravis
MI	myocardial infarction
MICU	medical intensive care unit
MNT	medical nutrition therapy
MOM	milk of magnesia
MRI	magnetic resonance imaging
MS	multiple sclerosis
MSOF	multiple system organ failure
MUGA	multiple gated acquisition
MVA	motor vehicle accident
MVI	multivitamins
MVP	mitral valve prolapse
MVS	mitral valve stenosis
NAD	no acute distress
NC/nc	nasal cannula
NCV	nerve conduction velocity
NICU	neonatal intensive care unit
NG/NGT	nasogastric tube
NH3	ammonia
NKA	no known allergies
NKDA	no known drug allergies
NOS	not otherwise specified
NPH	neutral protamine hagedorn (a modified insulin)
NPO	nothing by mouth
NS	normal saline
NSA	normal serum albumin
NSAID(s)	nonsteroidal antiinflammatory drug(s)
NTG	nitroglycerin
N/V	nausea and vomiting
O_2	oxygen
OCD	obsessive-compulsive disorder
OGTT	oral glucose tolerance test
OHCS; 17-OHCS	17-hydroxycorticosteroids
OR	operating room
ORIF	open reduction and internal fixation
OS	oculus sinister; left eye
OSA	obstructive sleep apnea
OT; OTR	occupational therapist, registered
OTC	over the counter
P	pulse
PAB	prealbumin
PACs	premature atrial contractions
$Paco_2$	partial pressure of carbon dioxide in arterial blood
PACU	postanesthesia care unit
PAF	paroxysmal atrial fibrillation
Pao_2	partial pressure of oxygen in arterial blood
$Paco_2$	partial pressure of carbon dioxide in arterial blood
Pap	Papanicolaou smear
PAP	pulmonary artery pressure
PBMV	percutaneous balloon mitral valvuloplasty
PCA	patient controlled analgesia
PCN	penicillin
PCP	primary care provider
PCP	*Pneumocystis carinii*
PCWP	pulmonary capillary wedge pressure
PD	Parkinson's disease
PE	pulmonary embolus
PEEP	positive end expiratory pressure
PEG	percutaneous endoscopic gastrostomy tube
PEN	parenteral enteral nutrition
Pen VK	penicillin VK
peri	perineal (related to perineum)
PERRL(A)	pupils equal round and reactive to light (and accommodation)
PET	positron emission tomography
PFM	peak flow meter
pH	negative logarithm of the hydrogen ion concentration—acidity/basicity of the blood
PHD	public health department
PHTH	portal hypertension
PICC	peripherally inserted central catheter
PID	pelvic inflammatory disease
PM	afternoon or evening
PMH	past medical history
PMI	point of maximal impulse
PO	by mouth

POD	postoperative day
postop	postoperatively
PPD	purified protein derivative (test for TB); packs per day (cigarettes)
PPS	postpolio syndrome
PR	progesterone receptor
PRC	packed red cells
preop	preoperatively
PRBC	packed red blood cells
PRN/prn	as needed
PSA	prostate specific antigen
PSH	past surgical history
PT/RPT	physical therapist; registered physical therapist
PT	prothrombin time
PTCA	percutaneous transluminal coronary angioplasty
PTH	parathyroid hormone
PTSD	posttraumatic stress disorder
PTT/aPTT	partial thromboplastin time; activated partial thromboplastin time
PUD	peptic ulcer disease
PVCs	premature ventricular contractions
PVD	peripheral vascular disease
PVR	post voiding residual
R	right
RA	room air; rheumatoid arthritis
RAI	radioactive iodine
RBC(s)	red blood cell(s)
RCA	right coronary artery
RD	registered dietitian
RDS	respiratory distress syndrome
rehab	rehabilitation
REM	rapid eye movement
RHD	rheumatic heart disease
RLQ	right lower quadrant (of abdomen)
R/O	rule out
ROM	range of motion
RPR	rapid plasma reagin (test for syphilis)
R/T	related to
RUQ	right upper quadrant (of abdomen)
SAH	subarachnoid hemorrhage
Sao_2	arterial oxygen saturation
SBO	small bowel obstruction
SBP	systolic blood pressure
SCC	sickle cell crisis
SCDs	sequential compression devices
SCI	spinal cord injury
Sed Rate/ESR	erythrocyte sedimentation rate
SES	socioeconomic status
SIADH	syndrome of inappropriate antidiuretic hormone
SICU	surgical intensive care unit
SL	sublingual
SLE	systemic lupus erythematosus
SNS	sympathetic nervous system
SOB	short of breath
S/P	status post
SQ/sq	subcutaneous
S/S	signs and symptoms
SSRI	selective serotonin reuptake inhibitor
S/T	secondary to
STAT	immediately
STD(s)	sexually transmitted disease(s)
T&A	tonsillectomy and adenoidectomy
tachy	tachycardic
TAH	total abdominal hysterectomy
T&C(M)	type and cross (match)
TCA	tricyclic antidepressant
TD	tetanus/diphtheria
TED	thromboembolic deterrent
TIA(s)	transient ischemic attack(s)
TICU	thoracic intensive care unit
TKO	to keep open
TM	tympanic membrane
TPA	tissue plasminogen activator
TPN	total parenteral nutrition
TUMT	transurethral microwave thermotherapy
TURP	transurethral resection of the prostate
Trig	triglycerides
TSH	thyroid-stimulating hormone
Tx	treatment
UA	urinalysis
UDA	urinary drainage system
UEs	upper extremities
UGI	upper gastrointestinal
UGIB	upper gastrointestinal bleed
UOP	urine output
UPPP	uvulopalatopharyngoplasty
USFDA	U.S. Food & Drug Administration
UTI	urinary tract infection
UVJ	ureteral vesicle junction
VA	Veteran's Administration
VDRL	Venereal Disease Research Laboratory (test for syphilis)
V-fib	ventricular fibrillation
V-tach	ventricular tachycardia
VT	tidal volume
$\dot{V}/\dot{Q}$ scan	ventilation-perfusion scan (of lungs)
VS	vital signs
WBC	white blood cell count
W/C	wheelchair
WHR	waist hip ratio
WNL	within normal limits
WNR	within normal range
W/O	without

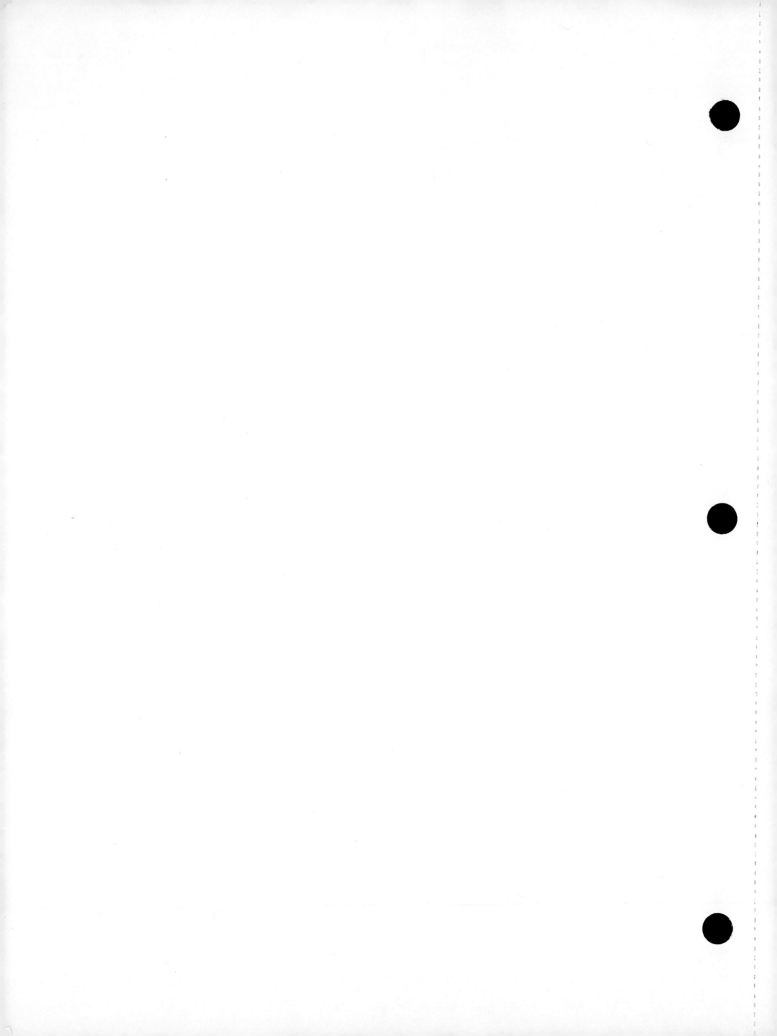

Roman M. Roman